Early Development of Children with Hearing Loss

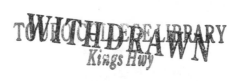

Brad A. Stach, Ph.D.
Editor-in-Chief for Audiology

Early Development of Children with Hearing Loss

Susan Nittrouer, Ph.D.

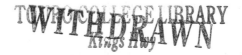
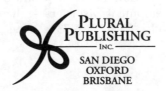
PLURAL PUBLISHING INC.
SAN DIEGO
OXFORD
BRISBANE

13219

KH

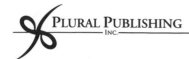

PLURAL PUBLISHING INC.

5521 Ruffin Road
San Diego, CA 92123

e-mail: info@pluralpublishing.com
Web site: http://www.pluralpublishing.com

49 Bath Street
Abingdon, Oxfordshire OX14 1EA
United Kingdom

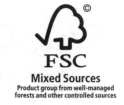

FSC
Mixed Sources
Product group from well-managed
forests and other controlled sources

Cert no. SW-COC-002283
www.fsc.org
© 1996 Forest Stewardship Council

Library of Congress Cataloging-in-Publication Data:
Nittrouer, Susan.
  Early development of children with hearing loss / Susan Nittrouer.
      p. ; cm.
  Includes bibliographical references and index.
  ISBN-13: 978-1-59756-323-9 (alk. paper)
  ISBN-10: 1-59756-323-4 (alk. paper)
  1. Hearing impaired children. 2. Child development. I. Title.
  [DNLM: 1. Hearing Loss—rehabilitation. 2. Child Development. 3. Child.
4. Infant. 5. Language Development Disorders—rehabilitation. 6. Rehabilitation
of Hearing Impaired—methods. WV 271 N733e 2009]
  HV2391.N58 2009
  155.45'12—dc22
                                                            2009010344

10/20/20

Contents

Preface

It is not unreasonable to suggest that the first step on this project was taken the morning of March 31, 1996. I had just returned from a trip to my sister's home in Calgary, Alberta, where I spent time with her family. My sister had two young children then, and I found myself wondering for the first time if I had made a mistake by not putting more effort into the goal of establishing a family. I loved children, and had met my share of eligible partners. But I just had never approached the goal of building a home life with the same determination that I brought to my work. On that morning, however, that would change as forces combined to set me on the path that would create my family, and eventually lead to the project reported here.

It was a Sunday. After getting in late the evening before, I looked forward to reading the *Omaha World Herald* in a leisurely manner that morning. I poured a cup of coffee and unfurled the paper to see that the front-page story was about a local woman who had gone to China to adopt a daughter. The next morning, April 1, I was waiting at the door of the adoption agency when it opened at 9:00 AM. Eight months later I was on my way to the town of Wuxi in eastern China to bring home my own daughter. My sister, the one who started it all by having such cute children, was naturally enlisted to accompany me.

Foreign adoption trips are very emotional experiences. At that time the adoption agency coordinated plans so that groups of several families traveled together. On this trip there were eight families, couples or other single women, who welcomed new daughters into their lives. We arrived in Shanghai late on a Saturday night and enjoyed a few days of sightseeing. That gave us time to rest, recovering from the long journey, before being thrust into the roles of new parents. Then, on Tuesday afternoon we found ourselves in a hallway at the Wuxi Holiday Inn, waiting for orphanage officials to deliver our daughters. My sister would later remark that she knew the trip would be like witnessing the birth of a child, but she was not prepared for it to be like witnessing eight births all at the same time. Most of us stood in that hall for what felt like hours while a few scouts went down to the lobby to watch for the arrival of the babies and the adults who would bring them. Not long after the scouts ran back upstairs to announce their sighting, the entourage from the orphanage emerged through the doorway at the top of the stairs and brought the months of waiting to a joyful end. After much hugging and crying we all returned to our rooms to begin our lives with our children.

But it was not long after the excitement in the hallway died down before I realized that there was something wrong with my daughter. At the time I wasn't sure what it was, especially since she had spent the first 9 months of her life in an orphanage. Perhaps it was just a temporary condition resulting from a lack of stimulation, I thought hopefully. Within months, however, I began to strongly suspect that she had a hearing loss. Unfortunately, it would take 2 more years before the loss would be confirmed because it was not a "clean" loss. The sensorineural component was present in only the high frequencies, and there was a significant conductive component overlaid on top of it. Many trips to visit our favorite audiologist at Boys Town National Research Hospital were required before we could identify the severity and nature of the loss. That delay provided me with 2 full years to contemplate what I would do if, as I strongly suspected, my daughter was found to have hearing loss.

I had worked with deaf children for several years before getting my PhD and so knew more than most parents who receive that diagnosis. I had taught in wonderful auditory-oral and total communication programs alike. I loved my experiences with American Sign Language, and greatly enjoyed every opportunity I ever had to interact with friends in the Deaf community. The arguments both for using sign language and for avoiding sign language with deaf children were familiar to me but acquired new significance as I considered what I would do with my own daughter if—or when—the diagnosis of hearing loss was made. As time went on without a firm confirmation of either the presence or absence of hearing loss, I realized that the designation of early identified was slipping away, and I worried about how that might affect any decision I would have to make. If the "window of opportunity" to start language development in a typical

time frame closes, does that mean it is more or less important to use sign language? Even with all my experience I felt I lacked sufficient evidence to make well-informed decisions about these important matters. And so my commitment to find a way to investigate these questions grew. I wanted to be able to provide data for other parents who would be facing the same decisions I was facing in those early years.

Three years after my daughter's hearing loss was finally diagnosed, the National Institute on Deafness and Other Communication Disorders issued a request for applications for projects to investigate intervention strategies for young children with hearing loss. My little family had moved to Logan, Utah, by then so I could take a position at Utah State University. I drafted my proposal and submitted it. Even as I was making the final adjustments to the proposal, I questioned my sanity at the idea of actually thinking of undertaking this project. It would involve children from all over the country, and numerous professionals as well. Nonetheless, I sent the proposal off to Washington, DC, and it was reviewed by a special panel of scientists knowledgeable about childhood hearing loss. Somewhat to my surprise, they approved of the methods and goals proposed.

Once funding was received for this project, the hard work began. The first lesson I learned was that not everyone was as enthusiastic about the goals of the research as the members of the review panel had been. Many obstacles were thrown in my path on the way to completing this project and some friendships were tested: The data have not confirmed everything everyone would like to have had confirmed. In the end, I believe that important information has been learned from this investigation that should help shape the way we approach treatment for children with hearing loss as we go forward into the 21st century. All the hard work involved and the difficulties encountered along the way will have been worth it if this book serves a useful purpose for even one family.

Typically, data generated by research projects like this one are published in brief reports, describing a very circumscribed outcome. I could have elected to handle dissemination that way, through a series of short reports, but I strongly believe it would have constrained the impact of the project as a whole. There is value to be derived from looking at trends both across time and across measures, and neither of those perspectives would have been possible with a series of brief articles. Presenting the entire project as an indivisible whole tells a very different tale than any collection of separate pieces could. However, the task of preparing a manuscript this length is very different from that of writing a journal article. The question of how to structure it was foremost in my mind as I tried to organize the massive amounts of data we had collected.

Some of the elements of structure finally decided on were these: As much as possible, similar analyses were performed on all measures. This should help readers follow outcomes as they progress through the chapters. It also means that this book is best read front to end.

I also tried to balance the requirements of providing a reference manual for other professionals with the desire to make this a document that nonprofessional readers, such as parents, could use as they approached very personal decisions regarding intervention for their children. To handle those competing goals I have presented as much data as possible, but relegated many of the data-laden tables to ends of chapters. If a figure is used to display outcomes, the accompanying table will be found at the end of the chapter; tables providing data not shown in figures are presented alongside the text.

An effort was made here to provide relevant background to this study. We all like to think that we are unbiased observers, asking questions and digesting information without preconceived ideas of what that information should reveal. In fact, the very questions we choose to ask are largely based on our accumulated experiences. We may lack even the ability to view problems from novel perspectives because of the ideas we grew up with. We encountered many examples of this notion of cultural "memes" on the adoption trip to China. Most of us believe that there are some inalterable principles that must be followed in raising children. The only problem is that ideas of what those principles are differ around the world, and every culture believes its own practices to be based on universal truths. In Western culture we worry about letting our children become overheated if we put them in too many clothes, yet while we were in China we were constantly admonished to put more layers on our babies. In North America we commonly provide infants with pacifiers to help them calm themselves, but that practice is taboo in China. Children regularly sleep with other family members in China, whereas American parents view that practice as something to be avoided at all costs.

Cultural biases also exist when it comes to the education of children with hearing loss. These are beliefs that emerged long ago, and largely go unexamined. For this reason the history of how we intervene with children with hearing loss is reviewed first in this book, along with an overview of what we know about human communication in general.

It is not until Chapter 5 that data from dependent measures are presented. I start by presenting information on the most general developmental outcomes, progressing through increasingly detailed measures of language development. Then in the final chapter, discussion returns to the basis of the document: How should this information shape our collective thinking about working with children who have hearing loss?

There is a great deal of data reported in these pages. It is a lot to work through for a nonprofessional. But in the end, I hope all readers will find the information gathered was worth the energy invested in reading it. It is my hope that this report helps a wide variety of consumers—parents, clinicians, educators, and scientists alike.

Acknowledgments

Although only one name appears on the cover of this book, many individuals contributed to the work. I want to thank all the people who made it possible. At the top of the list are those who served on the review panel that approved the initial proposal. I thank them for their belief that a study with this focus was needed and their faith in my ability to conduct this investigation in an objective and thorough manner. I trust that they will be satisfied with the final result.

The generous support of the National Institute on Deafness and Other Communication Disorders is gratefully acknowledged (NIH-NIDCD grant # R01 DC 006237). With sentiments similar to those above, I hope these results help us achieve our collective agenda to improve intervention services for children with hearing loss such that they can navigate the course of development unaffected by their sensory deficit.

Although obstacles were encountered during this work, there were many people who helped ease the way. Right after the NIH review panel, the first person whom I wish to thank is Kathleen Sussman, the director of the Jean Weingarten Peninsula Oral School. Kathy did a great deal to help get this project launched.

The next people whom I want to thank are two young men named Robert Packer and Christopher Chapman. An enormous amount of data was collected on this project. Keeping all of those data organized in an accessible manner was a tremendous undertaking. The fact that it was even possible was due to the ingenuity and dedication of Rob and Chris. Rob established the database when the project began at Utah State University, and Chris organized and reorganized that database as it grew and technology changed during our years at The Ohio State University. Similarly, I want to acknowledge the major contribution made by Christopher Holloman, who is responsible for the statistical modeling reported in Chapter 11.

Over the years several individuals worked to coordinate efforts on this project. They included Alma Burgess, Betsy Billman, Shana Moore, Amy Bartlett, and Joy Dransfield. These were the people who ensured that every detail of the project was attended to. They were the backbone of the study.

Many other people contributed as well by helping us recruit participants, organize a test site, devise test measures, or doing the actual data collection. These included Wendy Adler, Jill Bargones, Alisa Beard, Rhonda Bennight, Maura Berndsen St. Jacques, Lauren Branham, Pnina Bravman, Mary Evelyn Breland, Michelle Brinson, Betsy Brooks, Lisa Burton, Nate Burton, Annie Cardella, Robert Cook, Amy D'Alfonso, Monica Dorman, Michael Edwards, Tamara Elder, Apryl Eshelman, Heather Feekes, Laura Ferguson, Julie Flora, Cathy Frentz, Lauren Frock, Janice Gatty,

Anna Guenther, Abby Guerera, Janet Halley, Christy Hart, Marian Hartblay, Janet Holladay, Katie Imes, Julie Johanson, Cara Jordan, Kimberly Knight, Sara Kooima, Mary Ruth Leen, Joanna Lowenstein, Cebu Maybury, Mallory Monjot, Tara Montoney, Michael Moon, Ben Munson, Peggy Nelson, Anita New, Sarah Nicholson, Susan Norton, Danielle Paquin, Ashley Parker, Julie Pepper, Renee Polanco, Jennifer Polston, Laurie Preusser, James Quinlan, Carey Ratliff, Marsha Rawlin, Jennifer Ray, Ellie Rice, Daniel Robertson, Valerie Rodrigez, Shauna Rogers, Karen Rossi, Jane Ruddock, Lindsay Ruport, Erin Schuweiler, Samantha Sefton, Lynn Shea, Linda Sickman, Donal Sinex, Jerome South, Patricia Stelmachowicz, Chelsea Stephens, Jason Stephens, Ruth Stoeckel, Darcy Stowe, Carol Strong, Eric Tarr, Faruk Terzi, Patricia Truhn, Stephen Tueller, Mikki Tuma, Jennifer Uher, Carolyn Walthall, Elizabeth Wilkes, Amanda Wysocki, Comer Yates, and Abby Zoia.

I am especially grateful to Carol Fowler, Michael Studdert-Kennedy, and Antoine Shahin for reading various versions of chapters for me.

Finally, I want to thank two people who especially offered encouragement. Karl White, a friend and colleague at Utah State University, provided unflinching support during the establishment and conduction of the study. Brad Welling, chair of Otolaryngology at The Ohio State University, helped see the project through to completion.

To Emily and Allison

1

A Shared History: Putting this Book in Cultural Perspective

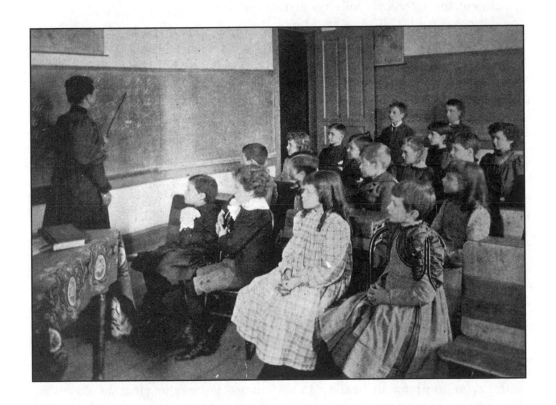

The purpose of this book is to report results of a study that measured developmental outcomes in children with moderate-to-profound hearing loss. These outcomes were compared to those of children with normal hearing. This work is timely, coming as it does at the start of the 21st century, because much has changed in the past 10 to 20 years regarding what we are able to do to help children with hearing loss. Until quite recently, we could teach deaf children about social studies, science, and other content areas. We could give them the technical skills needed to obtain jobs. But still these children would face the same obstacles that individuals with hearing loss had faced for all of human history. Communication with family, friends, and coworkers with normal hearing was difficult, due to problems in speech production involving voice quality, phonetic structure, and syntactic/grammatical organization. Speech perception was also tremendously restricted for most individuals with hearing loss, and reading abilities were generally limited to a third or fourth grade level.

That situation changed dramatically around 1990, largely owing to the development of cochlear implants and the Federal Drug Administration's approval of implants for children down to the age of 12 months. These devices have remarkably altered the lives of children with severe-to-profound hearing loss. Thirty years ago it was the rare child with hearing loss who possessed the spoken language skills needed to function in a classroom with normal-hearing peers. Those of us old enough to recall those earlier times cannot help but be stunned, constantly, by the pervasive changes in the communication abilities

of children with hearing loss. Many of these children appear to communicate as well as children with normal hearing. Voice quality and phonetic organization sound normal, syntax seems appropriate, and so on. On the surface it now appears as if the auditory functioning of children with hearing loss can be modified to allow them to acquire skills in spoken language equivalent to those of children with normal hearing. One goal of the research reported here was to examine whether that subjective impression that so many of us share is accurate.

Sign Language and the Early American Educational Experience

Of course, not everyone views the technological advances made available to children with hearing loss in the late 20th century as positive change. Many people feel that the state of having a hearing loss should not be viewed as an affliction to be cured, but rather as cultural variation to be appreciated. This point of view recognizes the legitimacy of a culture grounded in customs and traditions created by individuals with significant hearing loss. The empirical data reported here are not meant as a test of that perspective. Variability in cultures is something that should always be appreciated because that variability adds to the richness of the human experience in general. At the same time, the undeniable fact is that most children born with hearing loss have parents with normal hearing and little, if any, familiarity with Deaf culture. (Uppercase *D* is used here to designate the cultural aspects of deafness, rather than the physical state.) These parents naturally want their children to share their (the parents') cultural traditions, and to participate in mainstream society unhindered by the effects of hearing loss. The goal of the work reported here was to examine how the development of children with hearing loss has been impacted by recent changes in treatment options for these children. Not only have cochlear implants made it possible for us to provide some auditory stimulation to all children with hearing loss, but methods of screening hearing in newborns have allowed us to detect hearing loss very soon after birth, and legislative mandates have ensured access to intervention for all children with identified hearing loss starting at birth. This study examined whether these changes have brought children with hearing loss closer to the norms of children with normal hearing on measures involving spoken language, behavior, and cognitive development. It was not the purpose of this work to consider whether or not these potential changes would diminish the probability that these children would share the cultural bonds of Deafness.

Examination of the history of deaf education in Europe and America from roughly the start of modern times, around the 16th century, reveals changes that reflect trends in general educational conventions. Before the 19th century, education was a privilege of only the rich. Therefore, only deaf children of nobility were given any kind of instruction, and they were taught to communicate using whatever means were available and possible, facilitating speech skills as best as possible, but using gestures or written language to aid communication. Pedro Ponce De Leon, a Spanish monk in the 16th century, is usually credited with establishing the first "school" for the deaf. In fact, he tutored deaf children in the Monastery of San Salvador. His method was to first teach these children to write the name of an object, and then have them learn how to produce the spoken version of that name. Of course, not many people were able to read and write at that time, and so written language was not a generally useful communication tool. One could not, for example, go to the local market and make a purchase by handing the vendor a piece of paper with an order written on it.

Several other teachers of the deaf in Western Europe during the 16th and 17th centuries are commonly recognized in historical accounts of deaf education. These include Juan Pablo Bonet, also a Catholic priest, who published a book titled *Simplification of Sounds and the Act of Teaching the Deaf to Speak*. The approach advocated by this teacher was that deaf children should learn to represent words with a manual alphabet, and then learn to speak them. John Bulwer, who lived in the 17th century, was the first teacher of the deaf recognized in the English-speaking world. He was a physician in London, and believed that manual gestures were a natural language of all men, but especially of deaf individuals. He advocated the teaching of a manual alphabet to all deaf children. Once a child knew the spelling of an object, efforts were then made to help the child say it. All these early approaches were similar in that they prepared deaf children to live among the members of their community, most of whom had normal hearing. Teaching deaf individuals was an endeavor undertaken by men in the religious or healing professions, using a tutorial method. Schools as we now know them did not exist, and so there were generally no opportunities for large numbers of deaf people to come together.

A critical milestone in deaf education, especially for the eventual development of deaf education in America, occurred in France during the mid-18th century. It was there that Abbé Charles Michel De l'Epée met two little girls who could not speak. On learning that they were deaf, he was inspired to develop a standard system of signs that could be used to teach deaf children. Accounts differ of how he went about developing this system, with some accounts indicating that he observed the home signs of deaf individuals in Paris at the time, and other accounts suggesting that he built upon a framework of signs from Spain. Regardless of how he developed that system, he used it to help establish the Institution Nationale des Sourds-Muets de Paris, or the National Deaf-Dumb Institute of Paris, in 1754, the first school for the deaf in France. It would be at this school roughly 50 years later that Gallaudet would become close friends with Laurent Leclerc and learn De l'Epée's system of signs.

At roughly the same time that De l'Epée was establishing his school in Paris, efforts were underway in other parts of Europe to establish schools for deaf children, but none so structured in approach as that of De l'Epée. In particular, Thomas Braidwood, a Scotsman, began a private school for the deaf in Edinburgh. The eventual goal for the children in this program was that they be able to communicate with oral language, but the teaching staff allowed them to use whatever means was necessary. Among these means was the two-handed manual alphabet that is still used in England. Braidwood's approach would eventually become influential in early American efforts to teach deaf children to talk, although for quite some time advocates of the approach were guarded about sharing their methods.

While these rudiments of deaf education were evolving in Western Europe during the 16th to 18th century, there was nothing equivalent occurring in America. Settlers along the East Coast of what would become the United States had more immediate problems to think about. The emergence of public education in America greatly influenced the eventual establishment of institutions to teach deaf children, but public education emerged slowly. The most rigorous attempts at early education in America were conducted to teach religion to children. The colonies located in New England were largely settled by the Puritans, and these individuals were keenly interested in supporting education. These were people who had left England because they did not belong to the state church; they were seeking a place to live where they could follow their own religious convictions. They believed that salvation could be obtained only through understanding the Scriptures, and so all children needed to learn to read—boys and girls alike. They believed that illiteracy was a device of Satan meant to keep humankind from finding salvation. Evidence of their perspective on education could be found in an early pamphlet from New England titled *New*

England's First Fruits, published in 1643. It is copied here from Cubberley (1919):

> *After God had carried us safe to*
> *New England*
> *And we had builded our houses*
> *Provided necessaries for our*
> *livelihood*
> *Heard convenient places for God's*
> *worship*
> *And settled the civil government*
> *One of the next things we longed for*
> *And looked after was to advance*
> *learning*
> *And to perpetuate it to posterity*
> *Dreading to leave an illiterate*
> *ministry*
> *To the churches when our present*
> *ministers*
> *Shall lie in the dust.*

The first law requiring that children attend school was passed in 1642 in Massachusetts by these Puritan settlers. The Massachusetts Law of 1642, as it was known, did not provide public funding for education, but did allow government officials to determine if parents were fulfilling their obligation to teach their children to read the Scriptures. As had been the custom in England, the responsibility for education rested with the parents, or masters of orphaned apprentices who traveled to America, but officials were empowered to impose fines on those found to be neglecting their duties. It was not long, however, before it was ascertained that the Law of 1642 was not sufficient to ensure adequate education for all. Consequently, a new law was passed, the Massachusetts Law of 1647, which had no precedent in English tradition. This law directed that every town should levy taxes expressly to hire a teacher of reading and writing. Although arising from a primarily religious motive, this law established the precedent in North America of publicly funded education for all children.

Further south in the colonies, the approach to education was decidedly different, owing to the fact that settlers had emigrated from different areas of Europe, or had come for different reasons. Virginia had been settled not by dissenters from the Anglican Church, but by prosperous members of that church who came to America for further monetary gain. These settlers continued the English tradition in which the children of the wealthy were educated at home by tutors or at private, elite schools. Training in the trades was provided to orphans and children of the poor so that they could work for the wealthy.

The Middle Atlantic colonies were settled by still a different variety of European immigrant, from a broader base. Although all were Protestant, they were from different sects and different parts of Western Europe. New York was settled by the Dutch and English. In New Jersey, the English, Dutch, Swedes, Scotch-Irish, and Germans all mixed. William Penn founded Pennsylvania based on Quaker traditions, but other settlers soon followed. Because of this wider range of religions, there was no general appeal to the civil government for the support of education. These settlers were content to allow each church to provide its own form of education.

The War for Independence at the end of the 18th century decimated efforts to educate the European inhabitants of North America. In New England, towns were no longer able to afford to pay teachers. The parochial schools of the Middle Atlantic colonies and the private schools of Virginia were also forced to close. The original 13 colonies were faced with $75,000,000 of debt, an enormous sum by the standards of those times. It may have been frivolous under those circumstances to think of diverting public funds to education, but at the same time, it was necessary if the spirit of the Declaration of Independence was to be propagated. That spirit held that " . . . all men are created equal, endowed by their Creator with certain inalienable rights," and that " . . . governments are instituted among men, deriving their just powers from the consent of the governed." In order to promote equality among men and ensure that the citizenry had the intellectual capacity to consider the issues facing the collective population, it was necessary that an educational system be established. The inevitability of such a system was apparent from the start of the Republic, as this quote from Thomas Jefferson, writing to James Madison in 1787, illustrates:

> Above all things, I hope the education of the common people will be attended to; convinced that on their good sense we may rely with the most security for the preservation of a due degree of liberty. (Ford, 1905, pp. 374–375)

James Madison took those words to heart and wrote in a letter sent to W. T. Barry in 1822, "Knowledge will forever govern ignorance; and a people who mean to be their own governors must arm themselves with the power which knowledge gives" (Madison, 1865, p. 276).

Although it was clear from the start of our nation that education would have a mandate, instituting that mandate took considerably longer. And again, Massachusetts took a lead role in doing so. In 1837, Horace Mann was appointed the first secretary of the Massachusetts Board of Education. He pushed for mandatory attendance at school, and by 1852 Massachusetts had a law on the books requiring that attendance. It would not be until 1918 that all states had laws requiring school attendance. The goals of public education in the 19th century were no longer to provide religious education, as they had been before the War for Independence. Now the purposes of education were to create citizens capable of making decisions about their own governance, and to unite the new American society. In accordance with this second goal, focused efforts were placed on educating the youth of the 19th century to a new cultural and linguistic nationalism. Noah Webster was a leader in this movement, publishing three documents that together formed *A Grammatical Institute of the English Language* (1783–1785). This book contained guides to the pronunciation of words according to the new American English. It was expressly meant to eliminate the local dialects that had emerged as a result of people from several language backgrounds living in close proximity, and to establish a common American language. Webster's book sold millions of copies and tremendously influenced American education through the whole of the 19th century.

This rise of American public education coincided with the establishment of the first school in the United States for deaf children, the Connecticut Asylum at Hartford for the Instruction of

Deaf and Dumb Persons, which later came to be known as the American School for the Deaf. It was established in 1817 by Thomas Hopkins Gallaudet and Laurent Leclerc, and was the first institution in the United States to teach a consistent set of manual signs to deaf children. At the time the school was established these manual gestures were not referred to by the staff as a "sign language"; that would come later. Gallaudet had been sent to Europe by a prominent physician in the Hartford area, Mason Cogswell, and a number of other merchants in the community to see how deaf children were being educated there. The doctor's daughter, Alice, had lost her hearing as a toddler and had no way of communicating. Alice's family had tried unsuccessfully to teach her some symbolic gestures or written names of objects. Gallaudet met Alice when she was 9 years old, while visiting his parents in Hartford, Connecticut. Because he had been a sickly child, unable to keep up with other children in play, he was sympathetic to her condition of isolation, and became interested in trying to develop a way to help her communicate. Gallaudet met with some success. On observing his keen interest in solving this problem, Cogswell began the fund-raising effort that would send Gallaudet to Europe. Gallaudet's first stop was in London to visit a school that used the Braidwood method, but school personnel shrugged off his inquiries about those methods. Discouraged, Gallaudet moved on, and found his way to France. It was at the Paris School for the Deaf that Gallaudet was first exposed to the manual signs developed by Abbé De l'Epée. Unfortunately, funds were short, and so there was not enough time for Gallaudet to

master these signs. Instead, he convinced school administrators to allow one of their teachers, Laurent Leclerc, to return with him for 1 year to Hartford to aid in the establishment of the school. Leclerc was never to return to Paris. The combined efforts of Gallaudet and Leclerc established the first institution in America where deaf individuals could come together to learn and socialize with others who were also deaf. It was in this newly formed community that Deaf culture took root. We can only speculate as to how the history of deaf education in the United States may have been different if Gallaudet had been more successful at recruiting the help of proponents of the Braidwood method.

Not many years after the establishment of the American School for the Deaf, another father with another deaf child sought to establish a school where deaf children could be educated. That was Gardiner Greene Hubbard, of Boston, Massachusetts. His daughter, Mabel, had lost her hearing at 5 years of age from scarlet fever, and so had some spoken language. Hubbard wanted to help his daughter preserve the language that she had, but it was not until she was 10 years of age that a way to do so became apparent to him. He, along with some other parents of deaf children, convinced the Massachusetts legislature to start a school where deaf children would not have to learn sign language. The doors to Clarke School opened in 1867. In 1872, Alexander Graham Bell was hired to bring to the school the method of teaching speech to the deaf that his father had devised, known as Visible Speech.

Although an ardent supporter of teaching deaf children spoken language, it may well have been Bell who first formally recognized the sign system used at the American School for the Deaf as a true language. In 1898 he was asked to comment on an article by W. G. Jenkins, a teacher at the Hartford School for the Deaf, advocating the use of signs with deaf children. In the writings of these men it is clear that the debate boiled down to two issues: (a) Does the use of signs run contrary to the spirit and practice of teaching American English in the public schools? and (b) Is there a demonstrable benefit to using signs with deaf children? In fact, it is Jenkins (1897/2005) who argues that the sign system used at the American School is not a language at all, as he writes:

> It is customary among us to speak of the "sign-language," or the "language of signs," but language is that which belongs to the tongue, *lingua*; it is the utterance of vocal speech. (2005, p. 111)

Bell (1898/2005) responded to that statement by writing:

> . . . we are justified, I think, in claiming, not only that it [signs] is a "language" (in the correct and proper use of that term—not in a loose sense) but that it is a distinct language—as distinct from English as French or German, or any other spoken tongue. (2005, p. 112)

In the continued rhetoric it becomes quite clear that Jenkins was concerned that labeling the sign system used at the American School for the Deaf as a "language" would bring the use of that language into conflict with the strict adherence of the day to teaching only American English in schools. Furthermore, it is clear that Bell objected to the use of sign language, in part, for that reason precisely, as he writes:

> That such a language should be employed as a means of communication and instruction in our public schools is contrary to the spirit and practice of American institutions (as foreign immigrants have found out). (2005, p. 112)

Further disagreement is evident in the arguments of these two men regarding the potential benefits or harms of using signs with deaf children. Jenkins' claim is that using signs does no harm to the efforts of deaf children to learn spoken English; Bell retorts that such a meager claim is hardly justification for using it.

So it was that at the end of the 19th century there were two major institutions in New England dedicated to educating deaf children: one that used manual signs and one that did not. It is within that context that the debate over whether or not to use manual signs with children who were deaf began to incubate. Until then teachers and tutors of deaf children do not appear to have explicitly considered the issue of how the use of manual gestures might affect the development of deaf children. Their main goal had been to help deaf children communicate within the context of their hearing family and community. This was accomplished with whatever means necessary. But with the emergence of a Deaf community, the issue percolated.

Using Hearing to Educate Deaf Children

It would not be long before yet another perspective was brought to the debate in America about how to educate deaf children. In 1897 a young physician named Max Goldstein, shown in Figure 1–1, presented a paper titled "Advanced Method in Teaching the Deaf" to the American Academy of Ophthalmology and Otolaryngology, the organization he had founded. In that paper he argued for the need to use residual hearing in the education of deaf children, an idea with which he had become familiar during a visit to Germany. While in Germany (1894–1895), Goldstein worked with Adam Politzer and Victor Urbantschitsch in their clinic observing how to help deaf children learn to hear (Bailey, 2001). In his paper to the Academy Goldstein described in detail " . . . a systematic course of training of the auditory nerve by aid of the human voice" (p. 1675). This account describes the steps in

developing the hearing of deaf children, and these steps would be familiar to students of oral deaf education today: First it is necessary to train the child to respond to sound, next comes discrimination of two vowels, and eventually recognition of speech. At the time proponents believed that hearing actually improved, as indicated by the quote below from Fay (1893), describing the results of an experiment conducted at the Nebraska School for the Deaf at the end of the 19th century. There, a group of new students were trained exclusively in the "oral and aural" method, using an audiphone similar to that shown in Figure 1–2.

During the latter part of the year the use of the audiphones was almost

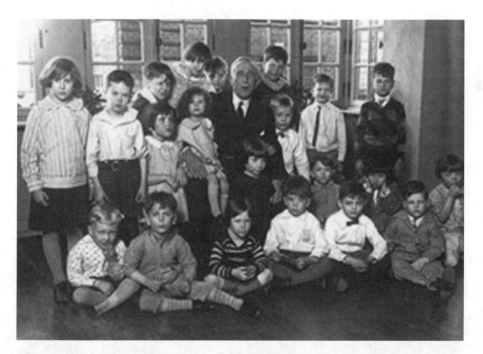

Figure 1–1. Max Goldstein and a group of students at the Central Institute for the Deaf, 1929. From *Deafness in Disguise*, by C. Sarli and E. Dubinsky, 2005: Central Institute for the Deaf (http://beckerexhibits.wustl.edu/did/mag/spv.htm). Copyright 2005, Central Institute for the Deaf. Reproduced with permission.

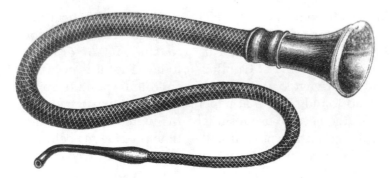

CURRIER'S CONICO-CYLINDRICAL CONVERSATION TUBE.

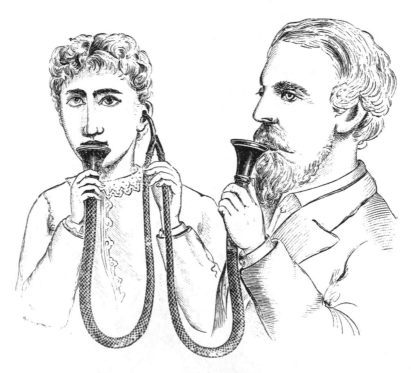

Figure 1–2. One version of the audiophone used with deaf students in the late 19th century.

wholly discontinued, from the fact that the pupils had discovered that without the audiophones they could really hear, and were happy to be relieved of the necessity of holding the instrument in position . . . (Fay, 1893, p. 3)

This method surely was the root of Auditory Verbal Therapy, as it is presently called (Kricos & McCarthy, 2007). Proponents of this method, such as Doreen Pollack and Helen Beebe, worked with Goldstein to develop the approach, and to extend downward the age at which it was started.

In 1914, Max Goldstein established the Central Institute for the Deaf in St. Louis, Missouri, according to his conviction that the education of deaf children should be approached with the joint efforts of teachers, physicians, and researchers. For the next century, this institution served as the center of oral deaf education in America. However, it would not be until the Second World War and the development of the transistor that we would have wearable hearing aids, and that was the first step in bringing truly useable amplification to deaf children. Transistors allowed control over the gain provided by the hearing aid. Then, with the development of digital filters later in the century, better frequency shaping was available in hearing aid fitting. Today deaf children have better access to acoustic hearing through hearing aids than ever before. Currently available hearing aids provide frequency-shaped gain according to a child's individual auditory thresholds. These aids also can direct the microphone in the direction of the source and reduce background noise. These characteristics should, presumably, enhance a child's ability to function in a regular public school classroom.

Getting Started Early

Many teachers of the deaf recognized the importance of starting a child's education as soon as possible. For example, Fay (1893) describes a private school in Chicago, started in 1883 by a teacher from Nebraska, Mary McCowen. The school was named, appropriately, the McCowen Oral School for Young Deaf Children. At a time when very few public schools had kindergartens, McCowen started one in her school. Before long, however, she decided that even starting deaf children in school at age 5 years involved too great a loss of teachable time, and so she began to accept students at 4 years, and eventually at age 3. The first kindergarten class at that school is shown in Figure 1–3. McCowen used the audiphone to train the children's "latent hearing," and she reported that the children who started earlier were more successful in developing adequate speech recognition and production skills than those children who started school at age 5 or 6 years.

At the time McCowen was teaching, hearing loss was generally not diagnosed much earlier than 3 years of age, and that situation did not change until we were able to develop methods of testing hearing without a child's cooperation. In fact, in 1988 the Commission on Education of the Deaf reported to the President and Congress that the average age of identification of hearing loss was about 2½ years of age, just what it had been 100 years earlier. It was at that point that efforts intensified to evaluate the efficacy and reliability of newborn hearing screening.

The first efforts at achieving the goal of identifying hearing loss during infancy had started much earlier, and were undertaken by Hallowell Davis around 1950. Hallowell Davis is often described as the father of neurophysiology in this country. The first brainwaves seen in North America were his own, recorded by his students in 1933. After he became director of research at the Central Institute for the Deaf in 1947, he developed an interest in finding

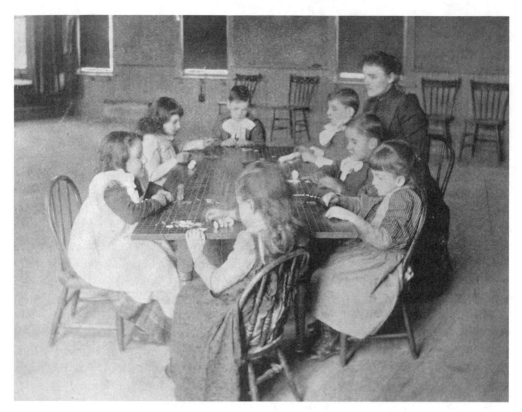

Figure 1–3. The first kindergarten at the McCowen Oral School for Young Deaf Children in Chicago, Illinois, 1883.

a way to test the hearing of individuals, including infants, who could not respond when they heard sound. For roughly 30 years he investigated the possibility of using evoked potentials, mainly the middle and late potentials, to evaluate hearing, but eventually concluded that those potentials were not sufficiently reliable. He became convinced that no evoked potentials would be reliable enough to do the job, and so abandoned his efforts. Meanwhile, others started to investigate the feasibility of using the early arriving potentials from the brainstem to obtain reliable measures of hearing (Jewett & Williston, 1971), and soon auditory brainstem responses emerged as a common tool for evaluating infants' hearing. Then in 1978, David Kemp discovered otoacoustic emissions from the cochlea, and attention was shifted to the possibility of using emissions that can be evoked for screening newborns' hearing. Today, more than half of the states in the country have laws requiring that newborns have their hearing screened before they leave the hospital. This emphasis on newborn hearing screening has led to the expectation that hearing loss can be identified by 1 month of age, amplification fit by 3 months, and intervention begun before a child is 6 months of age. In fact, this is the guideline recommended by the Centers for Disease Control.

The basis for these recommendations comes from several behavioral studies conducted around the turn of this century (2000) that all reported better speech and language outcomes for children who began intervention before 6 months of age, compared to those for whom intervention started later. Much of this work was done by a group of investigators in Colorado, headed by Christine Yoshinaga-Itano. This group did extensive analyses of the effects of age of identification on outcomes for children with hearing loss. For example, Yoshinaga-Itano, Sedey, Coulter, and Mehl (1998) reported on a comparison of the language abilities of 72 children whose hearing loss was identified before 6 months of age to that of 78 children whose loss was identified after 6 months of age. Although these groups were not explicitly matched on other variables, groups were similar in terms of gender composition, ethnicity, maternal education, and Medicaid status. Roughly half of the children in each group were in intervention programs that did not incorporate sign language instruction, and half were in programs that taught parents how to use signs in combination with spoken language input. When the children were 13 and 36 months of age, a caregiver completed the Minnesota Child Development Inventory (MCDI; Ireton & Thwing, 1974); the 1974 version was used because data collection was started before the 1992 version was published. Data were collected from children born over a several-year period. The Expressive Language subscale was used to index expressive abilities, and the Comprehension-Conceptual subscale was used to index receptive language. On both subscales, children whose hearing loss had been identified before

6 months of age were found to have standard scores of approximately 79, and the late-identified children had standard scores of approximately 64. Age of the late identification did not affect these scores; they were similar regardless of whether the child's hearing loss was identified between 7 and 12 months of age or between 25 and 34 months of age. This group of investigators published numerous reports, all reaching similar conclusions. The most extensive of these appeared in a monograph published by the Alexander Graham Bell Association, in the *Volta Review* (Yoshinaga-Itano & Sedey, 1998). Their major conclusion, that 6 months of age forms a natural boundary defining when intervention should begin for optimal outcomes, was replicated by several others (e.g., Calderon & Naidu, 1998; Carney & Moeller, 1998; Moeller, 2000; Robinshaw, 1996). Those findings serve as the basis of the recommendation of the Centers for Disease Control, and have remained largely unrefuted since the turn of the century.

But there has been one challenge to that common wisdom. It comes from research investigating the effects on language learning of the age of implantation for children who get cochlear implants. For these children it appears that the age of implantation, rather than the age of identification and initiation of intervention, explains the lion's share of variance in language outcomes, although there is disagreement about what the upper age limit is at which a child can receive a first implant and achieve maximum benefits. One report (Nicholas & Geers, 2006) claimed that the upper age limit is 12 months, whereas another study found that children demonstrated age-appropriate language skills as long as they received their implants before 24 months (Holt & Svirsky, 2008). It is perhaps not surprising that age of implantation would exert such a strong influence on language learning: These devices provide a signal to impaired auditory systems that is unmatched by what can be provided through a hearing aid. The age at which the sensory system begins to be stimulated may have significant, lifelong effects, at least according to the notion of critical periods.

Critical Periods

The notion of critical periods is used to bolster arguments in favor of several treatment options for deaf children. This notion, if accurate, makes it clear that early identification and initiation of intervention must be achieved if deaf children are going to acquire native abilities in a language. The work of Yoshinaga-Itano and colleagues seems to indicate that the first 6 months constitute this critical period, and so intervention must be started during that time. The idea of critical periods is also used to support suggestions that sign language should be introduced to deaf children as early as possible, as a way of getting language acquisition underway before children have access to auditory stimulation through cochlear implants (Mayberry, Lock, & Kazmi, 2002). Finally, the study by Nicholas and Geers (2006) is commonly cited as support for the suggestion that the 1st year of life represents a critical period for auditory stimulation: In that study, deaf babies performed better on language-related tasks 2½ years later if they received their

implants before 12 months, rather than after that 1-year birthday. So it seems that the increased risks of anesthesia to young infants, compared to that for older babies, are worth taking in order to get deaf babies implanted early enough to have maximum benefits.

Volumes have been written over the years on the various interpretations of critical, or "sensitive," periods. The original concept of critical periods arose from embryologic work showing that certain inputs to cells could exert an effect only at circumscribed periods in cellular development. In the 1920s, Charles Stockard was studying the effects of environmental toxins on the development of fish embryos. He found that when he introduced those toxins had different effects on embryonic development: The severity of the toxic effect was related to the time of exposure. The point in time when the embryo was most susceptible to damage he termed the *sensitive period*, or critical moment (Stockard, 1921). Thus, originally, the definition of the term was almost the inverse of what it is today: Rather than suggesting an age when something must occur in order for development to proceed normally, the term indicated a time when something deleterious had to occur in order to disrupt that normal development. Later, Hans Spemann and his colleagues studied embryonic development based on cellular context. They did this by transplanting cells from where they had begun development to a different part of the organism. What they found was that the future course of development was dependent on when the cell was transplanted. For example, a cortical neuron could be transplanted to the heart, and develop as a heart cell, if the transplantation occurred early enough. After a certain point in development, however, the cell was no longer capable of altering its developmental fate. Spemann (1938) termed this phenomenon *cellular induction*.

Konrad Lorenz extended this notion of cellular induction to early behaviors. In particular, his work showed that hatchlings of certain bird species "imprint" on the first large moving object they see, which is generally their mother (Lorenz, 1937). However, it can be other large, animate objects, as illustrated in Figure 1–4. There is only a brief period of time during which this imprinting can occur, according to Lorenz. It was not long after Lorenz's

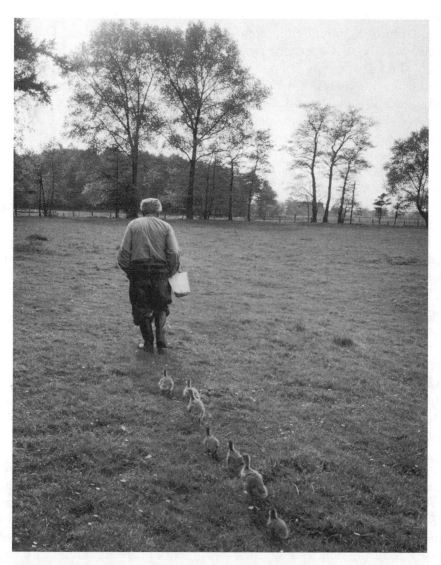

Figure 1–4. Konrad Lorenz with goslings following him. Thomas D. McAvoy/Getty Images. Reproduced with permission.

claim was made before this behavioral application of the notion of critical period, or induction, was extended to human development. In the 1940s it became accepted wisdom that children who were raised during their early years in orphanages would have difficulty forming attachments to adoptive parents (Goldfarb, 1945a, 1945b). Attachment between a child and parent refers to the feeling of security that a child has toward one loving adult, a concept often referred to as parent-child bonding. Behaviorally, it is apparent when children cling to parents in new or threatening environments, and/or when they check for the presence of a parent as they venture off with a new person or into a new situation. This relationship has long been viewed as being a critical basis for typical emotional development (Freud, 1938).

The development of sensory pathways in the nervous system has similarly been attributed to notions of critical periods. Without question, the work of Hubel and Wiesel (1970) with their "blind kittens" is the best-known example of this work. These investigators covered one eye of kittens at birth, and 6 weeks later when the patches were removed the kittens were blind in the occluded eye. This blindness seemed immutable to later visual experience.

Although these early studies on the phenomena of critical periods are well known, subsequent work that failed to replicate them is less familiar to most people. Inherent in all formulations of critical periods, be they related to cellular, behavioral, or sensory development, are the ideas that there is a relatively brief period during which some stimulus must be applied in order for typical development to unfold, and that the

effects of what happens (or does not happen) during these critical periods are permanent and irreversible. However, neither idea has stood the tests of time and repeated experimentation. It was not long after the publication of Hubel and Wiesel's blind kitten study that other investigators found that animals can be trained to use the previously covered eye, if they were forced to do so, such as by suturing closed the unaffected eye (Chow & Stewart, 1972; Harwerth, Smith, Crawford, & von Noorden, 1989). Regarding attachment, it has been demonstrated that the period during which orphaned children can develop strong bonds with new parents extends much longer into childhood than reported by investigators such as Goldfarb, and that many other factors influence the bonding process between child and parent (Ames & Chisholm, 2001). So, the development of both sensory pathways and of desirable behaviors may occur longer into an organism's lifespan than previously thought, and early deprivation may be mutable by later experience.

When it comes to the development of central auditory pathways, there is no doubt that certain developmental changes typically occur within the first few months of human life: Sininger, Doyle, and Moore (1999) provide a comprehensive review of these changes. For example, the nerve fibers in the auditory system are each tuned to carry information about very specific frequencies to the brain, and that tuning of fibers is typically completed by age 6 months in humans. Research with animal models shows that this development of neural tuning is interrupted when the auditory nerve is detached from the cochlea, and we may assume that congenital deafness has a similar effect on the central auditory pathways. But what we have lacked is an understanding of how mutable these effects are, at least until recently. Current research with children receiving cochlear implants during childhood is revealing that the auditory pathways are maximally plastic all the way up to the age of 3½ years (Sharma & Dorman, 2006); that means that the pathways can rapidly acquire normal characteristics if stimulation is provided to the auditory system. Regarding language, behavioral studies are demonstrating that language development may proceed typically in deaf children, even if it is not initiated within the first 6 months of life, as long as that intervention is appropriate and intense once it is initiated. For example, Nittrouer and Burton (2002) reported that children (8 to 10 years of age) with hearing loss who were not identified until 3 years of age seemed to have phonetic awareness similar to that of children with normal hearing, if they received intensive intervention from highly qualified teachers during the preschool years. Those results, for those children, differed from what was found for children with hearing loss who had their losses identified at the same age, but were placed in preschool classrooms within regular educational settings supervised by special education teachers with no explicit training in working with deaf children. Children in this latter group were found to have language skills (at 8 to 10 years of age) considerably poorer than either children with normal hearing or children with hearing loss who had been in preschool programs specifically for deaf children. The general conclusion of that study was that children

with hearing loss fare better when the teachers and clinicians working with them have been explicitly trained in how to work with deaf children.

Signs and Postmodern Parenting

Today we are clearly justified in our expectation that deaf children can develop spoken language skills that will serve them well throughout their lives. Deaf children can, if their parents choose, develop spoken language abilities that allow them to interact with family, friends, and coworkers without difficulty. However, debate persists concerning the best way to facilitate the development of those skills, with one critical issue being whether or not the use of sign language helps. For infants with some residual hearing, hearing aids should be fit as soon as the hearing loss is identified. But for those infants with hearing loss traditionally viewed as too severe to allow them to derive much benefit from hearing aids, the picture is more complicated. Cochlear implantation generally does not occur until children are at least 12 months of age, and so two concerns arise. First there is the question of how best to stimulate the acquisition of language while no auditory input is available. Even if parents' ultimate goal for their child is proficiency in spoken language, many professionals suggest that language input must start, somehow, before 6 months of age. According to this view, sign language can serve the function of providing that input until auditory stimulation is available. Often sign language is described as a "bridge" to spoken language: Having some vocabulary items stored in the lexicon as signs and the rudiments of a syntax and grammar makes the transition to spoken language easier once auditory stimulation is provided.

Another concern regarding the deaf child that is sometimes invoked to support the use of signs involves attachment. Some professionals believe that the language delays that arise from hearing loss and having to wait for an implant mean that children will fail to bond with their parents during the critical period for that process. This view persists in spite of the research with adopted children showing that the window for forming those attachments is longer than originally thought. The fear is that if a child is unable to bond effectively with a parent (or parents) during the critical period, the child may face a lifetime of emotional problems as a result (e.g., Vaccari & Marschark, 1997). So parents must sign with their deaf infants, according to this view, to facilitate an effective emotional attachment.

Both of these arguments for using signs with deaf children are supported by the current movement within the United States encouraging parents of children with normal hearing to sign with their children. One can hardly watch the morning news shows or read parenting magazines without finding entreaties for parents to sign with their infants. Programs designed to teach signs (frequently termed *symbolic gestures*) to infants are presented to parents of normally developing children as ways to "talk to your child before your child can talk" (e.g., Acredolo & Goodwyn, 1996). In these marketing campaigns it is commonly suggested that three advantages are accrued by teaching signs to one's infant: (a) the child will not experience the frustration that results from having thoughts constrained by the limits of vocal output; (b) cognitive skills will be improved; and (c) spoken language development will proceed at a more rapid rate. By providing the enhanced stimulation that signs give a child during the early, perhaps critical, period of development, these three benefits are provided to the child, and the positive effects are permanent and immutable. In other words, the child who is signed to during infancy will have superior language and cognitive skills to support his education later. Finally, the notion of early sign input serving as a bridge to spoken language is invoked frequently. For example, in their book, *Baby Signs*, Acredolo and Goodwyn (1996) explain the transition from signing to speaking this way:

> . . . as a veteran user of Baby Signs, he [the child] has already learned that communicating is fun, that things have names, and that people like to hear what he has to "say" about them. All that is left is to master the complexities of his vocal cords! (p. 95)

And so, the task of learning spoken language is made simple: Just add voice.

Although these arguments are appealing, evidence to support them is scarce. Regarding the suggestion that teaching signs to infants will accelerate the development of spoken language, the work of Acredolo and Goodwyn itself contradicts the suggestion. In 2000, Goodwyn, Acredolo, and Brown reported the results of a study in which they administered several standard assessments of language ability to children (ages 15 to 36 months) with normal hearing. Half of these children were signed to as infants and half were not. On average, the children who were being signed to were 1 month ahead in language development compared to the children not being signed to. However, this group difference was never statistically significant and always well within the general variability found for children in each group. In the end the authors were only able to conclude that " . . . [t]hese results provide strong evidence that symbolic gesturing does not hamper verbal development and may even facilitate it" (2000, p. 81). We may at this point invoke the retort of Alexander Graham Bell to W. G. Jenkins: Such a meager claim hardly justifies using signs—at least if parents' reasons for using it are to promote the development of spoken language.

Finally, one other argument offered for teaching signs to infants is that their vocal apparatuses are not ready to make phonetic gestures early in life (Acredolo & Goodwyn, 1996). Firm support for this assertion is usually not presented, other than to mention that first words generally appear later than first signs. Of course, studies of children's speech abilities do show that children's production differs from that of adults, and part of that difference can be traced to differences in vocal-tract anatomy. In particular, young children's tongues occupy more of their oral cavities than adults' tongues do, a trait that likely evolved because it helps with sucking. However, it also makes it difficult for children to form some cavities and constrictions needed for speech, such as the sublingual cavity associated with the lower frequency noises of /ʃ/ (McGowan & Nittrouer, 1988; Perkell, Boyce, & Stevens, 1979) and the retroflexed

constriction associated with American, rhotic /ɹ/ (McGowan, Nittrouer, & Manning, 2004). However, most young children manage to learn to talk in spite of these anatomical differences.

On the other hand, there is one way in which it could be hypothesized that early reliance on signs for communication might interfere with the learning of spoken language. Several investigators have suggested that the objects of speech perception are, in fact, phonetically relevant vocal-tract gestures (e.g., Fowler, 1986; Liberman, Cooper, Shankweiler, & Studdert-Kennedy, 1967; Surprenant & Goldstein, 1998). Although early versions of this notion, the original Motor Theory, were dismissed, recent evidence seems to be supporting the general position. For example, Fadiga, Craighero, Buccino, and Rizzolatti (2002) demonstrated that evoked potentials from the area of the motor cortex associated with tongue movements increased when listeners heard words that involve tongue gestures, but not when they heard words that do not involve tongue gestures. For the child facing the task of acquiring speech, the first task is learning how to move his vocal tract to produce the words or sounds in the ambient language (e.g., Nittrouer & Crowther, 2001; Studdert-Kennedy, 1987). Even among auditory scientists who were previously skeptical of the notion that listeners recover information about the moving vocal tract when listening to speech, there is a growing recognition that speech perception can only be understood when we view it as a sensorimotor activity (e.g., Todd, Lee, & O'Boyle, 2006). Accordingly, it can be hypothesized that an intervention approach focused on helping the child tune his perceptual attention to these vocal-tract gestures (whether through vision or audition) would be most facilitative for spoken language acquisition.

Changes in Laws and the Meaning of Public Education

Roughly a half century after public education became mandatory for all children in all states, the federal government passed a law extending the same obligations and privileges to children with special needs. In 1975, Congress enacted the Education for All Handicapped Children Act (Public Law 94-142). That law mandated that free and appropriate education be provided to all children with educationally significant handicaps between 3 and 21 years of age. In 1986, it was amended to include children from 0 to 3 years of age as well (Public Law 99-457). Provisions for the education of children with disabilities were modified once again with the passage of Public Law 105-17 in 1997, the Individuals with Disabilities Education Act (IDEA). With the passage of these laws, policy makers and educators began to investigate ways to provide intervention services to children with disabilities and their families from the time of the child's birth. It was a fortunate coincidence that the enhanced attention to early education generated by the IDEA transpired at the same time that methods for identifying hearing loss at birth were being developed. The simultaneous emergence of these events led to rapid increases in the numbers of programs, both public and private, available to infants, toddlers, and children with hearing loss. It is

fair to say, however, that research into methods of providing effective early intervention did not keep pace with the growth of these intervention programs.

The Effects of Cochlear Implants on Treatment of Deaf Children

In 1982, Laurie Eisenberg and William House reported on their initial experiences with children who had received cochlear implants. That device provided only a single channel of stimulation to the auditory nerve, but nonetheless led to great improvements in speech recognition for adults and children with severe to profound hearing loss. In roughly 1984, the Nucleus multichannel implant developed by Graham Clark and his colleagues in Melbourne, Australia, became available in the United States. These devices provided as many as 12 channels of stimulation to the auditory nerve, and quickly it became evident that more channels were better than one. In 1990, the Food and Drug Administration approved the use of cochlear implants with children as young as 12 months of age. As effective as they are, however, implants do not restore all the processing abilities of auditory systems with normal cochleae. In addition to providing tens of thousands of channels (i.e., separate and precisely tuned carriers of frequency information), the normal auditory system routinely provides an array of services that can be enlisted in the processing of acoustic signals, such as segregating the signal of interest from other signals in the environment and locating the source of the sound. Although implants do not appear to restore these aspects of auditory processing, they have radically changed the prognosis for children with severe-to-profound hearing loss because the one aspect of signal processing that they do the best involves speech signals.

The fact that cochlear implants are better at processing speech signals than performing other kinds of auditory processing is not an accident: Engineers and scientists have focused their efforts precisely on this function of audition. But they are severely limited in the numbers of channels of information they have to work with. If we consider each separate hair cell in the cochlea to be a separate channel for carrying information to the brain, individuals with normal hearing have as many as 30,000 such channels. Even multichannel implants can provide only about 20 channels of information. Because there are limits in the number of electrodes that can provide stimulation to the auditory nerve (reducing the numbers of channels of effective information that can be provided), only limited information can be presented with these devices. Initially, the approach taken to designing the external processor for the cochlear implant was to determine which acoustic properties of speech are most informative for recognition, then extract those properties and make them available through the implant. Several different processing schemes were tried and tested: Most presented the vocal pitch (i.e., fundamental frequency of the laryngeal source) along with one or two resonances of the vocal tract (formants). In the early 1990s, however, a different approach was tried. In this approach, the speech signal was divided into a few spectral bands, and the amplitude envelopes of those bands were derived and coded by the processor. According

to this method, no substantial amount of spectral information is provided. Nonetheless, the processing scheme met with success: Cochlear implant users could do quite well recognizing speech. That finding piqued the curiosity of scientists. What did speech sound like when only information about how amplitude changes over time was available, and could one really understand speech with such impoverished signals? At House Ear Institute, Robert Shannon and some of his colleagues decided to investigate. To do this they filtered speech signals consisting of sentence materials into several bands (one to four), and recovered the amplitude envelopes of those bands by half-wave rectifying the signals and low-pass filtering. Next, they used those envelopes to modulate bands of white noise divided as the original speech spectrum had been divided. Results showed that normal listeners could comprehend sentences processed in this manner (Shannon, Zeng, Kamath, Wygonski, & Ekelid, 1995). This result was difficult to explain using commonly accepted notions about how we perceive speech. To understand why it has been so hard to reconcile these findings with standard views of how humans recognize speech, it is necessary to appreciate the history of research into human speech perception.

A History of Speech Perception Research

Humans have long been interested in the phenomenon of speech communication. There are few behaviors that are so common across cultures as speaking, and so it has been the object of much study and speculation. In fact, oral educators of the deaf have figured prominently in more broadly based research on speech communication. For example, Alexander Melville Bell, Alexander Graham Bell's father, taught phonetics both in Great Britain and in America. His wife was deaf, and he had a strong interest in teaching the deaf how to articulate properly. As part of his work he developed a system of symbols, originally for the purpose of helping deaf students learn how to talk. That system was known as Visible Speech,

and Melville Bell described it in a book published in 1867 with the title of *Visible Speech*. Just one page from that document is shown in Figure 1–5. The system was quite involved, providing symbols for how to produce all the laryngeal and upper vocal-tract gestures one might imagine, for most of the major languages of the world.

As Melville Bell's work illustrates, most work on speech before the late 20th century involved trying to describe specific phonetic segments in articulatory and/or acoustic terms, and that

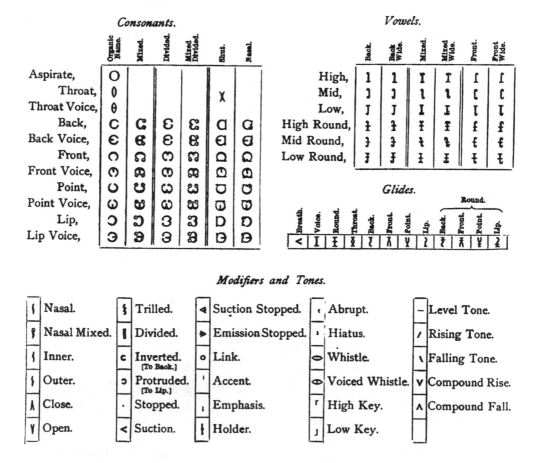

Figure 1–5. One page of the complete table of letters. From *Visible Speech* (p. 37), by A. M. Bell, 1867, London: Simpkin, Marshall & Co.

focus on the segment at that time made sense: For most of us the impression is strong that the phonetic segment is the basis of spoken communication, the "building block" of speech, as many textbooks define it (Hulit & Howard, 2002). Furthermore, before roughly 1950 our ability to study speech was largely restricted to written transcriptions of what speakers said and observations of how listeners responded to recorded signals. With the Second World War, however, came the technology to analyze sound into its component frequencies, and see how that frequency distribution changed over time. The first use of this technology was by scientists working for Bell Laboratories who wanted to develop a way of translating enemy communications recovered from radio transmissions on the battlefield into a readable form. The device that was built was known as a sound spectrograph. Potter, Kopp, and Green (1947) described the development of the spectrograph in a book titled, *Visible Speech*, after Melville Bell's 1867 book. They believed that the spectrogram generated by the device could be easily read by military personnel and deaf individuals alike, making it a valuable tool for many purposes. Of course, their belief was based on the assumption that phonetic segments are represented isomorphically in the acoustic signal.

The first spectrograph consisted of a magnetic recorder and playback that allowed a section of speech a couple seconds in length to be played repeatedly, a filter that would remain constant in bandwidth but scan the spectrum, and a stylus that recorded the energy in each frequency band onto photosensitive paper. An example is shown in

Figure 1–6. This device gave us a way to do a frequency × time analysis of speech signals. In addition to Bell Laboratories in New Jersey, two centers on the East Coast took a strong lead in the investigation of speech in the mid-20th century: the Acoustics Laboratory at the Massachusetts Institute of Technology and Haskins Laboratories, an independent group of research laboratories originally located in Manhattan, but later in New Haven, Connecticut. Both were focused on understanding the relation between the acoustic signal and phonetic structure. The goal of both groups

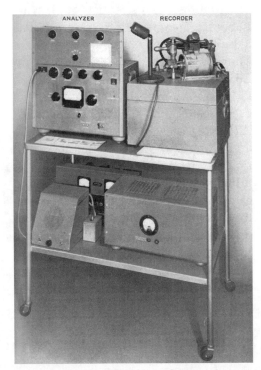

Figure 1–6. An early spectrograph at Bell Laboratories, circa 1947. From *Visible Speech* (p. 15), by R. K. Potter, G. A. Kopp, and H. C. Green, 1947, New York: Van Nostrand. Copyright 1947/1966, Dover Publications, Inc. Reproduced with permission.

was to explain how individual phonetic units are represented in the acoustic speech signal by specific spectral/temporal properties. Up until the time that the spectrograph became available, the view that these units are represented discretely was not questioned. Just as reading an alphabetic orthography involves scanning a string of separate visual symbols, it was presumed listening to speech must involve scanning a string of separate acoustic units—units that represent phonetic segments in an isomorphic manner.

The centrality of this view is evidenced from the goals that these early investigators established for themselves. The first task that scientists at Haskins Laboratories set out to accomplish was to build a reading machine for the blind. That work began in 1944 when Alvin Liberman joined Frank Cooper at Haskins Laboratories. Liberman describes these experiences in his book, *Speech: A Special Code* (1996). He writes that he and Cooper thought at the start that finding the relation between acoustic units and phonetic units would be the easy part of their work; the harder chore, they thought, would be designing an optical character reader. In fact, once the scanner had recognized the orthographic symbols on paper, they were not particularly concerned about translating those symbols into the actual speech sounds of English. It was their initial opinion that any acoustic alphabet should be learnable, as long as the sounds forming the alphabet could be easily discriminated from each other. They reasoned that listeners learned the acoustic alphabet of English (or some other language), and so they could learn a different, invented acoustic alphabet.

However, experiments quickly demonstrated just how wrong they were: If strings of these nonphonetic acoustic segments were presented at rates even approximating the transmission rate of phonemes in speech communication, they merged into incomprehensible blurs and no amount of training could improve that situation. Thus, they decided that speech must be a highly encoded signal, with each phoneme exerting an influence on the acoustic structure of adjacent phonetic segments. This notion is known as coarticulation, and was thought to explain one of the greatest problems daunting both scientists trying to understand human speech communication and engineers trying to build machines to recognize speech: the problem of segmentation. This problem explains the fact that it is difficult to draw lines on a spectrogram identifying where one phonetic segment ends and the next begins.

Nonetheless, scientists in human speech communication remained confident that there was an invariant connection between the acoustic structure of the speech signal and the phonetic structure of language; that connection simply needed to be uncovered and described. Efforts to do just that took the form of experiments in which highly stylized speech signals were generated, at first by drawing on photosensitive acetate that would be passed by a signal generator. The device that created these signals was known as the *pattern playback*, and is shown in Figure 1–7. Later, stimulus generation was accomplished by designating the parameters of the signal in digital form, and converting that to an analog sound signal for presentation to listeners. These sig-

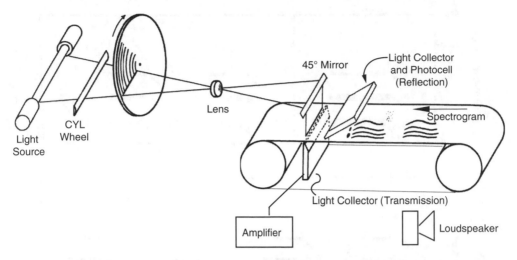

Figure 1–7. The pattern playback used at Haskins Laboratories from the 1940s to the 1970s. From *The Pattern Playback*, by P. Rubin and L. Goldstein, 1996, New Haven, CT: Haskins Laboratories (http://www.haskins.yale.edu/featured/patplay.html). Copyright 1996, Haskins Laboratories. Reproduced with permission.

nals were constructed so that all components remained constant across a set, save one, and that one was manipulated in discrete, equal-sized steps so as to create a continuum. The several stimuli along a continuum would be presented to listeners who reported whether they heard the speech syllable represented by one end of the continuum, or the syllable represented by the other end. This line of investigation can be illustrated with a common experiment involving the voicing of syllable-initial stop consonants.

The voicing feature for initial stops arises as a result of the time between the release of the closure somewhere along the vocal tract, and the onset of glottal pulsing. The time between these two articulatory events, often termed *voice onset time*, is brief for stops that we label in English as *voiced*, such as /d/ and /g/, and long for stops that we label as *voiceless*, such as /t/ and /k/.

One acoustic correlate of this articulatory phenomenon is the temporal property of when the first formant (F1) is excited, relative to the higher formants, a cue known as *F1 cutback*. This low formant is a resonance of the entire vocal tract, and so is not audible unless the vocal folds are pulsing. Figure 1–8 from Liberman, Delattre, and Cooper (1958) illustrates that the trajectories of the higher formants could be kept constant across a set of stimuli, with the timing of the F1 onset (relative to the onset of those formants) differing by varying amounts: Shorter F1 cutbacks generally signal voiced stops because they indicate that the vocal folds began vibrating shortly after the release of closure. Conversely, longer F1 cutbacks signal voiceless stops because they indicate that the vocal folds began vibrating after a considerable lag, relative to the release of the vocal tract closure. Figure 1–9 displays results of that experiment by

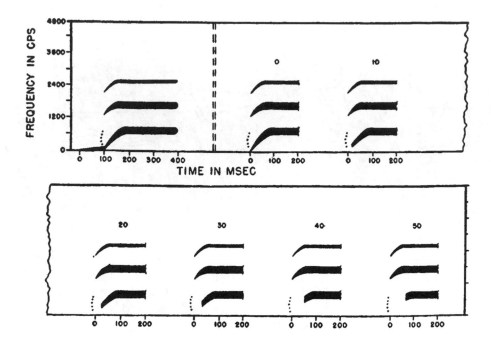

Figure 1–8. A schematic of stop-vowel stimuli used by Liberman, Delattre, and Cooper, 1958. From "Some Cues for the Distinction between Voiced and Voiceless Stops in Initial Position," by A. M. Liberman, P. C. Delattre, and F. S. Cooper, 1958, *Language and Speech*, *1*, p. 161. Copyright 1958, Kingston Press Ltd. Reproduced with permission.

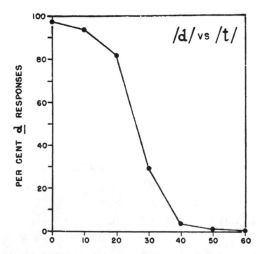

Figure 1–9. Results of a labeling experiment using stop-vowel stimuli, reported by Liberman, Delattre, and Cooper, 1958. From "Some Cues for the Distinction between Voiced and Voiceless Stops in Initial Position," by A. M. Liberman, P. C. Delattre, and F. S. Cooper, 1958, *Language and Speech*, *1*, p. 163. Copyright 1958, Kingston Press Ltd. Reproduced with permission.

Liberman et al. Here the proportion of voiced responses across a number of presentations of each stimulus is plotted. Given the constant change from step to step across stimuli, we might expect to see a linear function across the continuum: that is, equal sized changes in the proportion of d responses given for each step change in F1 cutback. Instead, we see a nonlinear function in which the listeners went from being quite certain that they were hearing a voiced initial stop, to rather abruptly being equally as certain that they heard a voiceless initial stop. In fact, there is only one stimulus where the listeners were uncertain about what they heard: the stimulus with the 30-ms F1 cutback.

Another example of this phenomenon comes from the group at the Massachusetts Institute of Technology. In this experiment the vocalic portion of the syllable remained the same across stimuli, and consisted of three synthetic formants that together were heard as /ɑ/. Aperiodic noise was placed in front of this vowel portion, but the spectral shape of the noise varied across stimuli. Specifically, the spectrum of the noise around 2500 Hz, where the third formant (F3) was located in the vocalic syllable portion, was varied in amplitude in the noise relative to the amplitude of that spectral region within the vocalic portion. When the amplitude of this region of the noise was a lot less than that of the vocalic portion, the syllable was heard as beginning with a /s/; when the amplitude of that region in the noise was greater than the same spectral region within the vocalic portion of the syllable, a /ʃ/ was heard. The top portion of Figure 1–10 shows stimuli from this experiment, and the lower portion of the same figure shows results of presenting the stimuli to listeners for labeling (Stevens, 1985). The fact that this experiment was conducted almost 30 years after the one described in the paragraph above indicates the pervasiveness of the approach and of the perspective that phonetic segments are recovered from the speech signal by extracting brief bits of spectral structure and knowing which segment that structure signals.

The nonlinear function found in the labeling responses of listeners in these experiments was termed *categorical perception* and for some time was assumed to be unique to speech perception. It was thought that listeners readily recover the acoustic cue(s) signaling each phonetic segment, and quickly translate the sensation into phonetic representations, losing the acoustic trace of what was heard. Decades of research have involved manipulating acoustic cues to see how each cue affected the categorical perception of those cues. To be sure, the specifics of this translation between acoustic cue and phonetic segment were hotly debated, with the loudest debate involving whether or not the process had to invoke reference to the articulatory movements that created the cue. But the focus of research across laboratories and across investigators remained steadfastly on these temporally brief, spectrally isolated sorts of properties.

The Motor Theory of Speech Perception evolved to try to explain how it is that listeners can so quickly and efficiently make phonetic decisions about stimuli that are variable in acoustic structure (e.g., Liberman, Cooper, Harris, & MacNeilage, 1963). This theory offered as solution the idea that speech production and perception share neurological processes, and those common processes mediate in speech perception. For example, the place of closure for a stop consonant is consistently targeted. Nonetheless, the acoustic correlates of stop place can vary across speakers and vocalic contexts. In spite of that acoustic variability, listeners accurately and reliably report stop place. This apparent mismatch led to the idea that the listener's own articulatory knowledge is harnessed in speech perception. The Motor Theory was used to explain how it is that speech signals are perceived categorically, and categorical perception was hypothesized by proponents of the Motor Theory to be unique to speech perception precisely because reference is made to one's own articulatory processes.

Both the notions of categorical perception and the Motor Theory came under harsh criticism during the last half

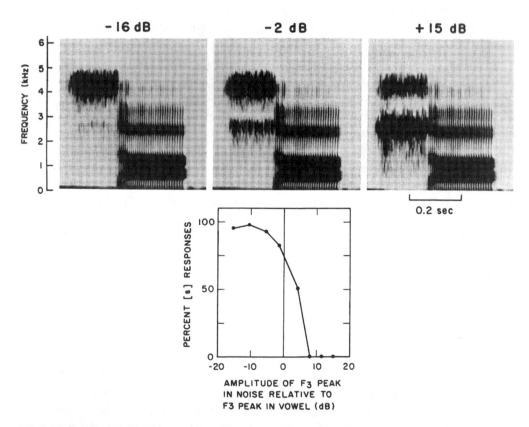

Figure 1–10. Fricative-vowel stimuli and labeling functions obtained by Stevens, 1985. From "Evidence for the Role of Acoustic Boundaries in the Perception of Speech Sounds," by K. N. Stevens, 1985. In V. Fromkin (Ed.), *Phonetic Linguistics: Essays in Honor of Peter Ladefoged*, pp. 243–255, Orlando, FL: Academic Press. Copyright 1985, Kenneth Stevens. Reproduced with permission.

of the 20th century by scientists who thought that listeners recover phonetic identity directly from the acoustic properties (e.g., Burns & Ward, 1978; Carney, 1977; Diehl & Kluender, 1989; Lane, 1965; Miller, Wier, Pastore, Kelly, & Dooling, 1976), and that categorical perception is ubiquitous to all auditory phenomena. But regardless of whether investigators thought that categorical perception was unique to speech or not, the methods described above were widely used in speech perception experiments: Discrete bits of either spectral or temporal structure were systematically manipulated, and the effect on binary labeling of stimuli by listeners was examined. In sum, the search for the acoustic correlates of individual phonetic segments was long and arduous and continues today. Undoubtedly, the reason for this protracted effort has to do with the fact that the acoustic structure of that portion of the signal temporally associated with any given segment varies so greatly across productions that it is impossible to find any one property that is consistently associated with a specific phonetic segment. The signal varies depending on whether the speaker is a man or a woman, a child or an adult. This speaker-related variability is illustrated in Figure 1–11, showing spectrograms of the word *cob* spoken by a man and by a child. It can be seen that the spectral structure of the noise associated with stop production is higher in frequency for the child's production (centered at roughly 2200 Hz) than for the man's production (centered at roughly 1600 Hz). This would make it difficult to identify an invariant correlate of the phoneme /k/.

The acoustic structure of any portion of the speech signal also varies depending on the surrounding phonetic composition of the utterance. For example, the spectral structure of the aperiodic noise associated with a /s/ varies depending on whether the following vowel is an /ɑ/ or an /u/: When /u/ is going to follow the fricative, as in the word *Sue*, we round our lips in preparation. Lip rounding lengthens the resonating cavity in front of the fricative constriction, and so the spectral composition of the /s/ is lowered. It is this kind of coarticulation that makes it impossible to define absolute acoustic correlates of any phonetic segment. That is the reason that it took so many decades of work, and so many scientists, to develop machines that can recognize speech, even when that speech is restricted to simple answers to proscribed sets of questions.

Around 1980 a group of scientists entertained the idea that the unfaltering focus of research efforts on discrete acoustic cues and their relation to phonetic segments could be misplaced. These investigators asked whether listeners might be able to understand speech without any of the traditional bits of signal properties that we label acoustic cues. To explore that possibility they decided to construct signals replicating speech, but without any of the traditional cues. Of course, devising a way to do that was not so easy. The method they settled on was to take a sentence, extract the trajectories of the first three formants, and represent them as simple sine waves. This approach is represented in Figure 1–12: The top panel shows the sentence, *Late forks hit low,* spoken by a man, and the bottom

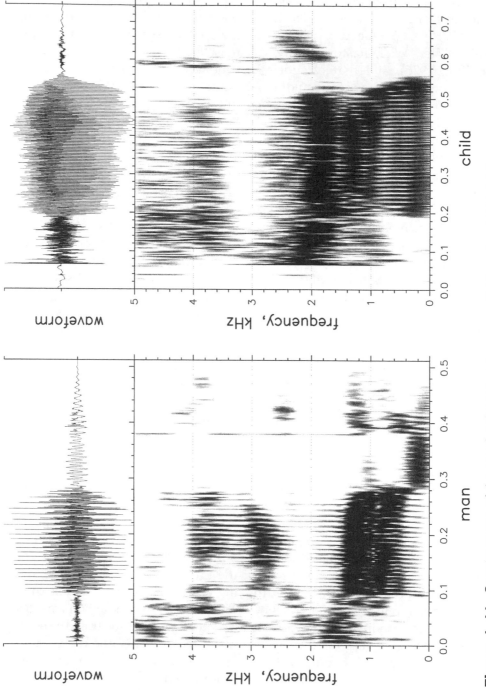

Figure 1–11. Spectrograms of the word *cob* spoken by a man (*left*) and a child (*right*).

panel shows its sine wave analog. In the sine wave signal there are no regions of aperiodic noise associated with stops or fricatives. Absent also is the pulsed structure of the vocalic portions, which arises from the vibratory pattern of the larynx. Formants lack their typically broad frequency bands. These are speech signals stripped down to their barest essence. Yet with a little training, listen- ers could understand what was said (Remez, Rubin, Pisoni, & Carrell, 1981). Such a finding had to have some significance, but it was not clear in 1981 what it was. Now we realize that the significance is to inform us that under- standing spoken language is not sim- ply the gathering of acoustic shards from the speech stream; the process is different in kind than earlier theories

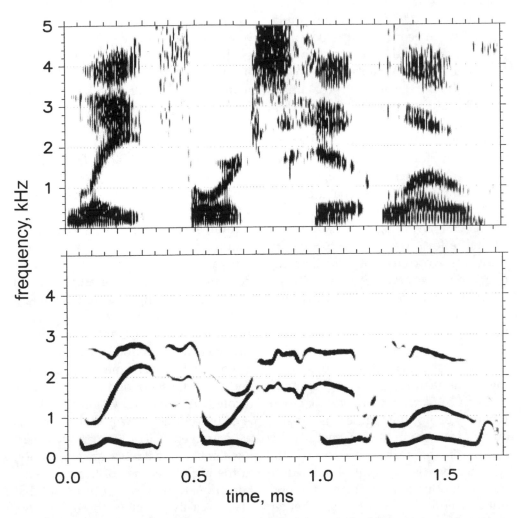

Figure 1–12. Spectrograms of the sentence, *Late forks hit low*, as spoken by a man (*top*), and as a sine wave analog of that production (*bottom*).

had proposed. This insight helps to explain the results that will be reported on these pages and helps to support the sorts of intervention strategies that are suggested.

Articulatory Features and Lipreading

Most of the work on speech perception done during the latter half of the 20th century sought to describe the correlation between acoustic properties of the speech signal and phonetic segments, but some examined another kind of linguistic structure: features. These entities describe characteristics of individual phonemes, and there are various kinds of features. There are the distinctive features of formal linguistics: In this system phonemes can be represented as sets of binary features that are either switched on or off (e.g., Chomsky & Halle, 1968). Although the taxonomy is formal, efforts were made to identify the acoustic correlates of these elements (e.g., Bondarko, 1969; Stevens, 1988).

Another kind of feature figures prominently in research with listeners with hearing loss: the articulatory feature. In this system phonemes (in particular, consonants) can be described according to the features of voicing, manner, and place. Voicing has to do with whether or not the segment is considered voiced or voiceless. Generally the setting on this feature has to do with whether there is laryngeal vibration during the production of a segment or not, but not entirely. As we saw, whether a syllable-initial stop consonant is considered voiced or voiceless depends on how long the onset of voicing is

delayed, relative to the release of the oral closure. So there is a period of time during which the vocal folds are not vibrating for both voiced and voiceless syllable-initial stops, but the length of time differs. Articulatory manner refers to how the segment is produced; examples include a complete closure in the vocal tract, as in stops, and a constriction narrow enough to create turbulence noise, as in fricatives. Finally, the place feature describes where the vocal-tract constriction is made. In speech perception research, questions for many years have focused on how the perception of one feature influences the perception of another feature (e.g., Miller, 1977), or on how information on the various features is integrated (e.g., Fitch, Halwes, Erickson, & Liberman, 1980).

Explorations of how individual features were recognized and integrated became a focal point of research on speech perception by deaf subjects, and a number of studies were conducted examining how well each kind of feature can withstand the effects of various degrees of hearing loss and different audiometric configurations (e.g., Bilger & Wang, 1976; Walden & Montgomery, 1975). In the experiments on audiovisual speech perception by deaf subjects, just one syllable at a time was presented, and subjects responded to that syllable through audition and vision combined. A common finding was that place was not perceived well by listeners with hearing loss because it relies on information in the higher reaches of the spectrum. Fortuitously, however, it turns out that place is easily perceived through vision. This finding helped to fuel hypotheses about the contributions of lipreading to speech recognition by listeners with hearing loss: A general perspective was that listeners with hearing loss can recover information about voicing and manner of consonant production through their limited hearing, and obtain information about place of production primarily through lipreading cues (e.g., Erber, 1975; Walden, Prosek, & Worthington, 1974.) This view influenced the way that lipreading skills were taught in aural rehabilitation programs for several decades, even though at least one study served as a serious challenge to the general perspective.

In 1976 a study on auditory-visual speech perception was conducted that called into question the perspective that consonantal features could be so easily separated in perception and assigned to different perceptual modalities. In that experiment McGurk and MacDonald (1976) presented subjects with auditory and visual stimuli, simultaneously. Unlike the experiments with deaf subjects, however, the two stimuli did not come from a single speech token. Instead, McGurk and MacDonald paired audio presentation of a /ba/ syllable with visual presentation of a /ga/ syllable. The commonly held perspective that consonant identity is derived by summing features had no prediction for what would happen if stimuli with conflicting features were simultaneously presented. Presumably one or the other setting for the place feature would win out, and the subject would hear either a clear /ba/ or a clear /ga/ percept. In contrast to that prediction, however, listeners reported hearing /da/. So the neat division of speech perception into auditory and visual features, with subsequent summing, was not supported. Instead, it appeared that a perceiver gets precisely the same information about the speech signal through both modalities.

The Speech Banana and Teaching Deaf Children to Talk

This review of the history of speech research is presented for a reason. The heavy emphasis during the latter half of the 20th century on acoustic cues and phonetic segments had strong effects on how we intervene with individuals, both children and adults, with hearing loss. The notion that there are discrete cues that signal individual phonetic segments led to a familiar icon of audiology: the *speech banana*. The banana, shown in Figure 1–13, is meant to show where the relevant spectral information is located for each phonetic segment. The goal of hearing aid fitting for much of the history of audiology has been to get the auditory thresholds of a patient into or above the speech banana, for as many frequencies as possible.

Our methods of teaching speech to deaf children have also been greatly influenced by the past half century of research on speech communication. Daniel Ling's highly influential book, *Speech and the Hearing-Impaired Child* (1976), contains 15 references to work by Alvin Liberman, 13 references to work by Frank Cooper, and numerous references to work by other investigators at Haskins Laboratories, such as Katherine Harris and Michael Studdert-Kennedy. Quite clearly, Ling's philosophy concerning how to teach deaf children to talk was based on the ideas emerging from the investigators at

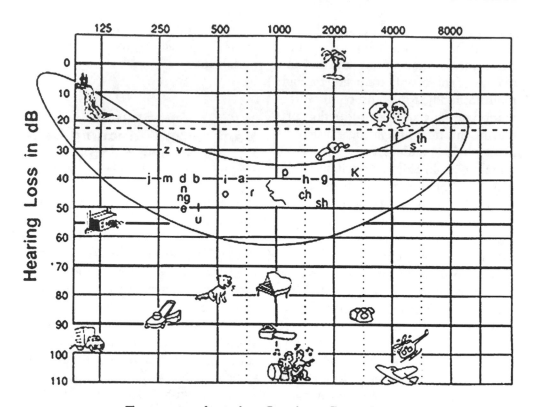

Figure 1–13. The speech banana, as commonly found on audiograms.

Haskins at the time, as evident in this passage in a section titled, "Motor Speech Ability and Auditory Skills":

> An encoded message must be decoded if the phonemes used are to be identified. It has been suggested by Liberman, Cooper, Shankweiler, and Studdert-Kennedy (1968) that this decoding process can only be achieved by means of auditory input. They also suggest that what we hear requires an intermediate decoding which involves some form of association with the articulatory process. In other words, other people's speech appears to be mediated in some way through reference to one's own speech system. (p. 26)

Here we see the foundation for viewing the phoneme as the building block of speech perception, an emphasis on auditory input only, and a reference to the Motor Theory—all notions that would guide our instruction of deaf children for years to come.

Chapter Summary

With both the science that we do and the intervention that we provide, most of us believe that we behave according to objective principles. In science we believe that we design experiments and interpret results without bias. Similarly, we believe we engage in clinical activities based on unbiased evidence concerning what constitutes best practices. Yet all of our science and all of our clinical practices come with traditions grounded in a long cultural history. It is only by trying to step out of the here and now to look at the past that we may start to appreciate how much of what we do comes from our shared history. This first chapter was meant to provide that kind of perspective. As data collection began for the study reported in the following chapters, many of the issues that were being debated at the turn of the last century, around 1900, were still influencing decisions about treatment for children with hearing loss. In 2002, as we started this project, we found ourselves engulfed, generally unwittingly, in many of the debates that had raged for decades. Hopefully, the data accumulated by this study will help to address some of the issues at the heart of those debates.

Of course, some things were different at the start of the 21st century, as we launched this project, than at the start of the 20th century. Advances in technology had led to the invention of devices that could serve children with hearing loss in ways that neither Alexander Graham Bell nor Thomas Gallaudet could have imagined. We can now identify children with hearing loss at birth, and so start intervention before 6 months of age. We can provide stimulation to the auditory systems of almost all deaf children, bringing their auditory sensitivities close to normal ranges. The government now mandates services for all children with special needs, down to birth.

On the other hand, we do not have Max Goldstein. We no longer have a facility like the Central Institute for the Deaf that combines professional training, education, and innovative research where students in all disciplines receive broad training. Instead, professionals have become highly specialized, causing service delivery for children with hearing loss to be compartmentalized: One person does the implant surgery, another person maps those implants, another fits hearing aids, another provides intervention, and still another does speech therapy. At the same time, training for professionals providing those services has expanded to areas unrelated to deaf children. A speech pathologist, for example, needs to learn about voice problems, the effects of strokes, swallowing problems, autism, childhood language, stuttering, and deafness to get certified. In our efforts to provide intervention for all children with special needs, we have lost some of our skill at helping children with specific needs.

The purpose of the study that will be reported in the pages ahead was to examine how we are doing now, at the turn of this century, in how we provide services to young deaf children, and to evaluate some of the thorny issues in the long-raging debates. To meet that goal, development in a variety of areas over the first 4 years of life for children with hearing loss was compared to developmental outcomes for children with normal hearing. The effects of three major independent variables were examined.

First, we examined potential benefits of identifying children with hearing loss as close to birth as possible. Roughly half of the deaf children in this study were identified with hearing loss, fit with hearing aids, and enrolled in intervention before (or close to) 6 months of age. The other half of the children with hearing loss were identified with hearing loss, fit with prostheses, and started in intervention between the ages of 12 and 30 months.

Second, we wanted to see if a benefit was obtained from the early use of signs. However, the purpose in this experimental manipulation was not to assess whether learning sign language for the purpose of being able to sign was desirable for children, either with or without hearing loss. One aspect of the American educational landscape that has shifted considerably over the past hundred years is our view of cultural diversity. When the IDEA of 1997 was written, wording was added explicitly supporting provisions for culturally relevant instruction. These provisions arose because minority children with disabilities were not making progress as rapidly as children who were not minorities. In general, however, these provisions reflect current societal values that all children should be free to grow up as members of their native culture. No longer is the goal of public education to raise all children to meet one cultural norm. Where deaf children are concerned, this shift means that educators are more sensitive to the desires of parents, either Deaf/deaf or hearing, who wish their children to grow up in Deaf culture. To actively participate in Deaf culture, an individual must be proficient in sign language. A child who is to grow up as a member of Deaf culture must learn that language. The work reported here did not address that function of sign language. Rather, this work examined the strengths of the arguments that early use of signs with children, either deaf or hearing, would facilitate the development of spoken language, enhance the bonding process

with parents, and decrease negative behaviors arising from feelings of frustration. The use of the term *sign language* will be avoided in this book out of a recognition that not all parents who support the input of spoken language to their children with signs are using formal American Sign Language. As will be seen, all the parents who participated in this study reported using signs expressly out of a belief that it would serve the functions listed above. There was a range in the kind and frequency of sign use among parents, from those who used a true sign language to those who supported their spoken English with some signs. This range reflects what happens in the real world among parents who choose to use signs with their children to support spoken language.

Finally, we explored the way that variability in prostheses affected outcomes. When this work was started in 2002, the expectation was that we would compare outcomes for children with bilateral hearing aids to those for children with one cochlear implant. It is an indication of how quickly treatments for deaf children have changed in recent years that instead we found many varieties of prosthesis combinations. Some children received bilateral implants at very early ages, some children received a second implant a couple years after receiving a first, and some children retained a hearing aid on the unimplanted ear. It was a challenge to examine all the possible combinations of prostheses, but we believe we were able to do so effectively.

In conclusion, the study to be reported in the following chapters sought to examine variability in developmental outcomes of three primary independent variables: age of identification of hearing loss, use of signs to support the acquisition of spoken language, and the effectiveness of various prosthesis combinations. Along the way we gleaned a lot of additional information that should serve us well in designing intervention programs for young children with hearing loss.

References

Acredolo, L. P., & Goodwyn, S. (1996). *Baby signs: How to talk with your baby before your baby can talk*. Chicago: Contemporary Books.

Ames, E. W., & Chisholm, K. (2001). Social and emotional development in children adopted from institutions. In D. B. Bailey, Jr., J. T. Bruer, F. J. Symons, & J. W. Lichtman (Eds.), *Critical thinking about critical periods* (pp. 129–148). Baltimore: Paul H. Brookes.

Bailey, B. J. (2001). Max Goldstein, MD: His continuing influences on our specialty. *Laryngoscope, 111*, 1675–1681.

Bell, A. G. (1898). The question of sign-language. *The Educator, V,* 3–4. [Reprinted in The question of sign-language and the utility of signs in the instruction of the deaf: Two papers by Alexander Graham Bell (1898), by M. Marschark, 2005, *Journal of Deaf Studies and Deaf Education, 10,* 111–121.]

Bell, A. M. (1867). *Visible speech*. London: Simpkin, Marshall & Co.

Bilger, R. C., & Wang, M. D. (1976). Consonant confusions in patients with sensorineural hearing loss. *Journal of Speech and Hearing Research, 19,* 718–748.

Bondarko, L. V. (1969). The syllable structure of speech and distinctive features of phonemes. *Phonetica, 20,* 1–40.

Burns, E. M., & Ward, W. D. (1978). Categorical perception—phenomenon or epiphenomenon: Evidence from experiments in the perception of melodic musical intervals. *Journal of the Acoustical Society of America, 63,* 456–468.

Calderon, R., & Naidu, S. (1998). Further support for the benefits of early identification and intervention for children with hearing loss. *Volta Review, 100,* 53–84.

Carney, A. E. (1977). Noncategorical perception of stop consonants differing in VOT. *Journal of the Acoustical Society of America, 62,* 961–970.

Carney, A. E., & Moeller, M. P. (1998). Treatment efficacy: Hearing loss in children. *Journal of Speech Language and Hearing Research, 41,* S61–S84.

Chomsky, N., & Halle, M. (1968). *The sound pattern of English*. New York: Harper & Row.

Chow, K. L., & Stewart, D. L. (1972). Reversal of structural and functional effects of long-term visual deprivation in cats. *Experimental Neurology, 34,* 409–433.

Commission on Education of the Deaf. (1988). *Toward equality: Education of the deaf: A report to the President and the Congress of the United States*. Washington, DC: Author.

Cubberley, E. P. (1919). *Public education in the United States: A study and interpretation of American educational history*. Boston: Houghton Mifflin.

Diehl, R. L., & Kluender, K. R. (1989). On the objects of speech perception. *Ecological Psychology, 1,* 121–144.

Eisenberg, L. S., & House, W. F. (1982). Initial experience with the cochlear implant in children. *Annals of Otology, Rhinology and Laryngology Supplement, 91,* 67–73.

Erber, N. P. (1975). Auditory-visual perception of speech. *Journal of Speech and Hearing Disorders, 40,* 481–492.

Fadiga, L., Craighero, L., Buccino, G., & Rizzolatti, G. (2002). Speech listening specifically modulates the excitability of tongue muscles: A TMS study. *European Journal of Neuroscience, 15,* 399–402.

Fay, E. A. (Ed.). (1893). *Histories of American schools for the deaf: 1817–1893*. Washington, DC: Volta Bureau.

Fitch, H. L., Halwes, T., Erickson, D. M., & Liberman, A. M. (1980). Perceptual equivalence of two acoustic cues for stop-consonant manner. *Perception & Psychophysics, 27,* 343–350.

Ford, P. L. (Ed.). (1905). *The writings of Thomas Jefferson* (Federal ed., Vol. 5). New York: G. P. Putnam's Sons.

Fowler, C. A. (1986). An event approach to the study of speech perception from a direct-realist perspective. *Journal of Phonetics, 14,* 3–28.

Freud, S. (1938). Three contributions to the theory of sex. In A. A. Brill (Ed. & Trans.), *The basic writings of Sigmund Freud* (pp. 553–629). New York: Modern Library.

Goldfarb, W. (1945a). Effects of psychological deprivation in infancy and subsequent stimulation. *American Journal of Psychiatry, 102,* 18–33.

Goldfarb, W. (1945b). Psychological privation in infancy and subsequent adjustment. *American Journal of Orthopsychiatry, 15,* 247–255.

Goldstein, M. (1897). Advanced method in teaching the deaf. *Laryngoscope, 2,* 349–357.

Goodwyn, S. W., Acredolo, L. P., & Brown, C. A. (2000). Impact of symbolic gesturing on early language development. *Journal of Nonverbal Behavior, 24,* 81–103.

Harwerth, R. S., Smith, E. L., III, Crawford, M. L. J., & von Noorden, G. K. (1989). The effects of reverse monocular deprivation in monkeys: I. Psychophysical experiments. *Experimental Brain Research, 74,* 327–337.

Holt, R. F., & Svirsky, M. A. (2008). An exploratory look at pediatric cochlear implantation: Is earliest always best? *Ear and Hearing, 29,* 1–20.

Hubel, D. H., & Wiesel, T. N. (1970). The period of susceptibility to the physiological effects of unilateral eye closure in kittens. *Journal of Physiology, 206,* 419–436.

Hulit, L. M., & Howard, M. R. (2002). *Born to talk: An introduction to speech and language development* (3rd ed.). Boston: Allyn & Bacon.

Ireton, H., & Thwing, E. (1974). *Minnesota Child Development Inventory.* Minneapolis, MN: University of Minnesota.

Jenkins, W. G. (1897). Question of signs. *The Educator, IV,* 216–220. [Reprinted in The question of sign-language and the utility of signs in the instruction of the deaf: Two papers by Alexander Graham Bell (1898), by M. Marschark, 2005, *Journal of Deaf Studies and Deaf Education, 10,* 111–121.]

Jewett, D. L., & Williston, J. S. (1971). Auditory-evoked far fields averaged from the scalp of humans. *Brain, 94,* 681–696.

Kricos, P. B., & McCarthy, P. (2007). From ear to there: A historical perspective on auditory training. *Seminars in Hearing, 28,* 89–98.

Lane, H. (1965). The motor theory of speech perception: A critical review. *Psychological Review, 72,* 275–309.

Liberman, A. M. (1996). *Speech: A special code.* Cambridge, MA: MIT Press.

Liberman, A. M., Cooper, F. S., Harris, K. S., & MacNeilage, P. F. (1963). *A motor theory of speech perception.* Proceedings of the Speech Communication Seminar, Royal Institute of Technology, Stockholm. Paper D3, Vol. II.

Liberman, A. M., Cooper, F. S., Shankweiler, D. P., & Studdert-Kennedy, M. (1967). Perception of the speech code. *Psychological Review, 74,* 431–461.

Liberman, A. M., Cooper, F. S., Shankweiler, D. P., & Studdert-Kennedy, M. (1968). Why are speech spectrograms hard to read? *American Annals of the Deaf, 113,* 127–133.

Liberman, A. M., Delattre, P. C., & Cooper, F. S. (1958). Some cues for the distinction between voiced and voiceless stops in initial position. *Language and Speech, 1,* 153–167.

Ling, D. (1976). *Speech and the hearing-impaired child: Theory and practice.* Washington, DC: The Alexander Graham Bell Association for the Deaf.

Lorenz, K. (1937). The companion in the bird's world. *The Auk, 54,* 245–273.

Madison, J. (1865). *Letters and other writings of James Madison: Fourth president of the United States* (Vol. 3). Philadelphia: Lippincott & Co.

Mayberry, R. I., Lock, E., & Kazmi, H. (2002). Linguistic ability and early language exposure. *Nature, 417,* 38.

McGowan, R. S., & Nittrouer, S. (1988). Differences in fricative production between children and adults: Evidence from an acoustic analysis of /ʃ/ and /s/. *Journal of the Acoustical Society of America, 83,* 229–236.

McGowan, R. S., Nittrouer, S., & Manning, C. J. (2004). Development of /ɹ/ in young, Midwestern, American children. *Journal of the Acoustical Society of America, 115,* 871–884.

McGurk, H., & MacDonald, J. (1976). Hearing lips and seeing voices. *Nature, 264,* 746–748.

Miller, J. D., Wier, C. C., Pastore, R. E., Kelly, W. J., & Dooling, R. J. (1976). Discrimination and labeling of noise-buzz sequences with varying noise-lead times: An example of categorical perception. *Journal of the Acoustical Society of America, 60,* 410–417.

Miller, J. L. (1977). Nonindependence of feature processing in initial consonants. *Journal of Speech and Hearing Research, 20,* 519–528.

Moeller, M. P. (2000). Early intervention and language development in children who are deaf and hard of hearing. *Pediatrics, 106,* E43.

Nicholas, J. G., & Geers, A. E. (2006). Effects of early auditory experience on the spoken language of deaf children at 3 years of age. *Ear and Hearing, 27,* 286–298.

Nittrouer, S., & Burton, L. (2002). The role of early language experience in the development of speech perception and language processing abilities in children with hearing loss. *Volta Review, 103,* 5–37.

Nittrouer, S., & Crowther, C. S. (2001). Coherence in children's speech perception. *Journal of the Acoustical Society of America, 110,* 2129–2140.

Perkell, J. S., Boyce, S. E., & Stevens, K. N. (1979). Articulatory and acoustic correlates of the (s-š) distinction. *Journal of the Acoustical Society of America, 65,* S24.

Potter, R. K., Kopp, G. A., & Green, H. C. (1947). *Visible speech.* New York: D. Van Nostrand.

Remez, R. E., Rubin, P. E., Pisoni, D. B., & Carrell, T. D. (1981). Speech perception without traditional speech cues. *Science, 212,* 947–949.

Robinshaw, H. M. (1996). The pattern of development from non-communicative behavior to language by hearing impaired and hearing infants. *British Journal of Audiology, 30,* 177–198.

Shannon, R. V., Zeng, F. G., Kamath, V., Wygonski, J., & Ekelid, M. (1995). Speech recognition with primarily temporal cues. *Science, 270,* 303–304.

Sharma, A., & Dorman, M. F. (2006). Central auditory development in children with cochlear implants: Clinical implications. *Advances in Oto-Rhino-Laryngology, 64,* 66–88.

Sininger, Y. S., Doyle, K. J., & Moore, J. K. (1999). The case for early identification of hearing loss in children: Auditory system development, experimental auditory deprivation, and development of speech perception and hearing. *Pediatric Clinics of North America, 46,* 1–14.

Spemann, H. (1938). *Embryonic development and induction.* New Haven, CT: Yale University Press.

Stevens, K. N. (1985). Evidence for the role of acoustic boundaries in the perception of speech sounds. In V. Fromkin (Ed.), *Phonetic linguistics: Essays in honor of Peter Ladefoged* (pp. 243–255). Orlando, FL: Academic Press.

Stevens, K. N. (1988, November). *Phonetic features and lexical access.* Paper presented at the Second Symposium on Advanced Man-Machine Interface through Spoken Language, Honolulu, Hawaii.

Stockard, C. R. (1921). Developmental rate and structural expression: An experimental study of twins, "double monsters," and single deformities and the interaction among embryonic organs during their origin and development. *American Journal of Anatomy, 28,* 115–275.

Studdert-Kennedy, M. (1987). The phoneme as a perceptuomotor structure. In A. Allport, D. G. MacKay, W. Prinz, & E. Scheerer (Eds.), *Language perception and production: Relationships between listening, speaking, reading, and writing* (pp. 67–84). Orlando, FL: Academic Press.

Surprenant, A. M., & Goldstein, L. (1998). The perception of speech gestures. *Journal of the Acoustical Society of America, 104,* 518–529.

Todd, N. D. M., Lee, C. S., & O'Boyle, D. J. (2006). A sensorimotor theory of speech perception: Implications for learning, organization, and recognition. In S. Greenberg & W. A. Ainsworth (Eds.), *Listening to speech: An auditory perspective* (pp. 351–373). Mahwah, NJ: Lawrence Erlbaum.

Vaccari, C., & Marschark, M. (1997). Communication between parents and deaf children: Implications for social-emotional development. *Journal of Child Psychology and Psychiatry, 38,* 793–801.

Walden, B. E., & Montgomery, A. A. (1975). Dimensions of consonant perception in normal and hearing-impaired listeners. *Journal of Speech and Hearing Research, 18,* 444–455.

Walden, B. E., Prosek, R. A., & Worthington, D. W. (1974). Predicting audiovisual consonant recognition performance of hearing-impaired adults. *Journal of Speech and Hearing Research, 17,* 270–278.

Webster, N. (1783). *A grammatical institute of the English language (1783–1785).* Hartford, CT: Hudson & Goodwin.

Yoshinaga-Itano, C., & Sedey, A. L. (1998). Language, speech, and social-emotional development of children who are deaf or hard of hearing: The early years. *Volta Review Monograph, 100*(5).

Yoshinaga-Itano, C., Sedey, A. L., Coulter, D. K., & Mehl, A. L. (1998). Language of early- and later-identified children with hearing loss. *Pediatrics, 102,* 1161–1171.

2

The Emergence of Language

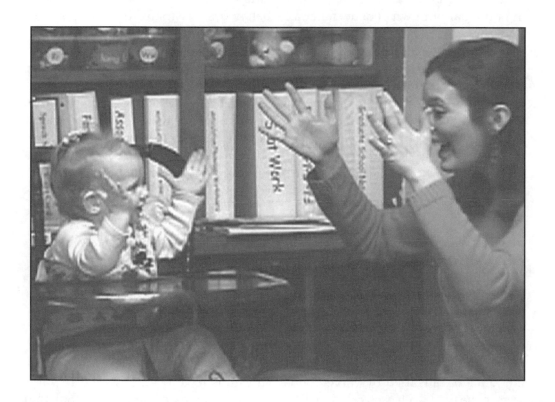

No behavior is more uniquely human than language. Other animal species communicate, but they do not possess language. Communication itself is an intriguing behavior because unlike many other behaviors selected through evolution, it involves cooperation. Most behaviors that have emerged through the evolutionary process involve competition among species and among members of the same species. Our intrinsic desire to perpetuate our species, and in particular our own genetic material, underlies this competitive motivation (Dawkins, 1976). So, why cooperate by communicating? The answer seems to be that there are times when cooperating increases the probability of survival for us and our genetic kin.

Why Communicate?

Communication among nonhuman animals has essentially three purposes. One primary function is to warn others of impending danger. This communicative function has been observed for several animal species, but most thoroughly in primates. Warning calls are specific in reference. For example, Seyfarth, Cheney, and Marler (1980) reported three different kinds of calls used by vervet monkeys in the wild, with each call signaling a different danger and evoking a different response. Long tonal units were observed to signal the presence of large, carnivorous mammals, and resulted in nearby monkeys running into trees for cover. A series of short, low-frequency chirps produced in rapid succession meant that an avian predator was in the vicinity, and caused monkeys to look up. Finally, a series of short, high-frequency sounds widely spaced in production signaled a snake in the grass, and caused monkeys to look down.

Another purpose of communication among nonhuman animals is to get needs met, but activities arising from this purpose seem to be restricted to immature individuals. For example, young primates communicate needs to their mothers through manual gestures and physical interactions such as the "nursing poke" (Blount, 1990). These behaviors dissipate, however, as an animal matures, and competition takes over as the motivating force behind interactive behavior. Once an animal reaches adulthood it would not serve him well to make public displays of the fact that he has needs, and specifically of what those needs are. Such displays could easily work against the adult by making him more vulnerable to his competitors.

The third purpose of communication among nonhuman animals is the establishment of social systems, including those of mating. Through the use of grooming behaviors, manual gestures, and vocal productions, primates within a group develop bonds with one another and establish power hierarchies (de Waal, 1998; Dunbar, 1996). The specific behaviors used to serve these social functions have been observed to vary across colonies of animals within the same species, suggesting that the identity of separate groups is shaped and made apparent to outsiders by the particulars of the communicative behaviors used within the group. These idiosyncrasies in communicative acts are one way that animals can separate "us" from "them." Because they exist, it means that the offspring within the group must learn these idiosyncratic behaviors from older members of the group; the emergence of communicative behaviors is not simply an ontogenetic process that unfolds without influences from the environment.

In humans there is clearly a genetic predisposition to acquire communicative abilities—a *language instinct*, as it is sometimes called (Pinker, 1994). The functions served by the ability to communicate with others are varied for humans, but not all that different from the functions served by communication among other species. Humans use language as a way of getting one's needs and wants met. We make requests of one another, asking that specific actions be performed or certain items be relinquished. Humans also communicate to form social networks, through gossip, vocal games, community rituals, and singing. Where acquisition is concerned, children practice communication and learn about language through nursery rhymes and pretend play, such as having dolls or stuffed animals talk to one another.

How We Communicate

While human communication may share many functions with those of other species, language, our main system of communication, differs greatly from systems used by other species. Language allows unlimited semantic scope; we can talk about objects and events that are not present, that happened in the past, or that will happen in the future. We can talk about things that are not even real. We can talk about abstractions, such as feelings and ideas. Language does not require external referents. The

form of language is independent of the objects or actions it references. Human language can be transduced into alternative modalities, such as written forms (Studdert-Kennedy, 2000).

The most significant way in which human language differs from the communicative systems of other species is in its structure. Language has what has been termed *duality of patterning* (Hockett, 1958): Phonemes combine to form words, but only in certain ways that are determined by a language, and words combine to form sentences, also according to language-specific rules. Individual phonemes are meaningless on their own, and in fact generally cannot exist independent of the syllable. However, this finite set of elements can be combined and recombined in countless ways to create lexical units of vastly differing meaning. Although individual words have meaning, when they are combined their summed meaning varies depending on word order and how the words are inflected. These two levels of structure, phonetic and syntactic/grammatical, provide us with unbounded abilities for communication. Human language is recursive in form. It is this complexity in linguistic structure that allows us to talk about things we have never experienced, to imagine things that have never been. Whether these linguistic properties evolved first and allowed humans to develop the great cognitive capacities that we possess, or whether the pressure of increasing cognitive abilities spurred the evolution of complexly patterned language systems is unknown. But clearly these two traits are uniquely human and support one another (Premack, 2004).

Human language also differs from the communication systems of other animals in that we use our vocal tracts to form resonating cavities, creating complex spectral patterns that are interpreted by listeners to derive meaning. The vocalizations of other primates lack the spectral complexity and dynamic patterning of human speech. That complexity and patterning are possible largely because at some time in the evolutionary process modern humans developed elongated pharynges. That is, the larynx descended in adult *Homo sapiens*, moving away from the soft palate, creating a substantial pharyngeal cavity. This difference between adult humans and other primates can be seen in the X-rays of human and chimpanzee vocal tracts, as seen in Figure 2–1. The lengthening of the pharyngeal cavity also meant that the tongue evolved to be longer in humans than in other primates, and has consequently become more agile. We are able to control the movements of separate sections

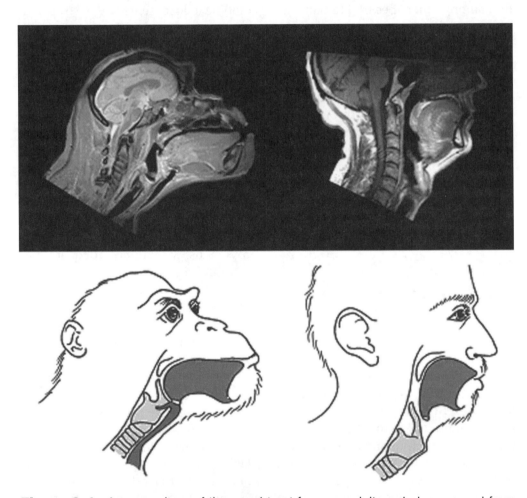

Figure 2–1. A comparison of the vocal tract from an adult, male human and from an adult chimpanzee. From "The Evolution of Speech: A Comparative Review" by W. T. Fitch, 2000, *Trends in Cognitive Sciences*, *4*, p. 260. Copyright 2000 Elsevier. Reproduced with permission.

of the tongue, which enables us to produce a wide range of phonetically relevant gestures.

Speech production is generally described by the source-filter theory (Fant, 1960), which posits that the asymmetrical opening and closing phases of the vocal folds (the opening phase is longer than the closing) create a harmonically rich acoustic source that is subsequently filtered by the supralaryngeal cavities of the vocal tract. If the larynx were positioned just behind the oral cavity, as it is in most animal species, the range of voiced sounds that we could produce would be tremendously limited. Because the larynx is lower, and so our supralaryngeal space is greater, we can produce more spectrally varied acoustic signals. That evolutionary process is frequently offered as a central reason for why human language emerged as it did (e.g., Lieberman, 1984; Nishimura, 2005), although the suggestion is not without its critics. There are those who point out that some evidence suggests the larynx may have descended in human ancestors long before symbolic expression emerged (Tattersall, 2007). Once humans did begin to use symbolic expression, according to this account, it started as speech. On the other hand, there are those who argue that the first languages were likely manual codes, emerging before the larynx had descended (e.g., MacNeilage, 1998). That position finds support in the fact that humans are primarily right-handed, and so motor control is in the left hemisphere, which is precisely where language is processed (Kimura, 1993). According to this view, human language eventually co-opted modern vocal-tract anatomy for linguistic purposes. But whether human language evolved as a result of the descended larynx, or the evolutionary process simply took advantage of this anatomical change, it is now the case that most languages are produced by gestures of the vocal tract, rather than of the arms and hands. Perhaps human language selected this production mechanism because of its efficiency: It requires less energy to move the lips and tongue than to move the arms. Perhaps it is because acoustic signals travel further, and can circumvent obstacles better than optical signals. This would provide a protective factor if early humans needed to communicate at distances, such as when they were hunting, or in the dark. In any event, perceivers of spoken languages are left needing to be able to interpret complex acoustic signals, shaped by moving vocal tracts. Clearly, this situation creates difficulties for those with impaired auditory systems.

These characteristics of human language—duality of linguistic structure and complexity of patterning in production and perception—make human language difficult to learn, requiring a protracted period of acquisition. Having a native level of skill with a language means rarely having to stop to think about how to inflect a word, or how to combine words to create a sentence. It means understanding syntactic and grammatical nuances well enough to know who lifted whom and who is holding the rope in each of the sentences, *The man whom the girl lifted held the rope*, and *The man who lifted the girl held the rope*, even though the three nouns (*the man*, *the girl*, and *the rope*) follow the same order of occurrence in the two sentences. Possessing native proficiency means having what might be called an "intuition" about proper structure in a language: Native speakers of English will recognize either of the following sentences as being grammatically correct:

(1) It was obvious the women baked the pies.
(2) It was obvious that the women baked the pies.

In English, the complementizer *that* may be present or absent in such sentences, although it is required in other languages. However, add a word or phrase and suddenly the complementizer becomes a requisite, as illustrated with this sentence:

(3) It was obvious to all that the women baked the pies.

Any native speaker would categorize the sentence as grammatically incorrect if the word *that* was missing, without ever having heard of a complementizer or knowing what such a device is. It is this kind of native familiarity that we wished to examine in the measures selected for the current study.

Comprehending Is Easier Than Generating

Communication happens not when someone produces a word, sentence, or gesture, but rather when another interprets the meaning of that communicative act. In human learning, comprehension always precedes production (Burling, 2000). This phenomenon is familiar to parents of young children who are able to issue commands that their children follow, even when their children can say only a few vocabulary items and have no expressive syntax (e.g., *Give it to me*, or *Put it down*). Even as adults, we understand dialects that we cannot reproduce. For example, it is not uncommon for a resident of Beijing, who speaks a Mandarin dialect of Chinese, to understand speakers of the Cantonese dialect, but not be able to speak Cantonese. The question that arises concerning these uneven roles of comprehension and production is the extent to which comprehension indexes the true mastery of a language. If one is able to perform actions that are requested, but cannot generate sentences with appropriate syntax and grammar, can we say that the individual has a deep and complete facility with the language? Is the line between comprehension and generative ability, in fact, the boundary between having a familiarity with a language and a true mastery?

Words Preceded Sentences in Evolution, but Not in Acquisition

It is generally agreed upon that in the evolution of specific languages, vocabulary preceded the emergence of syntax and grammar. That is, a fairly substantial set of words must have existed before rules could have started to be generated about how those words can be ordered and/or inflected (Bickerton, 1995; Studdert-Kennedy, 1998). Unfortunately, the child must sort it all out at the same time—vocabulary, syntax, and grammar. The acoustic speech signal being delivered to the child is complete in form; individual words are not separated in the signal. The task facing the child is at once to learn how to extract separate words, to discover how those words can and should be ordered, and to determine how they should be inflected to convey properties such as tense and case. As with measures that examine only a child's ability to comprehend language, measures that examine only a child's vocabulary, whether receptive or expressive, fail to tap into the child's real facility with that language.

Imitation, Teaching, and Theory of Mind

Reciprocity in human language far exceeds what is found in the communication of other species. For example, members of a primate colony may assume appropriately subordinate postures when confronted with a communicative gesture indicating superiority by a member of the group, but this response is largely reflexive, not voluntary. An animal would never, for example, ask for clarification of the communicative intent: Now, did you want me to roll onto my back, exposing my vulnerable underbelly, or run away in terror?

Animals of other species largely lack the capacity to imitate specific motor actions. They may select an object previously selected by another, a process sometimes termed *emulation*, but they do not imitate the specific actions used by the human model to obtain that object (Tomasello, 1999; Whiten & Custance, 1996). In fact, nonhuman primates raised by their mothers, without human interference, do not even demonstrate this level of imitation. It simply is not a behavior that occurs naturally among primates (Tomasello, 1999). Human infants and young children, on the other hand, readily and immediately imitate movements of others in general (e.g., Whiten & Custance, 1996), and movements of the face in particular (e.g., Meltzoff & Moore, 1997). This propensity to imitate extends to stimuli that are heard, as well as seen (Kuhl & Meltzoff, 1982). Such imitation apparently plays several facilitative roles in language learning. First, it provides practice for the child discovering how to make the gestures required for speech production. It is also hypothesized to be the first instance in which children dissociate linguistic structure from meaning (Studdert-Kennedy, 2000). By imitating directly the vocal productions of other speakers in the language community, the child can focus on the structure of language, rather than on its function. Of course, if language production remains consistently dissociated from its referents, then there will ultimately be a breakdown in communicative ability: The development of appropriate structure and function for linguistic forms must go hand in hand. And while imitation plays a crucial role in building vocabulary, it probably has little to do with the acquisition of syntax and grammar.

When the child produces a vocal utterance, a nearby adult often responds to that utterance with an expansion of what the child said, or a recast (i.e., producing an utterance with the same meaning, but a slightly different form). This type of teaching is unique to humans. Mature members of other species do not observe their young to ensure that actions are being produced correctly (e.g., Inoue-Nakamura & Matsuzawa, 1997), as shown in Figure 2–2.

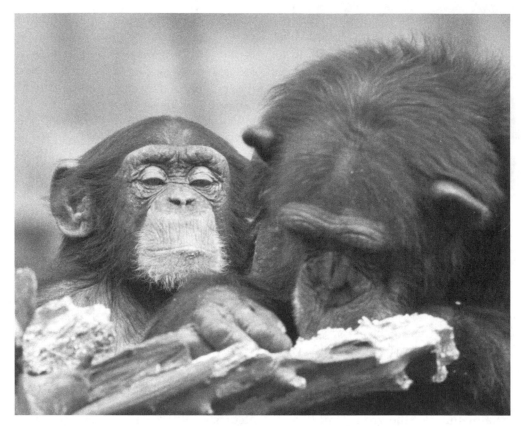

Figure 2–2. A juvenile chimpanzee observes a mature animal fishing insects from a log. From *Chimpanzee Politics: Power and Sex Among Apes* (p. 72), by F. de Waal, 1998, Baltimore: The Johns Hopkins University Press. Copyright 1998 Frans de Waal. Reproduced with permission.

This photo from Frans de Waal's thorough study of chimpanzee social systems shows an adult gathering insects from a rotted log. A juvenile chimpanzee observes, but the adult never checks or corrects his emerging skills. In sum, imitation and modeling are paired efficiently in humans in a way that does not exist in other species (Premack, 2004). When it comes to language, it is generally agreed that parents cannot directly teach their children syntax or grammar (Nowak & Komarova, 2001; Pinker & Bloom, 1990). However, the scaffolding of imitation by the child and modeling of new, related language by the adult work in concert to support language acquisition. To be effective, the child must respond to the adult's communication, and the adult must be sensitive to the child's communicative attempts.

Again, imitation is only a first step in learning language. It can help the child learn to produce the basic vocal-tract movements of speech production, and spur the acquisition of the first few vocabulary items, but it is not long into the language-learning process before a typically developing child begins to generate her own linguistic structures. This behavior on the part of individual children is part of a process that occurs in the evolution of cultures in which each generation elaborates upon what it acquires from the previous generation. The process is known generally as *ratcheting up* (Tomasello, 1999) and involves individuals using the skills and knowledge they gain from their elders as building blocks for further development of behavior and cultural traditions. Again, this growth of tradition is not observed among nonhuman primates, or any other species for that matter.

Just as adults in other animal species are unobservant of how their young are recreating actions that they must master, they are also insensitive to whether others appropriately understood what their communicative act meant. In other words, members of other species do not possess a Theory of Mind as humans do. In fact, there is no evidence that the communicative acts of animals are intentionally produced to convey meaning (Cheney & Seyfarth, 1990). If a vervet monkey signals that there is a snake in the grass, he does not check to ensure that the perceiver interpreted the message correctly—that he is looking down, rather than up.

Summary Statements on Language and Communication

Language, the preeminent form of communication among humans, has no equal among other forms of animal communication. It is recursive in struc-ture, with small components that may lack meaning on their own recurring in different orders to form longer sequences with variable meanings. It is this characteristic that allows humans to communicate on a wide, really unbounded, variety of topics. This recursive feature also creates systems that are highly complex linguistically. Similarly, the acoustic structure of human speech is complex, created by exquisitely coordinated gestures of the vocal tract. As a result of all these characteristics, language acquisition is a protracted activity, with mastery not being reached until adolescence (e.g., Chomsky, 1969; Hazan & Barrett, 2000). That mastery involves a deep appreciation of the grammar, syntax, and articulatory structure of one's native language that reveals itself as almost an intuition about what is permissible and what is not. Comprehension precedes generative mastery, and the learning of individual lexical items is started before any evidence of the acquisition of syntax and grammar is revealed.

In terms of learning devices, we find that young children will initially imitate older speakers in their language community. That behavior, however, needs to give way to practice in generating language in order for learning to be maximized. The trick for those of us interested in assessing how well and thoroughly language acquisition is progressing is to make sure that we tap into a deep enough level of proficiency, at developmentally appropriate ages. Evaluating higher order skills at ages that are too young or evaluating rudimentary skills at ages that are too old will lead to false conclusions about the course of acquisition.

What We Know about the Language Capabilities of Deaf Children

Human language is unique among communication systems in its complexity and patterning. For the most part, human language is produced by the organs of the vocal tract, and perceived through the auditory system. These latter characteristics likely arose because of the anatomical changes in hominid anatomy that occurred, but it is not a requisite that language be transmitted this way in order to have the recursive structure that it does. In societies where many or most individuals have hearing loss, language that is equally as complex in linguistic structure as any spoken language ultimately evolves, but in a manual form (e.g., Groce, 1985; Kegl, Senghas, & Coppola, 1999). The question of concern here is how well children with hearing loss learn a spoken language. Not long ago, the answer to that question clearly was that children with hearing loss generally did not learn spoken languages very well, if at all. But with the development of methods to screen hearing in newborns and to stimulate the auditory nerve directly, hopes were raised that children with hearing loss might acquire spoken language just as children with normal hearing do. The purpose of the study reported here was to evaluate how well we are meeting that expectation.

A couple trends regarding research methods are apparent in the literature on language acquisition in children with hearing loss. First, it is far easier to locate studies that have used measures of word recognition or of expressive vocabulary than those that have looked at syntax or grammatical competency. Likely that is because it is relatively straightforward to present a list of words or sentences to children for them to repeat, or to collect data on their vocabulary development. Word recognition tasks involve the child repeating words presented auditorily; the examiner records how many were repeated correctly. When it comes to evaluating vocabulary development, often parents are asked to make the judgments about which words their children have in their vocabularies. Therefore, the investigator has little involvement in generating the data. Reliability is generally quite high for these sorts of measures because of the ease of administration. However, these measures may only be examining the more superficial aspects of human language. That may be sufficient for comparing speech reception with one kind of auditory prosthesis versus another, which is a necessary and common goal of much research with deaf children. But to evaluate how well children are acquiring native proficiency with a language, different experimental methods are needed, methods that explicitly examine generative language.

Age at the time of testing is often quite variable for children with hearing loss in studies designed to examine their language abilities. That is because few centers have sufficiently large client bases to obtain adequate samples of children in particular age groups. Nonetheless, this factor is a confounding variable because the experiences that children have differ depending on when they were born. Technology is changing quickly, and the auditory prostheses that were available even a few years ago are giving way to newer technologies today. Even if children are served by the same intervention program, the methods used or teachers providing services may change over the course of a few years. Children's vocabulary development can be influenced by the books, television shows, and movies that are popular at different times. If the ages of children at the time of testing vary too much, say over a decade, outcomes may even be affected by changes in parenting styles. For example, it has only been within the past decade that it has become fashionable to support spoken language input with manual signs for children with normal hearing. That practice has changed the way that society generally views sign language, and so it may affect the cohort of children with hearing loss who are receiving sign support for their spoken language. A few years ago, it was generally children with poorer auditory thresholds and/or those who attended public institutions who were most likely to be taught sign language. Often parents who could afford to pay for their child's education sent them to private programs, which tended not to use sign language. Because of more accepting attitudes regarding sign language, more parents of children both with and without hearing loss are choosing to use signs with their children.

The majority of studies over the past 20 years have looked almost exclusively at language development in children with cochlear implants, or compared the development of these children to that of children with comparable auditory thresholds who were users of hearing aids or tactile aids. This design was appropriate because children with hearing loss were known to have significant delays in language abilities, prior to the availability of cochlear implants (e.g.,

Geers & Moog, 1978). Consequently, we had to establish that language skills are better when children receive cochlear implants, rather than when they use these other technologies, to support the continued treatment of childhood hearing loss with a relatively invasive procedure. However, it means that at the moment we have little data regarding how children with hearing loss are faring in general. How much have we been able to compensate for the effects of hearing loss on language acquisition? Are children with hearing loss learning language as well as children with normal hearing?

A few studies examining the language development of children with hearing loss help to exemplify trends on this topic over the past 20 to 30 years. In particular, the long and productive research program of Ann Geers, Jean Moog, and their colleagues needs to be recognized, as it has provided us with the most significant information regarding language abilities of children with hearing loss. During the 1970s, this team of investigators conducted some of the earliest work examining the syntactic and grammatical abilities of children with hearing loss. At that time, it was not reasonable to evaluate the syntactic and grammatical skills of children with hearing loss using tests designed for children with normal hearing. If toys or other materials were required to administer the test, they were selected to hold the interest of children with normal hearing much younger than the children with hearing loss to whom the test was to be given. That meant that the deaf children being tested were not interested in the test materials, and that can affect outcomes. In addition, it was not the case that the language of children with hearing loss was uniformly delayed across abilities. Probably because these children were receiving explicit instruction in language, they would often have learned the rudiments of complex syntactic or grammatical constructions, which would be evident in their productive language, but there would be numerous errors involving even simple aspects of syntax and/or grammar (Geers & Moog, 1978). Consequently, we could not quantify the language delay of children with hearing loss by the number of years they were behind. Instead, we needed to be able to describe how delayed they were in each area of language development.

An example of a language measure developed during the 1970s is the Scales of Early Communication Skills for Hearing Impaired Children (SECS; Moog & Geers, 1975). This tool required that the examiner observe the child and rate her language abilities using a list of specific skills. So, for example, at the earliest stages of language development it would be expected that the child knew to listen and watch the speaker. At later stages it was expected that the child knew irregular verb tenses. Each designated skill of receptive and productive language was rated separately in both a teaching situation and in an unstructured setting. The sum of points earned across skill areas served as the index of the child's language abilities. This method of summing points earned on observable skills was similar to measures developed to evaluate language abilities in children with normal hearing, such as the Developmental Sentence Score (DSS; Lee, 1974; Lee & Koenigsknecht, 1974). However, with the SECS, normative data regarding typical performance for children with hearing loss

was compiled, and subsequent studies compared outcomes to those data.

This team of investigators later modified and expanded the SECS to develop a tool titled the Grammatical Analysis of Elicited Language (GAEL; Moog & Geers, 1980, 1985). In this task, productions are elicited using toys and recorded onto audiotape. The language samples are then scored according to the grammatical devices that were used by the child. As with the SECS, scores were compared against normative scores obtained from children with hearing loss.

Even fewer investigations have examined the function of language for children with hearing loss than have examined the structure of their language. Evaluating communicative function of a child's language is perhaps trickier and more time consuming than evaluating the structure of the language produced. Yet it is important to understand because of the importance of language in developing social relationships. Again, human language and communication in other species share many of the same functions. In particular, communication helps to establish social systems. Where the infant is concerned, communication with one's mother helps to establish the bond that will enable the child to get needs met and to facilitate further learning. We have long had evidence that children with autism spectrum disorders (ASD) fail to use language for the same functions as children with typical language development. Children with ASD are less likely to respond to the communicative attempts of others and to initiate communication themselves (Wetherby & Prutting, 1984). These behaviors differ even from those of individuals with pervasive language impairments, but no signs of ASD (Loveland, Landry, Hughes, Hall, & McEvoy, 1988); this latter group uses language for similar purposes as the general population, but just not as competently. The diminished communicative functions in autistic children's interactions both exemplify their social separation and serve to perpetuate it.

Children with hearing loss have been found generally to initiate communication less than children with normal hearing (Duchan, 1988). When they do, the functions served by their communicative acts differ from those of children with normal hearing. As with children with ASD, deaf children respond less to communicative attempts on the part of their parents, and ask fewer questions themselves. However, children with hearing loss command their parents to behave in certain ways more frequently than do children with normal hearing (Nicholas & Geers, 1997). In particular, they will use one-word verbs in an effort to get specific actions performed (e.g., "Look" to indicate what a parent should be looking at; "Open" to indicate that something needs to be opened). This style of interaction was observed by Nicholas and Geers in 3-year-old children with hearing loss. Given the age of the children, it may very well indicate a discrepancy between the children's linguistic sophistication and their cognitive abilities. Younger children with normal hearing who are at the stage where they are using one-word utterances are generally labeling the things that they see, a developmental stage that typically occurs between 12 and 18 months. If a child is developing normally in the area of cognition, he is likely beyond wanting to label objects

by 3 years of age. Instead, he may wish to communicate more complex ideas, even if his language is not quite up to the task.

Varying perspectives on the question of whether language is fundamentally a motor behavior, with its neural representation in a form that is inherently perceptuomotor in nature, or is a cognitive process merely expressed by motor behavior have affected how we study language acquisition in deaf children, as well as how we intervene. As indicated in the first chapter, there are those who suggest that language intervention for children with hearing loss must start with sign language, as soon as possible (Mayberry, Lock, & Kazmi, 2002). That idea is predicated on the assumption that language is independent of modality of expression or perception. For investigators holding to that idea, it becomes imperative to find ways of assessing language capacities that are independent of the modality used either to express or to perceive it. An example of this approach is found in the work of Svirsky and colleagues, who purposefully assess language development in children with hearing loss through either signed or spoken forms. Their perspective on the dissociation of language and behavior is conveyed in the statement, "The option of conducting tests in these two modalities is important for measuring the children's underlying language abilities, as far as possible independently of their ability to understand spoken language or to produce intelligible speech" (Svirsky, Teoh, & Neuburger, 2004, p. 227).

The alternative to this view is that language is expressly a motor behavior, with the very elements it is comprised of being perceptuomotor in nature (e.g., Studdert-Kennedy, 1987). According to this perspective, language is not independent of the behavior that generates it, or the perceiving mechanism that interprets the signal generated by others. This view arises from the idea that language emerged from more general motor control. Human language is essentially a highly developed and refined motor activity. Support for this position is gathered from the fact that the left hemisphere controls both speech production and fine motor actions made by the (typically) dominant right hand (MacNeilage, 1997, 1998). Following from this perspective, the assessment of language should be tied to the system that produces and perceives it. That is the perspective that was adopted in this investigation.

Chapter Summary

Human language is the most complex of communication systems. Nonetheless, typically developing children with normal hearing acquire exquisite familiarity with the intricacies of this system within a very short time of life. It was our wish to examine this deep level of familiarity for children with hearing loss through the data collected on this project.

References

Bickerton, D. (1995). *Language and human behavior*. Seattle, WA: University of Washington Press.

Blount, B. G. (1990). Spatial expression of social relationships among captive *Pan paniscus*: Ontogenetic and phylogenetic implications. In S. T. Parker & K. R. Gibson (Eds.), *"Language" and intelligence in monkeys and apes: Comparative developmental perspectives* (pp. 420–432). Cambridge, UK: Cambridge University Press.

Burling, R. (2000). Comprehension, production and conventionalisation in the origins of language. In C. Knight, M. Studdert-Kennedy, & J. R. Hurford (Eds.), *The evolutionary emergence of language: Social function and the origins of linguistic form* (pp. 27–39). Cambridge, UK: Cambridge University Press.

Cheney, D. L., & Seyfarth, R. M. (1990). *How monkeys see the world: Inside the mind of another species*. Chicago: University of Chicago Press.

Chomsky, C. (1969). *The acquisition of syntax in children from 5 to 10* (MIT Research Monograph No. 57). Cambridge, MA: MIT Press.

Dawkins, R. (1976). *The selfish gene*. New York: Oxford University Press.

de Waal, F. (1998). *Chimpanzee politics: Power and sex among apes* (Rev. ed.). Baltimore: The Johns Hopkins University Press.

Duchan, J. F. (1988). Assessing communication of hearing-impaired children: Influences from pragmatics. *Journal of the Academy of Rehabilitative Audiology Monograph, 21*, 19–40.

Dunbar, R. (1996). *Grooming, gossip, and the evolution of language*. Cambridge, MA: Harvard University Press.

Fant, G. (1960). *Acoustic theory of speech production*. The Hague, Netherlands: Mouton.

Fitch, W. T. (2000). The evolution of speech: A comparative review. *Trends in Cognitive Sciences, 4*, 258–267.

Geers, A. E., & Moog, J. S. (1978). Syntactic maturity of spontaneous speech and elicited imitations of hearing-impaired children. *Journal of Speech and Hearing Disorders, 43*, 380–391.

Groce, N. E. (1985). *Everyone here spoke sign language: Hereditary deafness on Martha's*

Vineyard. Cambridge, MA: Harvard University Press.

Hazan, V., & Barrett, S. (2000). The development of phonemic categorization in children aged 6–12. *Journal of Phonetics, 28*, 377–396.

Hockett, C. F. (1958). *A course in modern linguistics*. New York: MacMillan.

Inoue-Nakamura, N., & Matsuzawa, T. (1997). Development of stone tool use by wild chimpanzees (Pan troglodytes). *Journal of Comparative Psychology, 111*, 159–173.

Kegl, J., Senghas, A., & Coppola, M. (1999). Creation through contact: Sign language emergence and sign language change in Nicaragua. In M. DeGraff (Ed.), *Language creation and language change: Creolization, diachrony, and development* (pp. 179–237). Cambridge, MA: MIT Press.

Kimura, D. (1993). *Neuromotor mechanisms in human communication*. New York: Oxford University Press.

Kuhl, P. K., & Meltzoff, A. N. (1982). The bimodal perception of speech in infancy. *Science, 218*, 1138–1141.

Lee, L. L. (1974). *Developmental sentence analysis*. Evanston, IL: Northwestern University Press.

Lee, L. L., & Koenigsknecht, R. A. (1974). *Developmental sentence scoring*. Evanston, IL: Northwestern University Press.

Lieberman, P. (1984). *The biology and evolution of language*. Cambridge, MA: Harvard University Press.

Loveland, K. A., Landry, S. H., Hughes, S. O., Hall, S. K., & McEvoy, R. E. (1988). Speech acts and the pragmatic deficits of autism. *Journal of Speech and Hearing Research, 31*, 593–604.

MacNeilage, P. (1997). Towards a unified view of the evolution of cerebral hemispheric specializations in vertebrates. In A. D. Milner (Ed.), *Comparative neuropsychology* (pp. 167–183). Oxford, UK: Oxford University Press.

MacNeilage, P. F. (1998). Evolution of the mechanism of language output: Comparative neurobiology of vocal and manual communication. In J. R. Hurford, M. Studdert-Kennedy, & C. Knight (Eds.), *Approaches to the evolution of language: Social and cognitive bases* (pp. 222–241). Cambridge, UK: Cambridge University Press.

Mayberry, R. I., Lock, E., & Kazmi, H. (2002). Linguistic ability and early language exposure. *Nature, 417*, 38.

Meltzoff, A. N., & Moore, M. K. (1997). Explaining facial imitation: A theoretical model. *Early Development & Parenting, 6*, 179–192.

Moog, J. S., & Geers, A. E. (1975). *Scales of Early Communication Skills for Hearing-Impaired Children*. St. Louis, MO: Central Institute for the Deaf.

Moog, J. S., & Geers, A. E. (1980). *Grammatical Analysis of Elicited Language—Complex Sentence Level*. St. Louis, MO: Central Institute for the Deaf.

Moog, J. S., & Geers, A. E. (1985). *Grammatical Analysis of Elicited Language—Simple Sentence Level* (2nd ed.). St. Louis, MO: Central Institute for the Deaf.

Nicholas, J. G., & Geers, A. E. (1997). Communication of oral deaf and normally hearing children at 36 months of age. *Journal of Speech, Language, and Hearing Research, 40*, 1314–1327.

Nishimura, T. (2005). Developmental changes in the shape of the supralaryngeal vocal tract in chimpanzees. *American Journal of Physical Anthropology, 126*, 193–204.

Nowak, M. A., & Komarova, N. L. (2001). Towards an evolutionary theory of language. *Trends in Cognitive Sciences, 5*, 288–295.

Pinker, S. (1994). *The language instinct*. New York: W. Morrow and Co.

Pinker, S., & Bloom, P. (1990). Natural language and natural selection. *Behavioral and Brain Sciences, 13*, 707–784.

Premack, D. (2004). Is language the key to human intelligence? *Science, 303*, 318–320.

Seyfarth, R. M., Cheney, D. L., & Marler, P. (1980). Vervet monkey alarm calls: Semantic communication in a free-ranging primate. *Animal Behaviour, 28*, 1070–1094.

Studdert-Kennedy, M. (1987). The phoneme as a perceptuomotor structure. In A. Allport, D. G. MacKay, W. Prinz, & E. Scheerer (Eds.), *Language perception and production: Relationships between listening, speaking, reading, and writing* (pp. 67–84). Orlando, FL: Academic Press.

Studdert-Kennedy, M. (1998). Introduction: The emergence of phonology. In J. R. Hurford, M. Studdert-Kennedy, & C. Knight (Eds.), *Approaches to the evolution of language: Social and cognitive bases* (pp. 169–176). Cambridge, UK: Cambridge University Press.

Studdert-Kennedy, M. (2000). Evolutionary implications of the particulate principle: Imitation and the dissociation of phonetic form from semantic function. In C. Knight, M. Studdert-Kennedy, & J. R. Hurford (Eds.), *The evolutionary emergence of language: Social function and the origins of linguistic form* (pp. 161–176). Cambridge, UK: Cambridge University Press.

Svirsky, M. A., Teoh, S. W., & Neuburger, H. (2004). Development of language and speech perception in congenitally, profoundly deaf children as a function of age at cochlear implantation. *Audiology & Neurotology, 9,* 224–233.

Tattersall, I. (2007). [Response to article by P. Lieberman (2007), *The evolution of human speech: Its anatomical and neural bases*]. *Current Anthropology, 48,* 57–58.

Tomasello, M. (1999). *The cultural origins of human cognition.* Cambridge, MA: Harvard University Press.

Wetherby, A. M., & Prutting, C. A. (1984). Profiles of communicative and cognitive-social abilities in autistic children. *Journal of Speech and Hearing Research, 27,* 364–377.

Whiten, A., & Custance, D. (1996). Studies of imitation in chimpanzees and children. In C. M. Heyes & B. G. Galef (Eds.), *Social learning in animals: The roots of culture* (pp. 291–318). San Diego, CA: Academic Press.

3

Development of Children with Hearing Loss: State of Our Knowledge

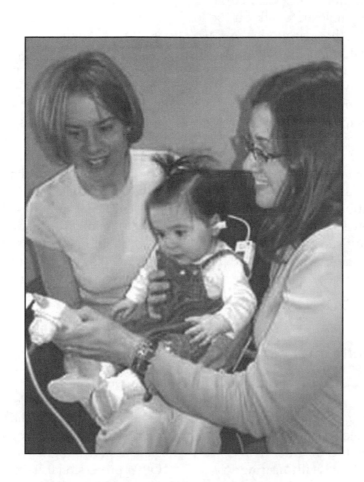

Parents have great dreams and ordinary expectations for their children. They may *dream* that one day their child will be the president of the United States, a starting pitcher for the Yankees, or a Nobel laureate. However, parents *expect* that their child will be able to tie his own shoes, climb the jungle gym, and talk. Unfortunately, physical or mental limitations sometimes shatter even the most ordinary of expectations. Until recently, severe-to-profound hearing loss was considered by most professionals to be a limitation that would curtail a child's ability to learn to talk, and so to interact with those around him. Two technological advances have changed that prevailing wisdom: (a) the development of ways to test hearing in infants too young to cooperate so that we may begin intervention early, and (b) the development and continued refinement of cochlear implants so that we can provide input to the auditory systems of all children with hearing loss, no matter how severe that loss is. However, even though the advent of earlier identification and cochlear implants offers new solutions to old problems, it also gives rise to a whole new set of questions.

Current Intervention Options

One critical question that arises from these technological advances concerns how we should be intervening with infants identified with hearing loss so very young. Because the capability to identify hearing loss shortly after birth was not available until fairly recently, it has not been long that we have had the opportunity to intervene at such a tender age. Consequently, we lack a collective account of what works and what does not work. Nonetheless, it seems that we should be able to determine what to do with infants found to have hearing loss, if only from our knowledge of basic human development. It seems as if the appropriate choice of treatment should be obvious. However, radically different solutions have been offered by various groups of clinicians, indicating that the answer must not be all that apparent.

Some professionals counsel parents to start using signs with their infants, even if their eventual goal is for their children to learn spoken language. This approach hinges on the belief that the representation of language in the central nervous system is amodal (i.e., linked to neither the auditory nor visual system) and without physical form. Accordingly, any input that stimulates language processing should be useful. Because it is sometimes difficult or even impossible to get adequate auditory stimulation to infants, the obvious choice for language input is through manual signs, according to this perspective. In fact, some advocates of this approach go as far as to say that instruction in spoken language should be delayed until certain milestones are achieved using sign language. Then the child can map the spoken forms, which are less clearly accessible to children with hearing loss, onto the salient representations that exist in the amodal form learned through signed input.

Other professionals recommend that the focus of early intervention should involve a systematic approach to developing listening skills. This perspective stems from the idea that language is an explicitly auditory task, with the representation of language in the central nervous system being auditory in form. Accordingly, the auditory system must be the focus of intervention. The treatment programs arising from this view generally have a structured hierarchy for the order in which listening skills should be acquired, and the tools marketed for use with deaf children resemble those marketed for use with children with language delay and/or auditory processing disorders. The steps in the recommended hierarchy usually follow the progression that the child must first be trained to respond to auditory stimulation with nonlinguistic sounds, then the child has to learn to discriminate between two sounds (again, not speech sounds initially), and finally the child can be expected to recognize what he is hearing. The reader should recognize these steps as similar to the auditory training course that Max Goldstein imported from Germany in the late 19th century, which was discussed in Chapter 1. In many of the current learning programs, however, nonlinguistic materials are used, whereas Goldstein focused on real speech. In the current programs, verbal stimuli are introduced only after the child reaches specified levels of auditory competence. Some professionals recommend that this kind of hierarchical instruction in listening skills should be combined with sign input: The child must learn to listen, using nonspeech materials, and learn language through manual signs. Only then will the child be ready to map spoken signals presented auditorily onto signed language.

Still other professionals suggest that high-quality amplification should be provided as soon as an infant is identified with hearing loss, and then parents should be instructed to speak to their infant just as parents typically do. Recommendations may be made to keep the background noise levels low and to try to engage in language stimulation more frequently than parents of infants with normal hearing do, but in general, no specific training regimen is suggested. This approach is based on the premise that if we identify children young enough, and provide adequate amplification, infants with hearing loss will develop just as infants with normal hearing do, without explicit training. The only challenge we continue to face with this approach is figuring out how to stimulate the auditory system early enough, with adequate power. It is this perspective that sparks the movement to implant infants at progressively younger ages.

The examples above are just a few of the approaches recommended for use with deaf babies, but they illustrate the range of diversity in current views. Clearly, there is no consensus on what we should be doing for newborns identified with hearing loss. The question of what constitutes appropriate intervention is important, although the answer is elusive. It is easy to imagine that if we do not provide appropriate intervention we will, at best, have wasted our efforts at identifying these babies at birth; at worst, we will do more harm than had we not identified them at all. It is not simply the case that any intervention is better than none at all. There are many aspects of normal development that could be affected by how we choose to interject ourselves in the typical course of development. Although those of us working with deaf children tend to focus on speech and language, a child is also developing the rudiments of social skills and personality during these early years. If we do not provide effective early intervention, or indeed provide intervention that interferes with typical development in any area, we could be doing harm. The purpose of this study was to examine even the basic belief that any intervention started shortly after birth provides benefits over similar efforts initiated at 1 or 2 years of age. In addition, potential effects of including, or not including, sign support to spoken language input were examined. This chapter reviews what we currently know about the development of children with significant hearing loss and describes how this knowledge shaped our selection of what to measure.

Language Development

The central focus of the current study is on the acquisition of spoken language by children with hearing loss. We wanted to know if deaf children's abilities to understand and produce spoken language have improved in recent years with the advent of early identification and cochlear implants. Of course, the history of evaluating language development in children with hearing loss younger than school age is brief. Until recently, even if children were identified early, expectations for spoken language before school age were minimal. Then, once children with hearing loss were in school, language assessment took the form of tools standardized on other children with hearing loss, as reviewed in Chapter 2. The work of Apuzzo and Yoshinaga-Itano (1995) was

the first to demonstrate the value of using language assessment tools developed for children with normal hearing with this population. Those investigators relied heavily on a behavior checklist that parents complete: the Minnesota Child Development Inventory (Ireton & Thwing, 1974). A great deal of research into the acquisition of language, both spoken and signed, by children with hearing loss has been done using standardized, commercially available instruments as dependent measures. Results of these investigations give us a picture of how children with hearing loss are developing, in general, compared to children with normal hearing.

In this study we made use of standard instruments, but also chose to examine language in a more open, natural manner. Although it is important to have standard measures of skills such as vocabulary, which can be evaluated with commercially available instruments, in the end it is how well a child uses language in his everyday interactions that really matters. Recognizing individual words and having words in one's own lexicon are important aspects of communication, but language involves much more than vocabulary or word recognition. In most languages, word order (or syntax) conveys information. The sentences, "The book was on the paper" and "The paper was on the book," have different meanings. One could of course change the meaning of the first sentence in this example by changing the word *on* to *under*. Nonetheless, in English we commonly make use of word order to convey meaning, and so syntax is an important aspect of language that children must discover. Similarly, morphological and grammatical devices are used to convey information to a listener, and every child needs to understand these linguistic devices. Inflectional endings such as -*ed* convey information about when something happened. We use personal pronouns to signal case and gender of the proper nouns they are replacing. Observing how often and appropriately a child uses these linguistic devices in his daily communication with others provides a much more sensitive index of language advancement than simply asking a parent to indicate if she thinks her child understands and can use these sorts of words. Consequently, we derived many of our measures from samples of the child's communication taken from videotaped interactions between a parent (generally the mother) and the child. In this way we were able to get very precise information about how the child developed the earliest rudiments of communication, how the child used language, and how the form of the child's language emerged over the course of this investigation.

For some language phenomena, however, there was no substitute for standard, commercially available tools. The standard instruments that we used for examining children's communication and language were selected carefully and with purpose. No measure was selected simply because it is commonly used in clinical practice or in research studies with deaf children. Rather, the range of language skills that we wanted to investigate was determined first, and then measures were selected based on how well they met our objectives, as well as how valid and reliable each was. In research, the notion of validity of a test instrument refers to how well it measures what it purports to be measuring. It is an unfortunate, but none-

theless true, aspect of research that the things we are most interested in knowing about are frequently the most difficult to measure in a precise fashion within a reasonable amount of time. Often the measures that are most convenient to obtain, and so are used most frequently, do not get at the heart of what it is we want to know. In this study we tried to use measures that examined language in an in-depth manner, asking how well the children were acquiring native ability with the spoken English they were purportedly learning. That meant that measures were required that are not so easily obtained.

Development of Personality

The term *psychosocial development* is generally used to describe how the personality develops and how one learns to interact socially with those around him. It includes aspects of personality such as whether one has fulfilling relationships with others or experiences isolation and whether an individual endures hardships with patience and humor or lashes out angrily at others when problems arise. Historically, it has been believed that the course of psychosocial development was determined largely by that first relationship in life, the one with Mom. This perspective was the basis of Freud's program for psychoanalysis, as laid out in a book published in 1940 (and translated into English in 1949). There he declared that the care a mother provides her infant forms " . . . the root of a mother's importance, unique, without parallel, established unalterably for a whole lifetime, as the first and strongest love object and as the prototype of all later love relations —for both sexes" (1949, p. 45). Similarly, Erikson (1963) wrote that the way a person interacts with the world throughout his life is determined by the quality of that first relationship: If an infant has an attachment to one caregiver, usually the mother, who is appropriately responsive to the child's needs, that infant will grow up to see the world as safe and inviting. If there is either no one individual to whom an infant can form an attachment, or if that one individual provides inappropriate or inconsistent responses to the infant's attempts to elicit responses, the development of personality could be inalterably and negatively affected. Although it has more recently been found that other influences also contribute to the development of personality (e.g., Sroufe, Carlson, Levy, & Egeland, 1999; Thompson, 1999, 2000), a child's early attachment to a responsive and consistent caregiver continues to be viewed as an important contributing factor to psychosocial development.

In designing this study it was considered critical to examine psychosocial development because the quality of that earliest attachment is highly dependent on the quality of communication between parent and child. If parents are unable to reliably ascertain their child's needs and wants, they will not be able to respond appropriately. Additionally, if the sophistication and specificity of a child's needs and wants develop faster than his skills at communicating them, frustration will result, which will ultimately affect the child's burgeoning personality. Thus, the child's ability to communicate may be one constraining variable in the development of his own psychosocial profile, albeit through an indirect route: A deficit in the ability to communicate can harm the quality of the parent-child bond, which in turn can influence the development of personality and social skills.

The notion that deficient communication between child and parent may hinder the development of typical personality traits and social skills receives strong support from studies on the Theory of Mind (ToM) in deaf children. In these studies, preschool children are typically asked about the beliefs of other individuals. For example, in an *unexpected contents* task, a child might be afforded the opportunity to discover that a crayon box actually contains a plastic spoon. When he is later asked what a friend thinks is in the box, he will answer with either his own current belief, or with that of the friend who was not given the opportunity to discover the unexpected content (Perner, Leekam, & Wimmer, 1987). In studies of young deaf children, those who have deaf parents fluent in sign language typically reveal an understanding of the other person's current belief; deaf children who have hearing parents not fluent in sign language tend to answer according to their own beliefs (e.g., Schick, de Villiers, de Villiers, & Hoffmeister, 2007). A common interpretation of these results is that deaf parents are able to discuss mental states with their children, whereas hearing parents are hobbled in their abilities to have conversations that abstract in nature with their deaf children because of a lack of adequate sign skill. In general, these results for ToM experiments help to explain an extensive and otherwise conflicting lineage of reports on the psychosocial development of children with hearing loss: The most critical factor determining psychosocial outcomes for children with hearing loss appears to be the extent of mismatch between the child's communication mode and abilities, and those of the ambient community. If a deaf child is in an environment where he can communicate adequately, the probability of psychosocial problems is lessened; if, on the other hand, there is a mismatch between the communication abilities of the child and those of people around him, the probability increases that the child will develop psychosocial and/or behavior problems. (Hindley [1997] provides a comprehensive review of this extensive literature).

One indicator of this effect is described by Musselman, MacKay, Trehub, and Eagle (1996). These investigators found a higher incidence of psychosocial disturbance among teenagers with hearing loss (mean age = 16 years, 7 months) in programs that use sign language (total communication) than among teenagers in programs that use oral communication. When they investigated further, however, they found a trend that at first appeared utterly contradictory to that general result: Among teens in the total communication programs, those with better spoken language actually had the higher incidence of psychosocial problems. The authors interpreted this trend as arising from the fact that the children in total communication programs with better spoken language had entered those programs late; they had spent a fair amount of their early years struggling in oral programs. Although these teens may have had good spoken language for students in total communication programs, their

oral skills were not completely adequate for participating in educational programs that provided no sign support, and so there existed a mismatch in communication styles for much of their young lives.

Several behavior problems especially concern us when dealing with children with hearing loss: problems of attention and hyperactivity, which are considered externalizing disorders because they are directed outwards, and problems of self-image, which can result in shyness and tendencies towards isolation or even self-harm. These latter difficulties are categorized as internalizing disorders. Across studies of psychosocial development in children with hearing loss, problems considered to be both externalizing (mostly attention and hyperactivity) and internalizing (problems of self-image, anxiety, and isolation) have been reported for children with hearing loss (Hindley & Brown, 1994). Within those general patterns, however, a couple trends emerge. First, when children with hearing loss have difficulty communicating with those in their environment, ratings of attention problems and hyperactivity increase (e.g., Sinkkonen, 1994). In addition, more problems of an internalizing nature, such as poor self-esteem, have been observed for children with hearing loss in educational settings located within regular schools than in schools for deaf children only (e.g., Hindley, 1993; Smith & Sharp, 1994). Children with hearing loss in regular schools have in the past reported feeling that they do not fit in. The predominance of that work, however, was conducted with children with hearing loss who did not receive early intervention and who did not have cochlear implants. It may be that children who are beneficiaries of these recent technological advances will fare better. This study was meant to investigate that possibility.

Of particular relevance, Nicholas and Geers (2003) reported that children who received cochlear implants before the age of 5 years demonstrated good psychosocial development. In their study, 181 children (8–9 years of age) were asked about their own self-competence, using a standard assessment that had been modified specifically for children with cochlear implants. At the same time, the parents of these children were asked to rate their children's social and emotional adjustment, using two instruments: one designed specifically for children with hearing loss, regardless of what prosthetic device they used, and another designed specifically for children with cochlear implants. Results showed that most of the deaf children with cochlear implants had positive self-images, and that their parents perceived them as well adjusted. These findings deviated from many of the earlier findings concerning psychosocial development in children with hearing loss, which tended to show some deficits in this area and that these deficits varied with the degree to which a child's communicative capacities were a mismatch to the ambient environment (e.g., Hindley, 1993; Hindley, Hill, McGuigan, & Kitson, 1994; Meadow, 1968; Polat, 2003). In general, the findings of Nicholas and Geers predict positive psychosocial outcomes for children with hearing loss, now that early identification and better amplification are available. Unfortunately, it is impossible to gauge whether the self-images of the 181 children in that study matched the images that children with normal hearing have of themselves because the measures used by Nicholas and Geers were explicitly designed for children with hearing loss (or even more specifically, for children with cochlear implants), and there was no control group of children with normal hearing. Consequently, we are left with an incomplete picture of how hearing loss influences the emergence of personality, and how that relation might be further affected by factors such as the use of signs or differences in prostheses. This study sought to fill that void.

Motor Skills Development

Both fine and gross motor development are important to the overall well-being of a child. In the classroom, age-appropriate fine motor skills are necessary for adequate functioning on tasks such as learning to write. Anecdotal reports from clinicians currently working with deaf children as well as some published reports on motor development in children with cochlear implants suggest that children with hearing loss, at least those with cochlear implants, may have delays in fine motor development. For example, Horn, Pisoni, and Miyamoto (2006) measured motor skills in children with cochlear implants using the Vineland Adaptive Behavior Scales (Sparrow, Balla, & Cicchetti, 1984), and found that children with cochlear implants were delayed compared to children with normal hearing. Of particular interest, the children with cochlear implants were found to be delayed in the area of fine motor development, but not in the area of gross motor development, and there was a mild correlation of this effect with language abilities. In discussing this result, the authors offered the hypothesis that the acquisition of motor speech skills may be related to the acquisition of fine motor skills in hand movements. The putative explanation for this relation is that fine motor tasks of the hands and motor speech tasks are controlled by the same cortical structures (e.g., Carello, LeVasseur, & Schmidt, 2002; Locke, Bekken, McMinn-Larson, & Wein, 1995), an idea discussed in Chapter 2. Because of this hypothesis, we examined fine motor development in the current study.

Anyone who has ever spent any time on a playground, either as a teacher or as a child, knows how important gross motor skills are to developing good social relations during childhood. If you can throw, hit, and catch a ball, it goes a long way towards making friends. Unfortunately, there is evidence that children with hearing loss are more prone to delays and disorders in gross motor development. For example, a study by Ittyerah and Sharma (1997) found that children with hearing loss, who relied on sign language, were clumsier and more accident prone than children with normal hearing. Nonsigning deaf children were not included in that study. The authors wrote that their results suggest there may be a relation between language development and neuropsychological development in general, other than that mediated by hand control. They did not elaborate further. Be that as it may, there is the very real fact that the vestibular system can be compromised when there is sensorineural hearing loss. Precisely because of that involvement of the vestibular system, children with hearing loss more frequently experience balance problems

than children with normal hearing (e.g., Cushing, Chia, James, Papsin, & Gordon, 2008). For these reasons, gross motor skills were examined in the current study.

Cognitive Development in Children with Hearing Loss

Ever since the advent of psychological science, debate has raged concerning the relation between thinking and language. In the early 20th century, two investigators, Edward Sapir and Benjamin Whorf, studied the language of Native Americans and reached the conclusion that the lexicon of a language reflects the way that people in the culture perceive the world, and in turn, one's own language constrains the way one can perceive the world (e.g., Whorf, 1956). Thinking, these authors argued, is fully determined by one's language. According to this perspective, if one has constraints on one's language abilities because of hearing loss or if one uses sign language, we might expect differences in how this individual thinks, compared to typical speakers of English.

Regarding children, traditional child psychologists such as Piaget have long emphasized the facilitative role of social interaction in some aspects of cognitive development, the outwardly directed activities, but have asserted that fundamental thinking and problem-solving abilities arise explicitly from a child's own sensorimotor manipulation of objects in the environment (e.g., Inhelder & Piaget, 1958; 1964; Piaget, 1959). Following on that perspective, Furth (1966) gave children with hearing loss (who used sign language) and children with normal hearing tasks to complete that were of a Piagetian nature and found no major differences in cognitive abilities. The deaf children exhibited some minor deficits precisely in the areas of thinking that require linguistic exchange with others, such as the compilation of facts. In the basic development of cognitive capacities, however, the deaf children were found to be remarkably unaffected by their lack of spoken language. That result has subsequently been replicated by others (e.g., Bond, 1987). Thus, the notion that there is a nonverbal core to cognitive abilities has persisted in our approaches to testing and education, for both children with normal hearing and those with hearing loss.

More recently, however, the perspective that thinking and language bootstrap onto each other in development has gained prominence and is reflected in the research on childhood language disorders. Several reports have suggested that "specific language impairments" are really not specific at all, but rather that children with these diagnosed impairments necessarily have other, perhaps "subclinical," cognitive impairments (Johnston & Smith, 1989; Leonard, 1989; Thal & Bates, 1988). Such ideas lead naturally to speculation about the development of cognitive capacities in children with hearing loss, who are commonly delayed in (spoken) language development. If the development of cognitive processing is at all dependent on language, then we would want to spur the onset of language development as soon as possible to support that development. This reasoning suggests that infants and toddlers with hearing loss should start language learning as soon as possible. Because sign language is more accessible for children with hearing loss, it should be the language of choice, according to this view. In fact, there are those who suggest that even children with normal hearing are given a "leg up" in cognitive development by being signed to as infants (Acredolo & Goodwyn, 2000).

Other studies that have been conducted on cognitive development in children with hearing loss have reached the conclusion that children with hearing loss due to genetic causes fare better than those with other etiologies (e.g., Kusche, Greenberg, & Garfield, 1983). However, the basis for inferring a genetic cause in those studies was that participants had deaf parents and/or deaf siblings. With recent advances in genetics, we are now aware that individuals with hearing loss may have a genetic cause for their hearing loss, but not have family members with hearing loss. Consequently, we question the conclusion of Kusche et al., and wonder if it may be the case instead that deaf parents of deaf children provide better environmental support for cognitive development. Just as a mismatch between the communication style and/or ability of the child and the environment might put a child at risk for psychosocial problems, so might the same mismatch put a child at risk for delayed cognitive development, particularly in areas that require linguistic exchanges.

Khan, Edwards, and Langdon (2005) evaluated the effects specifically of having cochlear implants on cognitive development in children using the Leiter International Performance Scale-Revised (LIPS-R; Roid & Miller, 2002). These investigators reported that full-scale IQs were lower for children with hearing loss without cochlear implants (HL-CI) than for children with normal hearing (NH) or with hearing loss and cochlear implants (HL+CI). However, the IQs of the children in the HL-CI group were well within the range of normal (mean = 103.3). Furthermore, the socioeconomic status of that group was reported to be lower than the socioeconomic status of children in the NH and HL+CI groups, which could certainly account for the discrepancy in full-scale IQs: Children in the NH and HL+CI groups had mean full-scale IQs of 112.7 and 114.4, respectively. The discrepancy in socioeconomic status among groups makes interpretation of results difficult. It seemed reasonable, given the results reported here, to investigate nonverbal cognitive abilities in children as part of this study.

The mean age of the children in the Khan et al. (2005) study was 4 years, but with a range from 2½ years to almost 6 years. The authors reported scores for all three groups (NH, HL+CI, and HL–CI) for all six subtests of the LIPS-R used in computing the full-scale IQ. Although these full-scale IQ scores were significantly different among groups, those differences were entirely accounted for by the Sequential Order and Classification subtests. Both of those tests, but not the others, showed significant effects of group, with Classification showing the greatest difference between the NH and HL–CI groups. That result could, in fact, reflect variation in overall language abilities: Being able to classify objects may be facilitated by the use of linguistic labels. We considered that hypothesis in selecting dependent measures related to cognition in this study.

Parenting Stress

At the start of the 20th century, psychologists worried that a secure attachment to a primary caregiver needed to be attained within a specific, or critical, period or else serious consequences would result. This view led to the widespread belief that later-adopted children would experience lifelong social and emotional problems (e.g., Bowlby, 1953). However, investigations toward the end of the 20th century revealed that children can achieve secure attachments to caregivers after the first year of life, which is after the proposed critical period for developing attachments. Some of the most informative work on this topic was done with children from Romanian orphanages who were adopted into Canadian families. In spite of some deplorable conditions in the orphanages from which they came, all of the adoptees were found to form attachments to their adoptive parents, although of varying quality (Chisholm, 1998; Chisholm, Carter, Ames, & Morison, 1995). It was found that the kind of parenting provided to these later-adopted children was more important to developing strong attachments than was the age of adoption. In particular, parents who interacted with their later-adopted children in especially nurturing ways were found to facilitate secure attachments. Stress on the parents' part was one factor that seemed to jeopardize the bonding process (e.g., Marcovitch et al., 1997). Of course, a lack of responsiveness from the child to the parents' efforts to nurture could be a source of stress for parents. In this case, parenting stress is a consequence of child detachment, rather than a cause. But regardless of the direction of effect, there seems to be a relation between parenting stress and the quality of parent-child attachment.

Where deaf children are concerned, the hearing loss itself can create communication barriers between parent and child. In addition to increasing the risk of psychosocial problems, those barriers may lead to increased stress on the parents' part. It is easy to see how a negative chain reaction could be established, set off either by behavior problems on the part of the child, such as increased aggression, hyperactivity, or shyness, or by stress on the part of the parent. Problems on either side of the parent-child relationship could initiate this kind of chain reaction. Regardless of its source, however, it could produce deleterious consequences for the child.

One event that can trigger an increase in parenting stress is the revelation that one's newborn may have a hearing problem. Citing evidence showing that positive screening results for other disorders can lead to enhanced parenting stress, Jack Paradise (1999) expressed reservations about the very idea of screening infants' hearing at birth. Paradise suggested that we might be better off leaving the diagnosis of hearing loss until later, after an appropriate bond has been formed between parent and child. Of course, that recommendation fails to take into consideration the possibility that a lack of responsiveness on the part of a deaf child, a form of detachment, could create stress in the parent. It might be that having an explanation for that lack of responsiveness, before it is even evident, can assuage a parent's feelings of stress

at the lack of responsiveness from her child. Pressman, Pipp-Siegel, Yoshinaga-Itano, Kubicek, & Emde (2001) examined how the emotional availability of both the child and parent influenced language development on the part of the child. Although emotional availability by both sides of this dyad had significant effects, parental availability seemed particularly important. Because of all the possible ways that parental availability and stress might be related to positive growth in language for children with hearing loss, we wanted to evaluate parenting stress in this study.

Parental Language Style

A well-replicated finding in the literature on child language development is that parents living in abject poverty talk to their children less than middle-class parents, and the form of their language input differs. A good example of this work comes from the studies of Hart and Risley, especially their report titled, *Meaningful Differences in the Everyday Experience of Young American Children* (1995). In that study, Hart and Risley followed 42 families, including some with low socioeconomic status (SES), from the time the children were 12 months old until they were 36 months old. Those investigators showed that the parents in the low-SES homes generally talked to their children less, and when they did they used fewer modifiers and fewer questions, and were less responsive and less encouraging to their children's communication attempts than were other parents. Hart and Risley were able to show that children from the low-SES households showed slower vocabulary growth and use than other children, with roughly 60% of the variance in those measures accounted for by how parents spoke to their children. That finding from a longitudinal study replicated similar findings by others for children from low-SES households (Hess & Shipman, 1965; Nittrouer, 2002; Schachter, 1979). In general, the way in which parents talk to their children and how frequently they do so influences language acquisition.

None of the families participating in this current study could be considered to be living in abject poverty, although there was a range of socioeconomic levels. However, we wondered if the very condition of living with a child with hearing loss could influence the way that parents communicate with their children. In addition, the necessity of having to incorporate signs into one's communication for some of these parents, none of whom were deaf, could have led to modifications in language style: Adults with normal hearing just are not used to signing when they talk. For these reasons, we wanted to evaluate the form and frequency of communicative behaviors used by parents.

Chapter Summary

When we began designing this study, our primary focus was on the development of spoken language in children with hearing loss. This focus was established because of the very real fact that it is spoken language that is most transparently affected by hearing loss. We were interested in the acquisition of human traits other than language that might directly or indirectly be related to language, but our sights were set most keenly on language.

Parents have a decidedly different view of their children. They are concerned with how their children are developing in their abilities to play with others, to solve mental puzzles, and to learn new information. Parents of deaf children, most of whom have normal hearing themselves, worry about ensuring that their children will grow up to be happy and productive, able to land good jobs, have lots of friends, and find loving spouses. What parents sometimes may not realize is how closely tied the achievement of these goals is to the development of language abilities. Children with language deficits, but with no hearing loss, have been found to have behavioral, social, and cognitive deficits (e.g., Beitchman et al., 2001; Cantwell & Baker, 1982, 1987; Cantwell, Baker, & Mattison, 1980; Redmond, 2002). Given the breadth of social and emotional traits that might be influenced by hearing loss itself or a consequent language delay, it was imperative that we examine all aspects of development for the children in this study.

In this chapter, current evidence regarding the development of children with hearing loss was reviewed. This evidence served as the basis for selecting dependent measures for this study. By artfully selecting measures based on current knowledge, we hoped to maximize the potential of the study to move the field of early intervention forward. Of course, it is equally important to consider independent sources of variability when designing a research study, and control these sources of variability. How we did that is the focus of the next chapter.

References

Acredolo, L. P., & Goodwyn, S. W. (2000, July). *The long term impact of symbolic gesturing during infancy on IQ at age 8.* Paper presented at the International Conference on Infant Studies, Brighton, UK.

Apuzzo, M. L., & Yoshinaga-Itano, C. (1995). Early identification of infants with significant hearing loss and the *Minnesota Child Development Inventory. Seminars in Hearing, 16,* 124–137.

Beitchman, J. H., Wilson, B., Johnson, C., Atkinson, L., Young, A., & Adlaf, E. (2001). Fourteen-year follow-up of speech/language-impaired and control children: Psychiatric outcome. *Journal of the American Academy of Child and Adolescent Psychiatry, 40,* 75–82.

Bond, G. G. (1987). An assessment of cognitive abilities in hearing and hearing-impaired preschool children. *Journal of Speech and Hearing Disorders, 52,* 319–323.

Bowlby, J. (1953). Some pathological processes set in train by early mother-child separation. *Journal of Mental Science, 99,* 265–272.

Cantwell, D. P., & Baker, L. (1982). Depression in children with speech, language, and learning disorders. *Journal of Children in Contemporary Society, 15,* 51–59.

Cantwell, D. P., & Baker, L. (1987). The prevalence of anxiety in children with communication disorders. *Journal of Anxiety Disorders, 1,* 239–248.

Cantwell, D. P., Baker, L., & Mattison, R. (1980). Psychiatric disorders in children with speech and language retardation. *Archives of General Psychiatry, 37,* 423–426.

Carello, C., LeVasseur, V. M., & Schmidt, R. C. (2002). Movement sequencing and phonological fluency in (putatively) non-impaired readers. *Psychological Science, 13,* 375–379.

Chisholm, K. (1998). A three year follow-up of attachment and indiscriminate friendliness in children adopted from Roman-ian orphanages. *Child Development, 69,* 1092–1106.

Chisholm, K., Carter, M. C., Ames, E. W., & Morison, S. J. (1995). Attachment security and indiscriminately friendly behavior in children adopted from Romanian orphanages. *Development and Psychopathology, 7,* 283–294.

Cushing, S. L., Chia, R., James, A. L., Papsin, B. C., & Gordon, K. A. (2008). A test of static and dynamic balance function in children with cochlear implants: The vestibular Olympics. *Archives of Otolaryngology—Head & Neck Surgery, 134,* 34–38.

Erikson, E. H. (1963). *Childhood and society.* New York: Norton.

Freud, S. (1949). *An outline of psychoanalysis.* New York: W. W. Norton.

Furth, H. G. (1966). *Thinking without language: Psychological implications of deafness.* New York: The Free Press.

Hart, B., & Risley, T. R. (1995). *Meaningful differences in the everyday experience of young American children.* Baltimore: Paul H. Brookes.

Hess, R. D., & Shipman, V. C. (1965). Early experience and the socialization of cognitive modes in children. *Child Development, 36,* 869–886.

Hindley, P. A. (1993). *Signs of feeling: A prevalence study of psychiatric disorder in deaf and partially hearing children and adolescents.* London: Royal National Institute for the Deaf.

Hindley, P. A. (1997). Psychiatric aspects of hearing impairments. *Journal of Child Psychology and Psychiatry and Allied Disciplines, 38,* 101–117.

Hindley, P. A., & Brown, R. M. A. (1994). Psychiatric aspects of specific sensory impairments. In M. Rutter, E. Taylor, & L. Hersov (Eds.), *Child and adolescent psychiatry: Modern approaches* (pp. 720–736). Oxford, UK: Blackwell Scientific.

Hindley, P. A., Hill, P. D., McGuigan, S., & Kitson, N. (1994). Psychiatric disorder in deaf and hearing impaired children and young people: A prevalence study. *Jour-*

nal of Child Psychology and Psychiatry, 35, 917–934.

Horn, D. L., Pisoni, D. B., & Miyamoto, R. T. (2006). Divergence of fine and gross motor skills in prelingually deaf children: Implications for cochlear implantation. *Laryngoscope, 116,* 1500–1506.

Inhelder, B., & Piaget, J. (1958). *The growth of logical thinking from childhood to adolescence.* London: Routledge & Kegan Paul.

Inhelder, B., & Piaget, J. (1964). *The early growth of logic in the child.* New York: Humanities Press.

Ireton, H., & Thwing, E. (1974). *The Minnesota Child Development Inventory.* Minneapolis: University of Minnesota.

Ittyerah, M., & Sharma, R. (1997). The performance of hearing-impaired children on handedness and perceptual motor tasks. *Genetic, Social, and General Psychology Monographs, 123,* 285–302.

Johnston, J. R., & Smith, L. B. (1989). Dimensional thinking in language impaired children. *Journal of Speech and Hearing Research, 32,* 33–38.

Khan, S., Edwards, L., & Langdon, D. (2005). The cognition and behaviour of children with cochlear implants, children with hearing aids and their hearing peers: A comparison. *Audiology & Neuro-otology, 10,* 117–126.

Kusche, C. A., Greenberg, M. T., & Garfield, T. S. (1983). Nonverbal intelligence and verbal achievement in deaf adolescents: An examination of heredity and environment. *American Annals of the Deaf, 128,* 458–466.

Leonard, L. B. (1989). Language learnability and specific language impairment in children. *Applied Psycholinguistics, 10,* 179–202.

Locke, J. L., Bekken, K. E., McMinn-Larson, L., & Wein, D. (1995). Emergent control of manual and vocal-motor activity in relation to the development of speech. *Brain and Language, 51,* 498–508.

Marcovitch, S., Goldberg, S., Gold, A., Washington, J., Wasson, C., Krekewich, K., et al. (1997). Determinants of behavioural prob-lems in Romanian children adopted in Ontario. *International Journal of Behavioral Development, 20,* 17–31.

Meadow, K. P. (1968). Early manual communication in relation to the deaf child's intellectual, social, and communicative functioning. *American Annals of the Deaf, 113,* 29–41.

Musselman, C., MacKay, S., Trehub, S. E., & Eagle, R. S. (1996). Communicative competence and psychosocial development in deaf children and adolescents. In J. H. Beitchman, N. J. Cohen, M. M. Konstantareas, & R. Tannok (Eds.), *Language, learning, and behavior disorders: Developmental, biological, and clinical perspectives* (pp. 555–570). Cambridge, UK: Cambridge University Press.

Nicholas, J. G., & Geers, A. E. (2003). Personal, social, and family adjustment in school-aged children with a cochlear implant. *Ear and Hearing, 24,* 69S–81S.

Nittrouer, S. (2002). From ear to cortex: A perspective on what clinicians need to understand about speech perception and language processing. *Language, Speech and Hearing Services in Schools, 33,* 237–251.

Paradise, J. L. (1999). Universal newborn hearing screening: Should we leap before we look? *Pediatrics, 103,* 670–672.

Perner, J., Leekam, S. R., & Wimmer, H. (1987). Three-year-olds' difficulty with false belief: The case for a conceptual deficit. *British Journal of Developmental Psychology, 5,* 125–137.

Piaget, J. (1959). *The language and thought of the child* (3rd ed.). London: Routledge & Kegan Paul.

Polat, F. (2003). Factors affecting psychosocial adjustment of deaf students. *Journal of Deaf Studies & Deaf Education, 8,* 325–339.

Pressman, L. J., Pipp-Siegel, S., Yoshinaga-Itano, C., Kubicek, L., & Emde, R. N. (2001). A comparison of the links between emotional availability and language gain in young children with and without hearing loss. *The Volta Review, 100,* 251–277.

Redmond, S. M. (2002). The use of rating scales with children who have language impairments. *American Journal of Speech-Language Pathology, 11,* 124–138.

Roid, G. H., & Miller, L. J. (2002). *Leiter International Performance Scale–Revised (LIPS-R).* Wood Dale, IL: Stoelting.

Schachter, F. F. (1979). *Everyday mother talk to toddlers: Early intervention.* New York: Academic Press.

Schick, B., de Villiers, P., de Villiers, J., & Hoffmeister, R. (2007). Language and theory of mind: A study of deaf children. *Child Development, 78,* 376–396.

Sinkkonen, J. (1994). *Hearing impairment, communication, and personality development.* Unpublished doctoral dissertation, University of Helsinki, Sweden.

Smith, P. K., & Sharp, S. (Eds.). (1994). *School bullying: Insights and perspectives.* London: Routledge.

Sparrow, S. S., Balla, B. A., & Cicchetti, D. V. (1984). *Vineland Adaptive Behavior Scales (Expanded Form).* Circle Pines, MN: American Guidance Service.

Sroufe, L. A., Carlson, E. A., Levy, A. K., & Egeland, B. (1999). Implications of attachment theory for developmental psychopathology. *Development and Psychopathology, 11,* 1–13.

Thal, D., & Bates, E. (1988). Language and gesture in late talkers. *Journal of Speech and Hearing Research, 31,* 115–123.

Thompson, R. A. (1999). Early attachment and later development. In J. Cassidy & P. R. Shaver (Eds.), *Handbook of attachment: Theory, research, and clinical applications* (pp. 265–286). New York: Guilford.

Thompson, R. A. (2000). The legacy of early attachments. *Child Development, 71,* 145–152.

Whorf, B. L. (1956). *Language, thought, and reality: Selected writings of Benjamin Lee Whorf.* Cambridge, MA: MIT Press.

4

Participants and Procedures: How Independent Sources of Variability Were Handled

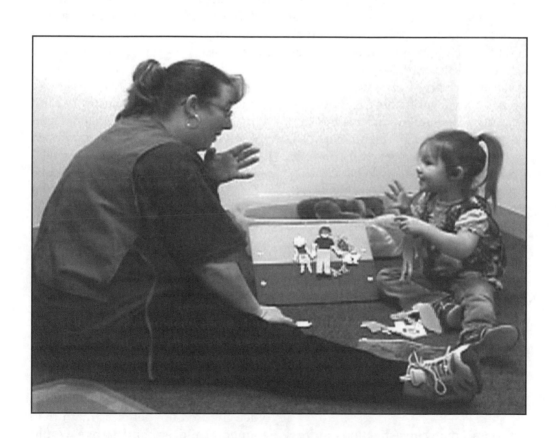

Variability is the stuff that research studies are made of. Any group of individuals will demonstrate variability in how they respond to any measure, no matter how well matched we believe they are on factors that can predict performance on that measure. For example, we might assemble a group of men, all born in Maryland in 1985, who are 6 feet, 5 inches tall and weigh exactly 195 pounds. All of them may have spent 4 hours per day, 6 days a week, swimming in their local pools since they were 7 years old. But only one of those young men would be able to swim fast enough to claim world records and go on to win eight gold medals in an Olympic competition in 2008. What is it about the physical makeup of that young man or his training regimen that produced that ability? That is the kind of question asked by scientific investigation, although we generally pose the problem more broadly: What explains the range of swimming speeds exhibited by this group of individuals? The overarching question addressed in the research study reported here concerned the factors that might explain the variability in developmental outcomes, particularly those involving language, for young children with hearing loss.

Examining Sources of Variance

Of course, many investigations address the issue of variability in yet a different way, asking if a well-specified factor that serves to define two or more groups is associated with significant differences among the groups on a dependent measure. So, using another example, we might ask if fourth graders in the United States and in Canada differ in their math abilities; the factor that defines the groups in this example is country of residence. To answer this question, we would draw random samples of fourth graders from both countries, and administer a test of math ability. We could compute mean scores for both groups, and compare those scores. In these kinds of analyses, differences across group means are compared with reference to the amount of variability that is found within groups. We are asking if the difference between (or among) group means is greater than what we would expect based on typical within-group variability. With that in mind, the country with the highest scoring fourth graders on the math measure would win as long as we know that we had not somehow inadvertently drawn two samples that differ on some other, relevant variable. That situation would be a problem if it were, for example, the case that children start school a year later in one or the other country. If so, then fourth graders in the country with the later starting children would be slightly older than fourth graders in the country where children begin school at a younger age. Any observed difference in scores might then be explained by that age factor, rather than by how the educational systems in the two countries approach math instruction. We are likely not interested in asking if older children are better at math than younger children, and so we would want to ensure that children in the two groups are similar in their ages. That is a factor that we would want to control by restricting the age range of children in the study: We would exclude all children from participation who were not within a well-defined range of ages typical of fourth graders in both countries.

But what about the amount of time children in the two countries spend in math instruction? Time spent in instruction might also be a factor that could influence math scores. On the other hand, perhaps sheer instructional time does not matter. Perhaps instead the kind of instruction explains more of the variance in outcomes. Determining the extent to which each of these two factors, time and kind of instruction, affects outcomes is important to determining policy regarding how math is taught, and so we would not want to control these factors by restricting participation to children receiving one amount or kind of instruction. To do so would eliminate all potentially significant clinical interpretations that could be gained from the study. Instead, we would want to keep careful records of the amount of time each child spent in math instruction, and the kind of instruction each child received. We could then evaluate if indeed the two groups differed on one of those factors, and if the country providing more time in instruction or a particular kind of instruction had better fourth-grade math scores than the other country. If so, the conclusions reached would involve how amount or kind of instruction is related to math outcomes. In addition, we could do regression analyses to see how strongly math scores across individuals correlate with amount or kind of experience. That information could have important educational implications. For example, if it was found that one instructional method was generally associated with better outcomes than another method, but the better method is quite a bit more expensive to implement, we would want to know the amount of variance in outcomes explained by both instructional method and time spent in instruction. It might be more cost-effective to hire an extra teacher for each school in order to provide more time in instruction for each child, rather than to purchase the more effective, but costly, instructional method for all schools.

Independent Variables

Factors such as country of residence, amount of time in math instruction, and kind of instruction from the example above are independent variables. In the current study there were many independent variables related to the research participants that needed to be carefully considered. Those variables that were not a focus of this investigation could be controlled by having exclusionary criteria for participation —criteria that would make specific children or families ineligible to participate. For those independent variables that were a focus of this study, about which we wished to make statements regarding clinical significance, we kept careful records. We were able to determine if groups differed significantly on these variables. If groups differ on a relevant independent variable, we need to worry that it might explain any differences between groups that are found on the dependent variables. Subsequently, we used several statistical methods to evaluate the extent to which variability on those independent variables accounted for variability in scores on the dependent measures. It is possible for two groups to be well matched on an independent variable, and so that variable cannot explain any group differences that might be measured. At the same time, within-group variability on that particular independent variable could account for some of the within-group variability on scores for the dependent measure. In the example above, it might be the case that children in the samples from the United States and Canada might have spent the same amount of time in math instruction, according to group means. If a significant difference in group means on the math measure was obtained under that condition, we would be unable to attribute it to amount of time spent in math instruction. Rather, some other factor related to the samples from the two countries would need to be invoked to explain the significant group difference. However, our regression analysis could reveal that amount of time spent in instruction explains some of the variability within each of the two groups of participants. This finding might suggest that more instructional time would be useful for students.

This example illustrates a basic principle of human behavior: Each behavior in which we engage has multiple underlying factors that explain it. The ultimate goal of research into human behavior is to provide a thorough accounting of how much of the variability in each dependent variable is explained by all possible independent measures. This type of thorough accounting of the factors explaining a specific behavior is difficult to provide in brief research reports. Studies designed to ask very specific questions, the kinds that can be answered in brief reports, necessarily must control all relevant independent factors so that they cannot have con-

founding influences on the dependent measures being examined. The purpose of the study described here, on the other hand, was to examine a wide range of sources of variability in developmental outcomes for children with hearing loss. This goal mandated that results be published in this format, as a book, rather than in a series of separate research articles.

Exclusionary Criteria

All children who participated in this project were born within a narrow time window. We originally targeted children born in the year 2003, but permitted some leeway on each end of that range. As it turned out, the oldest children in this study were born in August 2002, and the youngest children were born in June 2004. Restricting birthdates of participants in this way ensured that variability on several factors that were not of interest to us was controlled. It meant that the treatments these children received were more similar than they would have been had we collected data from children who spanned a wider range of birthdates. In the separate programs from which they came, there was likely to be consistency in intervention methods. Trends nationally in intervention approaches remained constant within this short time window. The kinds of auditory prostheses with which they were being fit likely did not vary as much as they would have, had there been a broader range of birthdates. In particular, the model of implants and processors that children received, if they received cochlear implants, were all of the same vintage. The kinds of hearing aids being used by children who wore hearing aids were similar.

There are several factors related to the treatment of children with hearing loss that we decided were simply beyond our ability to examine, given the type of study we had planned. In particular, we did not wish to examine how cognitive or physical disabilities influenced outcomes for children with hearing loss. Children with a range of disabilities may have hearing loss, but the way in which each disability interacts with hearing loss differs: A pervasive developmental delay would impact all outcome measures, but to varying degrees depending on the extent of the delay. A visual impairment might have a milder impact, overall, but differentially affect various aspects of development. For example, a visual impairment might not impact language development, but it could delay the development of personal living skills. These inconsistencies in affected behaviors and magnitude of effect would make the goal of examining sources of variability in developmental outcomes for children with hearing loss very difficult to achieve. Consequently, children were excluded if they had any disability that could reasonably be expected on its own to lead to difficulties in any aspect of development. For example, children were excluded if they had visual impairments that could not be completely corrected with glasses. Children were excluded if they had obvious motor difficulties or developmental delays. In addition, we excluded children if they had significant risk factors for cognitive or physical disabilities that might affect development. In particular, all children in the study needed to have been full term at the time of delivery (i.e., more than 35 weeks' ges-

tation), with no prenatal or perinatal complications.

Another factor that we felt we could not address in this study was the issue of how exposure to more than one spoken language might influence the acquisition of a primary spoken language (in this case, English). It was an explicit goal to examine the contribution to developmental outcomes of receiving sign support in addition to spoken language input, and it would be difficult to accomplish that goal if the language environment was complicated by the inclusion of yet another language. Consequently, all children needed to come from homes where the parents spoke only English to each other and to their children. As with the presence of disabilities, we realized that bilingual home environments are something that clinicians face regularly. However, we worried that our ability to estimate the strength of contributions from other independent variables would be diminished too greatly if we included this additional factor in this study.

Finally, all of the children whose data are reported here had parents with normal hearing. Every year the Gallaudet Research Institute collects and reports data on children with hearing loss, and every year it is found that over 90% of children with hearing loss have two parents with normal hearing, if they come from a family with two parents, or have one parent with normal hearing, if they come from a single-parent household. Therefore, requiring that parents in this study have normal hearing meant that we were testing children in the most typical situation for children with hearing loss. It also ensured that all children were receiving good speech models in the home.

Our Participants

Data are reported for 205 children: 87 of these children had normal hearing, and 118 had moderate-to-profound hearing loss. Of these participants, 9% of parents described themselves and their children as Hispanic, 3% as Native American, 8% as Asian, and 8% as African American. The other 72% were White. Descriptions of the children who participated are provided, but care is taken to protect the confidentiality of all children. For that reason, specific information is not given if it would permit the identity of any one child or family to be recognized.

Quantifying Hearing Loss

All of the children with normal hearing passed a hearing screening at birth. Additionally, at 3 years of age these children also passed an audiological screening of the frequencies 500, 1000, 2000, and 4000 Hz presented at 20 dB HL to each ear separately. To participate as a child with hearing loss, a child needed to have an unaided pure-tone average for the frequencies 500, 1000, and 2000 Hz (i.e., three-frequency average) in the better ear of poorer than 50 dB HL. This factor will be labeled as the better-ear pure-tone average (BE-PTA) in this report. We requested copies of audiograms each time a child had a new hearing test. The BE-PTAs reported here are from the most recent audiogram that we had on file when the child stopped participating in the study. Only 11% of the children who received cochlear implants had unaided thresholds measured after they received

an implant. For the children who did not have unaided thresholds measured once they got implants, we used the last threshold values obtained. No child in the study showed evidence of having progressive hearing loss, and children were not included if they were diagnosed with auditory neuropathy.

It has recently started to become common to see four-frequency averages reported to describe auditory sensitivity in children with hearing loss, with either 3000 or 4000 Hz included as the fourth frequency. That practice actually arises from work with adult stapedectomy patients where it is known that the auditory gains in high frequencies obtained by middle-ear surgery account for the lion's share of improvements in speech reception for adults. Changes in sensitivity in the lower frequencies, such as those included in the calculation of the three-frequency PTA, do not correlate well with changes in speech perception for these patients. For that reason a committee convened by the American Academy of Otolaryngology-Head and Neck Surgery recommended using this four-frequency metric, rather than the previously common three-frequency PTA (Committee on Hearing and Equilibrium, 1995). That recommendation has subsequently been shown to provide more accurate indices of benefits obtained in such surgeries (de Bruijn, Tange, & Dreschler, 2001). For describing the losses of individuals with moderate-to-profound sensorineural hearing loss, there is no obvious benefit to using either a three-frequency or four-frequency PTA. However, PTAs for the same ears are generally poorer if the four-frequency average is used, rather than the three-frequency average, for the simple reason that most hearing loss becomes more severe at higher frequencies. That is indeed the case for the participants with hearing loss in this study, and so it should be remembered that PTAs would have been poorer for these individuals if we had chosen to report four-frequency PTAs.

Age of Identification

One independent factor in which we were keenly interested during the conduction of this work was the age of identification of children's hearing loss. Hearing loss is being identified shortly after birth for many children, and treatment in the form of amplification and/ or intervention is being started before 6 months of age for many of those children. Does this early start lead to developmental patterns that more closely match what is observed for children with normal hearing? That was a central question in this investigation. It is an important question because it is much trickier and involves a much greater outlay of resources to identify hearing loss at birth than it does to wait for a year or so and see if a child is learning to talk. To answer the question, we sought to recruit children with hearing loss who were identified at three discrete ages: before 6 months of age, between 12 and 18 months of age (i.e., at 1 year), and between 24 and 30 months of age (i.e., at 2 years). We largely excluded children whose losses were identified between 6 and 12 months or between 18 and 24 months in favor of having discrete categories. Nonetheless, the matter of appropriately characterizing a child's age of identification of hearing loss turned out to be tougher than first imagined, owing to the fact

that the age when a child's loss is identified may not indicate precisely when steps are taken to treat that hearing loss. The age at which something starts to be done about a child's hearing loss is more likely to affect developmental outcomes than the age at which that loss is recognized. For these reasons, this variable, age of identification, came to be defined by three related events: the age at which a child was identified as having a hearing loss, the age at which the child was first fit with an auditory prosthesis, and the age at which intervention commenced. A child classified as having been identified with hearing loss before 6 months of age in this study also had to at least have been fit with a prosthesis before 6 months to participate in the study. Generally speaking, those children also started receiving intervention before 6 months of age as well, but in some cases that did not happen until the child was slightly older than 6 months. However, for the latter two age groups (1 year and 2 years of age at the time of identification), there needed to be more wiggle room in the temporal proximity of these events if we wanted adequate sample sizes. If a child was identified shortly before the specified age bracket, but did not receive amplification or initiate intervention until the specified window, that child was included in the study. In fact, there were a couple children in the study who failed their newborn hearing screening, but no follow-up was provided until the child was more than a year old. Those children are included in the 1-year age-of-identification group. There are other children who started receiving some speech therapy between 18 and 24 months of age because their parents thought they were language delayed, although they had not been identified as having hearing loss. These children had not been given newborn hearing screenings, and no one tested their hearing until they were older than 2 years of age. Because of these situations, we decided to characterize group membership using a mean of the three age measures: age of identification of the hearing loss, age of first amplification, and age of first intervention. Figure 4–1 shows this measure for these 118 children with hearing loss. It can be seen that there is clear separation of the three groups of children depending on this derived value. From here on the label *ID-Age* will be used to refer to the mean of these three time values. This variable provides a measure that is continuous in distribution. The term *age of ID* will be used to refer to the categorical variable of group membership.

Signing

Seventy-seven of the children in this study were exposed to signs: 33 of the children with normal hearing and 44 of the children with hearing loss. We were interested in how the parents of these children learned sign language. One child with normal hearing and two children with hearing loss each had one deaf relative, other than a parent, and so their parents learned sign language from family members. In those cases the parents were highly familiar with sign language, although they could not be classified as being native signers. All other parents who provided sign input to their children learned signs expressly to provide support for their spoken language input. This is the typical situation for children who receive sign support for the purpose of facilitating spoken

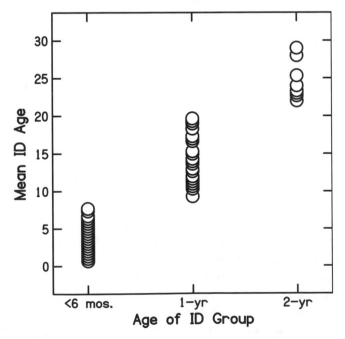

Figure 4–1. The continuous variable of ID-Age (in months) plotted for each child with hearing loss according to Age of ID group.

language development; their parents have no prior experience with signs.

We kept track of how parents learned signs. We asked parents to indicate if they learned signs from books and/or videotapes, from classes, or from all of those sources. Table 4–1 indicates the numbers of parents of children with normal hearing and of children with hearing loss who reported learning signs from each of those sources.

We also asked parents to estimate the percentage of the time they accompanied their spoken language input to their child with signs. This question was generally asked each time the child was tested. However, if a family did not enter the study until an older test age, we asked parents to think back to when their children were younger and estimate the amount of time they spent signing to their children at each of those earlier ages. Because the time span we were asking parents to recall was generally not more than a year, we trusted these estimates to be correct. We have data from each 6-month age range for children with hearing loss, starting at 12 months for children whose losses were identified before 6 months of age, and starting at 30 months for children

whose losses were identified after 1 year. Figure 4–2 provides those results separately for children whose losses were identified early (i.e., before 6 months of age), and for children whose losses were identified late. In this figure, any child whose loss was identified after 12 months of age is included in the late age-of-ID group. Results are plotted for the mother and father separately. We also asked parents to estimate the percentage of time that children accompanied their spoken language production with sign language; these estimates are shown as well. Standard deviations are quite large across participants for all three of these estimates: on the order of .30 across test ages.

It is clear from Figure 4–2 that the amount of time that all family members spent signing generally decreased as the child got older. Was this because the children were adequately acquiring a mastery of spoken language, and so the signs became unnecessary? If that were the case, it would mean that the early use of signs had fulfilled the goal of using them (i.e., to facilitate the development of spoken language). Or was it the case that parents simply tired of trying to sign with their children,

Table 4–1. The numbers of children with parents who learned signs from each of the methods listed.

Group Number of Participants	NH+S 33	HL+S 44
Book/Video	8	8
Class	18	12
Book/Video/Class	4	14
Relative	1	2

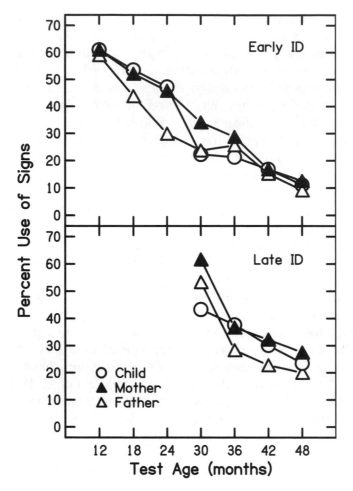

Figure 4–2. Estimates of the percentage of time that parents of children with hearing loss, and the children themselves, accompanied their spoken language with signs.

much as many of us tire of our New Year's resolutions come February? Those questions could hopefully be answered by comparing measures of children's language development to these estimates of time engaged in signing.

We initially asked parents of children with normal hearing to report on the frequency of their sign use, as well as that of their children. However, by 24 months of age all parents of children with normal hearing, as well as the children themselves, had ceased using signs altogether. Consequently, we discontinued asking.

The data traced on Figure 4–2 may appear bleak to proponents of using signs to facilitate the acquisition of spoken language: Parents who reportedly were supporting their spoken language input with signs were doing so generally less than half of the time. There were wide ranges on these values, but generally speaking, parents were not consistently using signs. These proportions for use of signs in the homes decreased as children got older, even though many children at 36 months of age began attending preschool programs that routinely used signs. Nonetheless, we have every reason to believe that these numbers reflect the reality for children with hearing loss. The Gallaudet Research Institute conducts an annual survey of children with hearing loss and asks about sign use in the home. The most recent data available at the time of this writing were from 2006, and were provided for 37,352 children nationally. Forty-seven percent of those children were in school programs that used signs, either alone or in combination with spoken language. However, only 24% of parents reported that family members regularly signed at home, and that percentage included deaf parents. If we assume that close to 10% of deaf children have deaf parents, we may conclude that roughly only 15% of hearing parents of deaf children regularly sign at home. No definition is provided of what it means to "regularly sign," but regardless, these numbers suggest that hearing parents of deaf children generally do not sign everything that they say to their children, even when they have the best of intentions.

Before leaving the topic of signs, it should be mentioned that we were interested in what types of signs parents were using with their children. These parents all reported using signs to supplement spoken language input, rather than to teach their children sign language itself, and so we had assumed that most parents would be using a version of manually coded English. However, when we asked parents what kinds of signs they were using, slightly more

than half (28 out of 44) of the parents of children with hearing loss reported that they used signs that could appropriately be considered American Sign Language. The parents of the remaining 16 children who received sign support stated that they used some version of a manually coded English system.

Audiograms

From the audiograms that we received from children's audiologists, we were able to compute composite audiograms across groups of children. Figure 4–3 shows composite unaided audiograms for early- and late-identified deaf children, grouped by the kind of prosthesis they wore and by whether they used signs or not. Children within the signing and nonsigning groups were well matched, as were early- and late-identified children. The only factor differentiating mean auditory thresholds was whether children wore hearing aids for the entire time they were in the study or received a cochlear implant. Figure 4–4 shows composite aided audiograms, and illustrates that even the effect of type of prosthesis worn by children disappeared when aided thresholds are considered.

Geography

The children in this study were recruited from communities in 20 different states: New Hampshire, Massachusetts, New York, Pennsylvania, Ohio, Tennessee, Georgia, Florida, Illinois, Mississippi, Missouri, Minnesota, Nebraska, Kansas, Oklahoma, Texas, New Mexico, Utah, Washington, and California. In a few

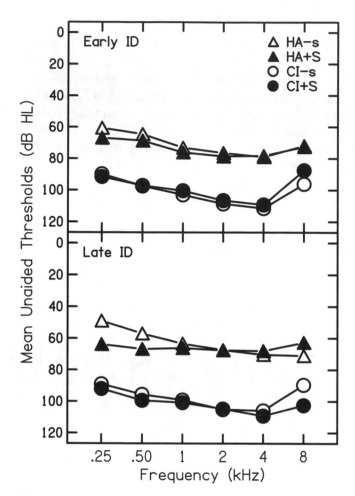

Figure 4–3. Composites of mean unaided auditory thresholds in the better ear for early- and late-identified children with hearing loss, grouped by the type of prosthesis they had (HA = hearing aid; CI = cochlear implant) and by whether they used signs or not (–s = no signs; +S = signs).

cases, testing was done at more than one location within a state. In some cases, children traveled to a test site from a different state. The specific communities where we set up data collection had to meet several criteria. Most importantly, they needed to have at least two early intervention programs that provided services to families of children with hearing loss at least once per week. One program had to provide signing instruction to its clients and one had to provide some version of auditory-oral intervention. This criterion did not ensure that families from both sorts of programs in any one community enrolled in this study; it simply meant that there was the opportunity to recruit from both sorts of programs. There also needed to be professionals

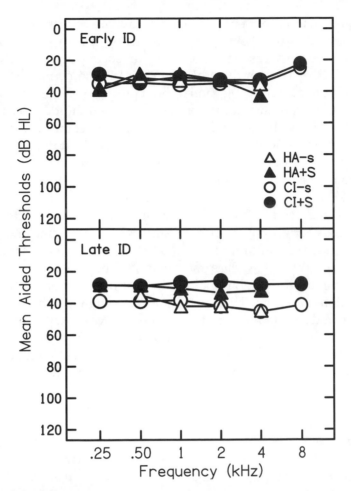

Figure 4–4. Composites of mean aided auditory thresholds for early- and late-identified children with hearing loss, grouped by the type of prosthesis they had (HA = hearing aid; CI = cochlear implant) and by whether they used signs or not (–s = no signs; +S = signs).

in the vicinity who were willing to distribute recruitment brochures to parents of children with hearing loss meeting our criteria for participation. Finally, there had to be at least one professional willing to collect data for us. An important aspect of the design of this project was that data collection would be decoupled from specific intervention programs. The data reported here were

never collected as part of the clinical procedures of any intervention program.

Having test sites distributed so widely meant that our samples included children from a variety of programs. In this way we ensured that we were not examining possibly idiosyncratic characteristics of individual programs in specific locations. In particular, if data collection were restricted geographically it might be the case, by chance, that either the signing program or the nonsigning (auditory-oral) program was preferable in some way. Perhaps one or the other program was private, attracting families of higher socioeconomic status, for example. Or perhaps the individuals providing the intervention were better educated and more experienced at one type of program or the other. By including a broad array of geographic areas we hoped to distribute idiosyncratic variability across our groups in such a way as to minimize its contributions to tests of group equivalence. At the same time, we gathered information about the intervention programs in which these children and their families participated, and examined contributions to overall outcomes of certain aspects of those programs. That information is discussed later in this chapter.

Demographics

Table 4–2 shows demographic information for all participants. An important independent variable that we were interested in was socioeconomic status. This descriptor generally refers to the social and educational ranking of a family. Especially in an egalitarian society, as we have in the United States, it is difficult to design a scale of social and educational ranking that validly indexes this trait. Precisely because we believe in providing easily accessible public education, we place few restrictions on who can attend college. This differs from other societies in which only the wealthy are able to attend. At the same time it means that there are individuals in our society who have attended col-

lege, but are nonetheless living in conditions of poverty. Similarly, there are in our society individuals who have not had much formal education who hold prestigious professional positions. This makes it difficult to explain developmental outcomes completely by the socioeconomic status of a child, and there are those who worry that developmental research in this country has been poorly served by using socioeconomic status as a predictor variable in such work (e.g., Duncan & Magnuson, 2003). In spite of those concerns, a substantial body of research has shown that both the language style of parents and the language abilities of children generally vary with family socioeconomic status. The most well-known of these studies was conducted by Betty Hart and Todd Risley. Their report, titled, *Meaningful Differences in the Everyday Experience of Young American Children* (1995), described results for 42 families, including some with low socioeconomic status (SES). Hart and Risley followed their young participants from the time the children were 12 months old until they were 36 months old. Those investigators showed that parents meeting the criteria of having low SES generally interacted less, and did so differently from parents with middle or high SES. Children from the low-socioeconomic households showed slower vocabulary growth than other children, with roughly 60% of the variance in those measures accounted for by how parents interacted with their children. This finding was similar to findings reported by other investigators for children from low-socioeconomic households (Hess & Shipman, 1965; Nittrouer, 2002; Schachter, 1979). Because of this well-replicated

Table 4–2. Means of descriptive statistics for the 205 participants in the study, with standard deviations in parentheses. Socioeconomic status is given using the two-factor index described in the text. Occupational and educational rank is determined using the eight-point scales described in the text. Family income is rated using a four-level scale, described in the text.

Age of ID Group			<6 Months		1 Year		2 Years	
	NH–s	NH+S	HL–s	HL+S	HL–s	HL+S	HL–s	HL+S
Number of Participants	54	33	48	29	20	8	6	7
SES	32.78 (11.13)	34.36 (14.87)	29.73 (13.57)	31.45 (12.59)	31.30 (14.51)	30.63 (15.62)	31.00 (9.88)	43.00 (13.58)
Occupational rank of father	4.91 (1.38)	5.48 (1.60)	4.60 (1.63)	4.86 (1.64)	4.50 (1.76)	4.88 (1.81)	4.83 (1.17)	6.14 (1.68)
Educational rank of father	5.48 (1.37)	5.64 (1.56)	5.19 (1.79)	5.38 (1.57)	5.25 (1.71)	5.00 (1.69)	6.33 (0.52)	6.43 (1.40)
Occupational rank of mother	3.69 (1.80)	3.45 (1.87)	3.48 (1.77)	3.83 (1.98)	4.40 (1.54)	3.75 (1.75)	2.00 (0.00)	4.29 (2.21)
Educational rank of mother	5.93 (1.03)	5.79 (1.27)	5.52 (1.54)	5.17 (1.71)	5.95 (1.50)	5.75 (0.71)	5.83 (0.75)	6.00 (1.00)
Family income	3.41 (0.84)	3.30 (0.95)	3.21 (1.17)	3.45 (0.99)	3.80 (0.52)	3.63 (0.74)	4.00 (0.00)	4.00 (0.00)
Number of siblings	1.41 (0.79)	1.15 (0.51)	1.38 (0.94)	1.48 (1.53)	1.00 (0.46)	1.38 (1.06)	1.33 (0.82)	1.43 (0.79)
Proportion of males	.54	.48	.48	.52	.50	.25	.17	.57
Proportion of two-parent households	.89	.85	.85	.79	.75	.63	.67	.57

demonstration of a relation between SES and children's language acquisition, which appears to be mediated by how parents talk to their children, it was deemed important to collect information on the SES of the families of children in this study.

August Hollingshead, a professor at Yale University, is credited with developing the two-factor scale that is traditionally used to index SES. He created this scale in the late 1950s, with the first draft of the document available in 1957. He modified procedures slightly, and sometimes one will see *The Two Factor Index of Social Position* cited as becoming available in 1965. Regardless of what date is given, Hollingshead never published this index, although it is used widely. Methods involve ranking the head of household's occupation according to a scale of how socially prestigious it is, and similarly ranking the individual's educational level. A weighted sum of these two factors serves as the socioeconomic score for the family.

When the relation between SES and language acquisition was to be examined for the first time in the author's laboratory (Nittrouer, 1996), it was evident that Hollingshead's rankings were outdated. For example, his rankings included occupations that no longer exist, such as hod carrier and porter, but did not include newer occupations related to technology, such as network manager and data entry personnel. As a result, we decided to update those scales. To do so we had individuals categorize the occupations shown in Appendix A into eight levels of social status, with *1* as the lowest and *8* as the highest. We used the means of those rankings to establish an occupational scale. A similar eight-point scale is used to rank the

highest educational level achieved by the individual being assigned a socioeconomic ranking. In the current study, we collected data regarding both the mother's and father's occupations and educational levels. The scores from the highest income earner were used to index the family's overall SES. This value is computed by multiplying the obtained values for occupation and educational level for that individual. This procedure works well, but it needs to be noted that the scale is not linear because the separate scores are multiplied. As a result, equivalent differences on one of the scales (occupation or education) will result in unequal differences in overall statuses, depending on whether individuals fall toward the lower or higher end of the other scale. For example, if two individuals receive educational codes of 2 but one receives an occupational code of 1 and the other receives an occupational code of 2, they will obtain SES metrics of 2 and 4, respectively. Those two individuals differ by two points on the SES scale, based on the one-point difference in occupational ranking. However, if two individuals both receive educational codes of 8, but one receives an occupational code of 7 and the other receives an occupational code of 8, they will obtain SES scores of 56 and 64, respectively. In this case, a one-point difference in occupational ranking translates into an eight-point difference in overall SES. Thus, a one-point difference on either of the scales results in different overall scores, depending on which end of the other scale the individual falls onto.

The first row on Table 4–2 shows mean SES for children in each of our groups, calculated based on values derived from the parent with the highest income. A one-way analysis of variance (ANOVA) was performed on these SES metrics, with group as the between-subjects variable. No significant difference across the eight groups was found. The average child in this study came from a family in which the primary income earner had a college education and an occupation commensurate with that educational level. However, we did have a range of socioeconomic levels represented. That range permitted us to examine SES as a predictor variable in this study: We could ask what proportion of variance on our dependent measures was explained by this independent variable. Rows 2 through 5 give occupational and educational rankings for each parent separately.

In addition to collecting information on occupational and educational factors, data were collected about annual family income, and was coded using a four-point scale: (1) less than $20,000; (2) between $20,000 and $30,000; (3) between $30,000 and $45,000; and (4) greater than $45,000. Row 6 shows mean annual income for each group, using these category labels. Again, a one-way ANOVA was performed, and again no difference across groups was observed. Although the values listed on Table 4–2 show the mean annual income across participants to be in the $30,000 to $45,000 range, roughly half of the children in this study came from families whose annual income was above $45,000. In the case of both SES and annual family income, data were collected when a child enrolled in the study and was not updated later.

Rows 7 to 9 on Table 4–2 display mean scores for other independent variables that might be of interest to readers. On row 7 we see the mean number

of siblings that participants had. Most came from families of two or three children. Row 8 shows that there was an even distribution of boys and girls in the study, and row 9 indicates that most children had two parents living in the home. Data on the number of siblings a child had and the number of parents living in the home were updated as each situation changed. The most recently reported data are shown.

In summary, we find that participants were similar across our eight groups. Of particular interest, we had some within-group variability on the metric of SES, although most participants would accurately be portrayed as middle class. Nonetheless, the effects of SES on developmental outcomes were examined closely.

Further Description of Children with Hearing Loss

Table 4–3 provides information specific to participants with hearing loss only. Line 1 lists mean three-frequency BE-PTAs, in dB HL. These are the values that were obtained most recently at the time of writing from the children's audiologists. It is quite apparent from Line 1 on this table that, for children whose hearing losses were identified before 6 months of age, BE-PTAs were similar regardless of whether the children received sign support or not. A one-way ANOVA performed on these values for all children revealed that mean BE-PTAs were similar for five groups, with significantly better BE-PTAs for the children with hearing loss identified at 2 years of age who did not use signs. However, when the two groups of children whose losses were identified

Table 4–3. Means of descriptive statistics for the 118 participants with hearing loss, with standard deviations in parentheses. All age-related values are given in months; all pure-tone thresholds are given in dB HL.

Age of ID Group	<6 Months		1 Year		2 Years	
	HL–s	HL+S	HL–s	HL+S	HL–s	HL+S
Number of Participants	48	29	20	8	6	7
BE-PTA	92 (20)	94 (24)	99 (18)	84 (23)	66 (15)	91 (31)
Aided PTA	33 (11)	31 (10)	37 (14)	29 (8)	41 (11)	26 (6)
Age of ID	2.08 (1.58)	1.55 (1.84)	12.35 (4.48)	13.00 (3.59)	24.17 (2.93)	23.86 (2.27)
Age of first prosthesis	3.75 (1.68)	3.59 (1.72)	13.45 (3.85)	15.38 (3.29)	25.83 (2.93)	25.57 (3.10)
Age of first intervention	3.88 (2.40)	4.28 (3.84)	15.60 (4.49)	15.88 (5.94)	23.17 (5.81)	23.86 (2.27)
ID-Age	3.24 (1.67)	3.14 (1.91)	13.80 (2.95)	14.75 (3.27)	24.39 (2.53)	24.43 (1.99)
Proportion of participants with: HA	.29	.38	.05	.50	.83	.43
CI	.71	.62	.95	.50	.17	.57
Age of first implant	14.32 (4.78)	14.94 (6.55)	19.89 (5.38)	18.50 (3.11)	37.00 (0.00)	30.50 (4.43)

later than 6 months of age are combined (as they generally are in reporting the data), we find that there were no significant differences in BE-PTA: Children whose losses were identified late (at 1 or 2 years of age) and received sign support had a mean BE-PTA of 87. For children with late-identified losses who did not receive sign support, mean BE-PTA was 92.

Line 2 on Table 4–3 shows mean aided PTAs obtained by free-field testing. We find that children in all groups were well-matched on this variable. It is interesting that the children with hearing loss identified at 2 years of age who did not use signs had the poorest aided thresholds, given that they had the best unaided thresholds. Looking at children with hearing aids and cochlear implants separately, we find that mean aided PTAs for children with hearing aids was 30 dB HL (standard deviation = 7 dB); the mean for children with implants was 33 dB HL (standard deviation = 12 dB).

Line 3 on Table 4–3 indicates the mean age of identification of children's hearing losses, line 4 shows the mean age of first amplification, and line 5 indicates the mean age of first intervention. Line 6 shows the mean ID-Age for each group. Again, this is the mean of age of identification, age of first amplification, and age of first intervention.

Line 7 shows the proportion of participants in each group who wore hearing aids for the duration of the study. Across all groups, there were 38 children with hearing aids. With one exception, they all wore bilateral hearing aids.

Line 8 gives the proportion of participants in each group who received cochlear implants at some point in the study (total = 80), and line 9 indicates

the age at the time of receiving that first implant. Naturally, these values increase with increasing age of identification. No distinction is made here among children who had one implant, two implants, or an implant and a hearing aid. If a child had at least one implant, she was counted in this tally. Of the children who had cochlear implants, 61% were from Cochlear Corporation, 35% from Advanced Bionics, and 4% from Med El.

A total of 73 children used hearing aids for a substantial period of this study, either bilaterally or in combination with a cochlear implant. Fifty-five percent of these were Phonak aids, 19% were Oticon, and 18% were Widex. The remaining 8% of aids were Unitron, AVR, or Starky. Sixty-three percent of the hearing aids used by children could be programmed with low-frequency cutoffs at 200 Hz or lower, which is important in considering how hearing aids and implants might function together.

We asked parents whether or not their children had access to FM systems. Half of the parents of children with hearing aids and 26% of parents of children with cochlear implants said that their children had access to FM systems, but overwhelmingly this was only during preschool. Even if they owned FM systems, very few parents reported using them regularly with their children.

Parents were queried regarding the etiology of their children's hearing losses, but in 68% of the cases they did not know. Another 29% of the parents reported that there was a genetic cause associated with the hearing loss, generally involving connexin 26. Etiology for the remaining four children was evenly split between cytomegalovirus and Mondini malformation.

We were very interested in characteristics of the interventions these children received, as well, and so collected precise data on their intervention programs. Table 4–4 presents this information, for intervention provided between 12 and 35 months of age, and for intervention provided from 36 to 48 months of age separately. There is a natural break in intervention services at 36 months of age because the child's services move from Part C to Part B of the Individuals with Disabilities Education Act. In particular, we were interested in whether the intervention programs the children were in focused more on interacting with the child (child-focused), with the parent (parent-focused), or if professionals in the programs split their attention roughly equally between child and parent. We also were interested in whether the family traveled to a center for intervention (center-based), or if the interventionist traveled to the child's home (home-based), or if some of the time the family traveled and some of the time the interventionist traveled (both). The data on Table 4–4 indicate that when children reached 36 months of age, their intervention changed so that it was more frequently centered on the child and it more frequently took place in a center. These trends reflect the fact that most children began attending preschool programs.

For those children not receiving sign support with their spoken language input, we were interested in whether the family attended a program that considered itself auditory oral or one that was auditory verbal in approach. To be considered auditory verbal in approach, the center had to have certified auditory-verbal therapists providing the intervention. Finally, we collected data on how often the child received intervention. The numbers shown on Table 4–4 indicate the mean numbers of times in a month that children in each group generally received intervention; these numbers do not reflect the duration of each visit. When children were infants, the numbers listed on this row of Table 4–4 likely indicate 1-hour visits with an early intervention specialist. By 36 months of age, the visits likely represent 4 to 6 hours of preschool. The mean number of visits per month before the age of 36 months appears to differ depending on age of ID, but this trend reflects the fact that the number of visits generally ramped up as children got older. The means for children identified with hearing loss at later ages were more heavily weighted towards those periods of more frequent visits.

Procedures

Recruitment

A primary consideration in this study was that we wanted to keep data collection and analysis as unbiased as possible. In particular, we did not want the collection of data on the dependent measures to be tied to children's interventions. The measures reported here were not gleaned from the children's clinical records; rather, they were obtained through careful and consistent methods of data collection, separate from their customary assessments.

In order to achieve our goal of maintaining a separation between this project and children's intervention programs,

Table 4–4. Proportions of participants receiving intervention that met each of the following criteria: *Who* refers to whom the intervention was focused on; *where* refers to where it took place. *Type* of intervention is given for children not receiving sign support, and refers to whether the intervention was auditory oral or auditory verbal. *Mean number of visits* is given as visits per month, with standard deviations in parentheses.

Age of ID	<6 Months		1 Year		2 Years	
Group	HL–s	HL+S	HL–s	HL+S	HL–s	HL+S
Number of Participants	48	29	20	8	6	7
12–35 months						
Who Parent	.07				.33	
Child	.47	.65	.57	.63	.33	1.00
Both	.47	.35	.43	.38	.33	
Where Child's Home	.20	.26	.07	.25		
Center	.42	.09	.79	.38	.33	.67
Both	.38	.65	.14	.38	.67	.33
Type Auditory Oral	.69		.71		1.00	
Auditory Verbal Therapy	.31		.29			
Mean number of visits	8.39 (6.19)	7.61 (4.49)	9.94 (5.31)	11.97 (8.25)	20.78 (5.21)	14.60 (4.86)
36–48 months						
Who Parent	.03				.33	
Child	.90	.89	.80	.83	.50	.71
Both	.08	.11	.20		.17	.29
Where Child's Home	.03		.05		.17	
Center	.92	.94	.95	.83	.50	.86
Both	.05	.06			.33	.14
Type Auditory Oral	.77		.70		1.00	
Auditory Verbal Therapy	.23		.30			
Mean number of visits	15.60 (8.59)	16.06 (6.74)	16.19 (6.20)	19.20 (4.97)	18.34 (6.09)	17.43 (5.94)

we obtained help recruiting participants from a variety of sources, not only from programs that provided early intervention services. In this way we were able to avoid having only preselected children involved in the study. Programs that helped in the recruitment of participants included schools, daycares, classes for teaching parents how to use signs with their infants, audiology centers, otolaryngology clinics, pediatric clinics, and early intervention programs. Brochures describing the project were made available at these facilities through procedures such as displaying them in waiting areas. In addition, personnel at these facilities handed the brochures to parents of children with normal hearing and to parents of children with hearing loss. If interested, the parent tore off a postage-paid postcard attached to the brochure and mailed it to the central facility. Public service advertisements were also played on the radio in the communities where participants were being recruited. Parents could call a toll-free number at the central facility, and a brochure was mailed to them. Once the postcard from the brochure was received, parents were contacted by someone at the central site to provide them with more information about the project, and to answer their questions. Then they were sent a form to complete that asked for information about the child and family in more detail. At that time, a consent form was also sent for the parents to sign. Parents of children with hearing loss were also sent a release form to sign so that audiological records could be obtained from their children's audiologists. Data gathered from the information forms served as independent variables, and included information on family income,

SES, the child's general health history, and intervention programming. At a later time, requests for more information were sent to the intervention agencies that parents reported using, without revealing the names of participants. In this way, staff at the central facility kept track of all independent variables. The people doing the actual testing did not have access to this kind of information. (In this report, the term *central facility* or *central site* refers to the laboratory where the author was located. For the first 2 years of the project, the central site was Utah State University; for the last 3 years, it was The Ohio State University.)

Examiners

All data were collected by individuals who did so independently of their professional positions. The individuals who did the actual data collection were termed *examiners*. All of these examiners had at least a bachelor's degree in an area relevant to early intervention with deaf children, such as deaf education, communication sciences and disorders, speech-language pathology, audiology, and psychology. Some examiners were doctoral students in related fields; some were already working in their chosen field. Thirty-nine examiners in all helped to collect the data reported here. Of those 39 testers, 31 had master's degrees or PhDs. The other eight had bachelor's degrees.

With data collection occurring at so many sites, it was important that consistency in procedures be maintained across those sites. That consistency was achieved by training all examiners to follow the same procedures. At the start of the project, a 2-day training session was conducted in Logan, Utah, at Utah State University. Procedures were reviewed in detail, and examiners practiced in small groups. Figure 4–5 shows a group of examiners practicing how to set up the video cameras. After training, each examiner returned home and ran a practice participant. That session was videotaped from start to finish, and evaluated by the staff at the central facility. Comments were provided on ways to modify the testing, if necessary, and practice participants were run until each examiner was able to do the testing in conformance with general procedures. If a new examiner missed that first training session, she visited the central facility and received individual training. A second training session was

held when participants started turning 36 months of age, both as a refresher and to introduce the procedures that changed at 36 months of age.

Examiners collected data outside of their normal working hours. They were minimally involved in recruitment of participants, and were given no information about the children and families whom they tested, other than names and phone numbers. In some cases, participants received services from the facility where the examiner was employed, but in no case was the examiner the one directly providing the services. Examiners kept no data at their test sites, nor were they involved in scoring the materials generated in the test session. When a participant in their area was

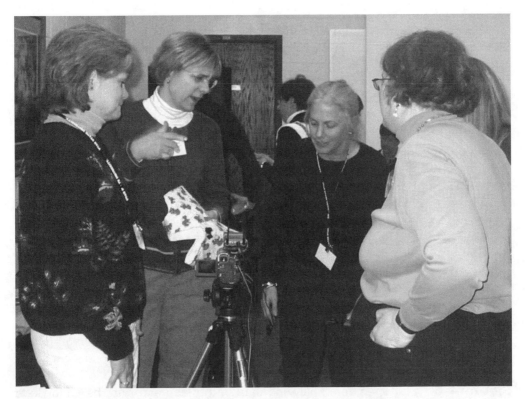

Figure 4–5. A training meeting for test examiners in Logan, Utah.

2 months away from a 6-month birthday, the examiner was sent a packet of information. A test session was then scheduled that was within the window of 1 month before to 1 month after the 6-month birthday. All materials necessary for testing were included in the packet. The order in which various tasks were to be administered during the test session was consistent across sites. So, for example, each child was given the Auditory Comprehension task first, followed by the tasks to be videotaped, and so on. After completing a test, all materials were immediately mailed back to the central facility. In these ways, we kept to a minimum the opportunities for testers to influence and know about results.

Scorers

A number of individuals helped to analyze the data, as well. These individuals worked at the central site, as shown in Figure 4–6. Some scorers were project staff, and some were graduate students. Each scorer was extensively trained, and weekly meetings were held to discuss any problems that arose.

General Procedures

One perspective that has been missing from our general picture of how children with hearing loss are faring is a good sense of how they are developing

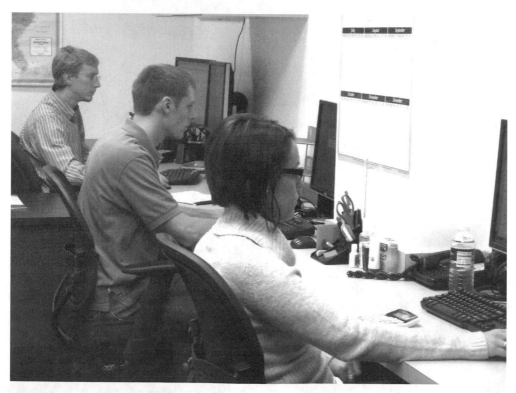

Figure 4–6. Staff members analyzing data in the laboratory at The Ohio State University.

across time. For many kinds of dependent measures, we have information from discrete ages, or even across a few ages. There have been a few studies that have followed some children with hearing loss over a period of a year or two, but none that has followed children from the same populations for several years. This situation introduces several constraints on our understanding of how children with hearing loss are developing, how we should be intervening, and how we should be assessing their progress.

The paucity of data on the same measures across time has left a gap in our collective understanding of the development of children with hearing loss because dependent measures vary in how sensitive they are at different ages. A measure that fails to capture change between groups at a young age may do so very well at a later age. This happens when measures index behaviors that do not begin to emerge in typically developing children until a certain stage in development. Similarly, some dependent measures may index group differences at very young ages, but become insensitive to those differences later on. That situation arises for measures of behavior that all children eventually acquire, even if it is in a delayed time frame. A study that fails to find differences between children with normal hearing and children with hearing loss, or between children who are exposed to signs and those who are not, may just be using a measure that is insensitive to potential differences at that point in development. It is precisely because of this variability in sensitivity of measures that data were collected over a 3-year period for children with and without hearing loss in this study.

In a sense, this focus on collecting data across a relatively long period dictated that the research project be longitudinal in design. After all, we were interested in how children develop, and if there might be differences in the developmental patterns of children depending on whether or not they have hearing loss, whether their spoken language input is supplemented with signs, and the age at which their hearing loss was identified, if indeed they had hearing loss. In keeping with that focus, this study was designed to collect data on children every 6 months between 12 and 48 months of age, on their 6-month birthdays (+/− one month). But there are strengths and weaknesses to strictly longitudinal designs, most of which are related to variability on independent measures among participants. On one hand, if an investigator can ensure that she has groups matched on all independent measures, except those of interest to the study, then such designs can provide the desired data. But how can we ever know that? How can we, in fact, know what all the relevant independent variables might be prior to doing the experiment? Coming back to the example of the study comparing math skills in Canadian and American children, what if it turns out that the time of day that math instruction is provided has an influence on a child's ability to grasp the material, and the experimenter never collected data on that factor? In that case we might reach erroneous conclusions, if it just so happened that time of instruction was unevenly distributed across the two samples.

Partly because of that concern—that a strictly longitudinal sample could introduce unnoticed variability on unspecified independent variables—the design of this study was not kept strictly longitudinal. Another reason for not insisting on a strictly longitudinal design was the recognition that it is very difficult to retain the same participants across time. People move away, get sick, or become busy with work, school, or hobbies. Sometimes people learn of a study in which they may participate only after it has started. If an experimental design dictates that all participants must provide data at each test time, or else that individual's data will be removed from the analysis entirely, there could be a lot of effort wasted in collecting data that eventually get discarded.

The other extreme in sampling methods would be to obtain new samples of the same populations at each test age. If we were interested in how math skills emerge for children living in Canada and the United States, we might test children in both countries once per year, at each year between first and fifth grade. If we were worried about having biased longitudinal samples, we could obtain different samples of children who nonetheless fit the criterion of living in one or the other country each year. Of course, in this case we run the risk of incurring a different sort of bias. What if, for example, we just happened to obtain progressively smarter children in one of the countries each year? In that case it could appear as if children in that country learned math at a more rapid rate.

To deal with these concerns regarding sampling methods, we asked parents of our participants to continue in data collection at each test age, once they were enrolled in the study, but we were thoroughly understanding if something came up that prevented them from participating. Table 4–5 displays the numbers of participants in each group who participated at each test age. Table 4–6 indicates how many participants, out of the total number of 205 participants, attended four or more test sessions, or three or less. Slightly more than half of all participants contributed data to at least four sessions, or more than half of the time.

Finally, we kept track of the reasons for families failing to participate in a test session, once they were enrolled. The primary reasons were these: First and foremost, children failed to provide data at test ages before they were enrolled in the study. More children enrolled as their parents heard about the project and decided to participate.

For children with normal hearing, participation by some families was stopped by us. Test sites were added over the course of the first year of testing, as indicated by the fact that the number of participants nearly doubled between the 12-month and 18-month test ages. We wished to have some participants with normal hearing at each test site. In that way, every examiner would have experience testing children with normal hearing. Also, we wanted a way of checking the consistency of test methods across sites. If scores were roughly equivalent on these measures for children with normal hearing across test sites, we reasoned, there would be a basis for asserting that testing was being conducted in a consistent manner across sites. Indeed, in all cases we found that children with normal hearing from the various sites across the country performed similarly at each test age.

Table 4–5. Numbers of participants with data included at each test age.

Number of Participants	NH–s	NH+S	< 6 Months		1 Year		2 Years		Total
	54	33	HL–s 48	HL+S 29	HL–s 20	HL+S 8	HL–s 6	HL+S 7	205
Test Age									
12	29	12	11	5	0	0	0	0	57
18	43	28	24	13	2	0	0	0	110
24	32	25	30	11	5	2	0	0	105
30	25	27	37	14	11	4	1	0	119
36	31	30	37	14	12	6	3	3	132
42	27	26	35	12	18	6	5	4	139
48	26	25	34	18	20	6	6	6	141

Table 4–6. Numbers of participants tested at four or more test ages (longitudinal) or at three or less test ages.

Number of Participants	NH–s	NH+S	< 6 Months		1 Year		2 Years		Total
	54	33	HL–s 48	HL+S 29	HL–s 20	HL+S 8	HL–s 6	HL+S 7	205
Four or more	29	26	32	13	10	3	1	7	114
Three or less	25	7	16	16	10	5	5	7	91

When the central facility for this project relocated from Utah State University to The Ohio State University, a glitch in administrative oversight occurred. Every research project has to follow procedures to ensure that adequate steps are being taken to protect the safety and welfare of participants, and oversight of those procedures is handled by Institutional Review Boards. There was a 3-month period during the transition when there was no oversight in place by an Institutional Review Board, and so data could not be collected. This was mainly at the 18- and 24-month test ages.

Some families did indeed move away from a community where there was an examiner to collect data, and so those participants were not in the entire study. Sometimes families simply could not find a time during the 2-month window around the child's 6-month birthday to attend a test session. The most frequent reason for this problem was that a new baby had been recently born, and so it was hard for the child's mother to get out of the house. In three cases, parents changed their minds about wanting their children with hearing loss to have spoken language as their primary communication mode; instead, they decided American Sign Language would be their children's primary language. Those children discontinued participation once that decision was made.

Statistical Considerations

Once data were entered, statistical analyses of those data proceeded in a structured manner. First, the data were checked to make sure variability within each group of participants was reason-ably similar across all groups. Again, the question asked by inferential statistics is whether the variability in mean performance across groups defined by independent measures is greater than what would be predicted based on the amount of variability we would expect to see among participants, just because people vary. The estimate of variability among participants is derived by computing a measure of variability within each group, and taking a sort of average across the groups. For that reason it is important that within-group variability is fairly similar for all the groups. That was never a problem in this study: all groups showed similar within-group variability on all measures.

It is also important that scores are normally distributed within groups (i.e., the residuals are normally distributed) if we are to have sensitive statistical tests. When that is not the case, the data can be transformed so that they conform to a normal curve. Rarely was it necessary to use a transformation with these data.

Once that screening of the data was completed, inferential statistics were used to examine whether the main effects in which we were interested were significant. Then regression analyses were performed to determine the extent to which the independent variables of interest accounted for outcomes on each dependent measure at the final test age. Those procedures are discussed in the following sections. Finally, hierarchical modeling was done to examine questions of a broader nature. In these procedures, performance on individual measures can be combined to form a composite, or latent, variable. In this study, we combined several measures of specific language functions to create a global measure of language ability and asked how the development of that ability was affected by our independent variables. Procedures and outcomes for those analyses are reported separately in Chapter 11.

For all dependent measures, raw scores were used in the statistical analyses and are reported in the following chapters. This use of raw scores may present some difficulty for readers who are accustomed to looking at standard scores, but there are good reasons for using raw scores. For one, our samples of children with normal hearing provide more appropriate comparisons than the normative samples used in most commercially available tests. Generally speaking, individuals who volunteer to participate in research studies, such as this one, tend to be slightly better educated than the overall population. Authors of clinical instruments strive to obtain normative samples that are representative of the population in general because those instruments are used across a wider range of individuals. It is for that very reason that scores on standardized instruments can underestimate the magnitude of the delay or disorder a child is experiencing due to a hearing loss. That is, if a child is from a middle class background, as most children in this study were, we would expect his language skills to be slightly better than the mean values obtained on standardized instruments. Using the Preschool Language Scales–4, from which we derived our measure of auditory comprehension of language, we find that only 23% of the children in the normative sample came from homes in which the primary caregiver had attended college. In this study, 59% of the children, both with and without hearing loss, had fathers who graduated from college and 70% had mothers who were college graduates.

Another reason for not using standard scores in statistical analysis has to do with how raw scores and standard scores are matched across ages: Standard scores tend to be insensitive at younger ages. Again, using the Preschool Language Scales–4 as an example, we find that at 1 year of age a difference of 1 point in raw scores on the auditory comprehension subscale corresponds to a difference of 9 or 10 points in standard scores: For 12-month-olds the difference between 20 and 21 points in raw scores corresponds to the difference of 99 and 109 in standard scores. This lack of sensitivity would decrease our ability to find statistically significant differences, if indeed they existed. At older ages the correspondence is better, but not perfect. At 48 months, for example, the difference between 50 and 51 points in raw scores corresponds to the difference of 101 and 104 in standard scores. This lack of sensitivity aside, magnitude of effect transfers across the two scales: If there is a difference of ½ of a standard deviation between two groups in terms of raw scores, there will be a difference of ½ of a standard deviation between those two groups on standard scores.

Inferential Statistics

We followed the same procedures for all of the inferential statistics, regardless of dependent measure. The term ANOVA refers to the commonly used statistical test, analysis of variance, and this was the test most frequently used. This test computes a ratio, F, of the amount of variance among group means to the amount of variance within groups. We can compare that ratio to what we would expect it to be due to sheer chance. If it is significantly larger than expected, we conclude that the group differences measured likely represent true differences among the populations.

The first step was to examine outcomes without the data from the children whose hearing losses were identified late (after 6 months of age). The general expectation going into these analyses was that children whose losses were identified shortly after birth would be faring the best of the children with hearing loss; certainly, we would not expect children with late-identified losses to fare any better. Therefore, we included only children with normal hearing and those with early-identified hearing loss in this first step. The independent variables of interest, or main effects, were hearing status (normal hearing or hearing loss) and whether or not signs were used to support spoken language input. This analysis will be termed simply the *FIRST ANOVA* in the following chapters.

Next, outcomes for children with hearing loss were examined, without data from children with normal hearing. The very first ANOVA done with these data examined differences among children with hearing loss identified at 1 and 2 years of age separately from the children with hearing loss identified before 6 months of age. In no instance did we find a difference in effects for children identified with hearing loss at 1 versus 2 years of age. Whenever age of ID was found to have significant effects, those effects could be traced to differences in outcomes for children identified before 6 months of age and for those identified later. Because it was never the case that differences were observed between children identified with hearing loss at 1 versus 2 years of age, these groups are combined under the general label of late-identified from here on.

The term *SECOND ANOVA* in the following chapters refers to tests without children with normal hearing, in which the independent variables were age of ID and whether or not signs were used. In these analyses, age of ID was treated as a binary variable: Children were simply categorized as having had their hearing losses identified early, if it occurred before 6 months of age, or as late, if it occurred after 12 months of age.

Lastly, several analyses were performed to unravel more precisely the effects of age of ID, signs, and prostheses for the children with hearing loss. This was done by testing these effects within specific groups. For the prosthesis variable, children were grouped by whether they wore hearing aids for the duration of the time they were in this study or received a cochlear implant at any time during their participation. Except for one child, all the children categorized as wearing hearing aids had bilateral aids. All the children categorized as having cochlear implants had at least one implant. At this stage in the analyses, children were not further grouped based on whether they had one or two implants, or had a hearing aid on the unimplanted ear. Detailed analyses of the effects of using two implants, one implant, or combining an implant and a hearing aid will be reviewed in Chapter 9. Table 4–7 shows how many children with hearing loss were tested at each age according to age of ID, sign use, and prosthesis.

Table 4–7. Numbers of participants with hearing loss tested at each age, according to age of ID, sign use, and type of prosthesis worn. Children with hearing loss identified between 12 and 30 months of age are grouped together under *Late Identification.*

	Early Identification				Late Identification			
	No Signs		Signs		No Signs		Signs	
	HA	CI	HA	CI	HA	CI	HA	CI
Test Age (Months)								
18	10	14	4	9		2		
24	13	17	4	7		5		2
30	12	25	5	9	1	11	1	3
36	11	24	5	7	4	11	5	4
42	13	25	7	8	5	18	3	7
48	11	23	8	10	5	21	4	8

Regression Analyses

Regression analyses were done on data collected at 48 months of age. The goal of this study was to examine the contributions to outcomes of various independent measures, and for this study, scores at 48 months were the final "outcomes."

The independent measures that were of interest were: BE-PTAs, ID-Age, whether or not sign support was received, frequency of intervention, and SES. Simple Pearson product-moment correlation coefficients are reported. So, although no distinction was made in the inferential analyses for children with hearing loss identified late based on whether the precise age was closer to 1 or 2 years, in these regression analyses we more precisely evaluated the effects of ID-Age.

Chapter Summary

The primary goal of the research reported in this book was to explain the sources of variability in developmental outcomes for children with hearing loss. We were primarily interested in variability that might be controlled by treatment options, things such as prosthesis and intervention effects. For those reasons, we sought to limit sources of variability over which we had no control, and which could introduce enough variability themselves to diminish our ability to examine more pertinent sources. To that end, children and their families were excluded from participation if the child had a disability that could have delayed development, or if parents spoke a language other than

English to each other and to their children. Variability that could have been introduced by differences in how the data were collected was carefully controlled by training all examiners to collect data in a consistent manner. Similarly, data were analyzed in a consistent and reliable manner. Inferential statistics were performed on the resulting data to gather a general picture of how these children with hearing loss were faring, compared to children with normal hearing. Regression analyses were also performed to determine the extent to which various factors contributed to outcomes, either positively or negatively. Finally, appropriate modeling was done to obtain a sense of how all the variables, both independent and dependent, interacted. In the following chapters we report on these outcomes.

References

Committee on Hearing and Equilibrium. (1995). Committee on Hearing and Equilibrium guidelines for the evaluation of results of treatment of conductive hearing loss. *Otolaryngology–Head and Neck Surgery, 113,* 186–187.

de Bruijn, A. J., Tange, R. A., & Dreschler, W. A. (2001). Efficacy of evaluation of audiometric results after stapes surgery in otosclerosis: I. The effects of using different audiologic parameters and criteria on success rates. *Otolaryngology–Head and Neck Surgery, 124,* 76–83.

Duncan, G. J., & Magnuson, K. A. (2003). Off with Hollingshead: Socioeconomic resources, parenting, and child development. In M. H. Bornstein & R. H. Bradley (Eds.), *Socioeconomic status, parenting, and child development* (pp. 83–106). Mahwah, NJ: Lawrence Erlbaum.

Gallaudet Research Institute. (2006). *Regional and national summary report of data from the 2006–2007 Annual Survey of Deaf and Hard of Hearing Children and Youth.* Washington, DC: Gallaudet University, GRI.

Hart, B., & Risley, T. R. (1995). *Meaningful differences in the everyday experience of young American children.* Baltimore: Paul H. Brookes.

Hess, R. D., & Shipman, V. C. (1965). Early experience and the socialization of cognitive modes in children. *Child Development, 36,* 869–886.

Hollingshead, A. B. (1957). *Two Factor Index of Social Position.* Unpublished manuscript, Yale University, New Haven, CT.

Nittrouer, S. (1996). The relation between speech perception and phonemic awareness: Evidence from low-SES children and children with chronic OM. *Journal of Speech and Hearing Research, 39,* 1059–1070.

Nittrouer, S. (2002). From ear to cortex: A perspective on what clinicians need to understand about speech perception and language processing. *Language, Speech and Hearing Services in Schools, 33,* 237–251.

Schachter, F. F. (1979). *Everyday mother talk to toddlers: Early intervention.* New York: Academic Press.

5

Behavior, Personality, and Cognition

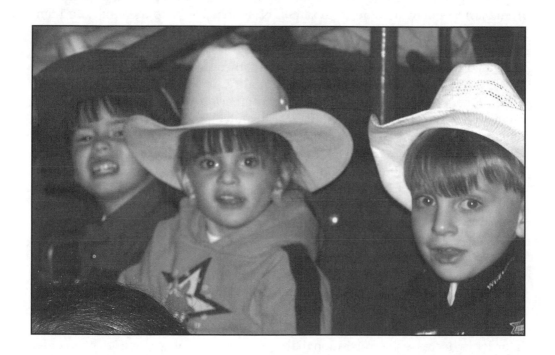

Although the focus of this study was largely on language, there is more to child development. It is easy for those of us who work with deaf children to lose sight of that fact because we focus so strongly on language. But parents worry about all aspects of their children's development. They want to know that their children will grow up to be happy, competent in their social skills, and able to function in the workplace. In this chapter, the first to present data from the dependent measures, we examine the development of the children participating in this study in areas largely unrelated to language.

We were interested in assessing the development of skills unrelated to language because we wanted to know whether hearing loss or factors related to that loss influence how children develop in general. In addition to the hearing loss, factors related to the intervention that children were receiving could possibly have influenced their general development. For example, the use of signs with infants, both those with normal hearing and with hearing loss, is promoted as providing benefits in areas other than language. Parents are encouraged to use signs with an infant in order to decrease the frustration that the infant might experience as a result of not having the language skills to communicate what he wants to. Using signs with infants is also promoted as a way to facilitate cognitive development.

Finally, parents' interactions with their children could be affected by the knowledge of their children's hearing loss in ways that would influence development. If parents are less effective in their efforts to form attachments with their infants due to the hearing loss, some professionals suggest, children might be more likely to develop behavioral problems that in turn can create long-term personality disorders.

In selecting dependent measures, we wanted to make sure we could directly compare outcomes for children with hearing loss to outcomes for children with normal hearing. For that reason, assessment tools designed only for children with hearing loss were never used. The commercially available instruments that we selected were ones that had all been designed for broader populations. Now that we have the ability to identify hearing loss at or close to birth in many cases, and to provide auditory prostheses previously unmatched in quality, it was our goal to evaluate whether or not we are able to guarantee outcomes for children with hearing loss similar to those of children with normal hearing.

The Development of Behavior

In order to evaluate the development of behavior, personality, and social skills, the Child Behavior Checklist (CBCL; Achenbach & Rescorla, 2000) was used. This instrument is a revision of an older one designed just for 2- to 3-year-olds (Achenbach, 1992). The updated version used by us is appropriate for children between 18 months and 5 years of age. The CBCL examines 100 separate behaviors such as *Afraid to try new things*, *Cries a lot*, and *Hits others*. It is presented to parents as a questionnaire to complete. The test authors do not provide information about how well parents have to read in order to complete this form, but do state that it is appropriate to read the items to parents if necessary. All the parents in this study were able to complete the form themselves, reflecting the fact that we had no families participating who could be considered to be in abject poverty. To complete the CBCL a parent must respond to each item by circling a number from 0 to 2, indicating whether ascribing the behavior to one's own child would be *not true (0)*, *somewhat or sometimes true (1)*, or *very true or often true (2)*. A weighted sum across items is obtained, and results load on seven clusters: Emotionally Reactive (I), Anxious/Depressed (II), Somatic Complaints (III), Withdrawn (IV), Sleep Problems (V), Attention Problems (VI), and Aggressive Behavior (VII). The sum of scores on clusters I through IV serves as a general internalizing index, and the sum of scores on clusters VI and VII serves as a general externalizing index. Scores for each cluster can be reported as standard scores, or T scores, with a mean of 50 and a standard deviation of 10. Any score more than 1.5 standard deviations above the mean (i.e., over the 90th percentile) is considered clinically significant by the test authors. For our purposes, we always used raw scores in statistical analyses. Because the CBCL is not standardized on children younger than 18 months, we were unable to use this instrument at the first test age (12 months). Data is missing from seven children for test sessions at 18 months or older because the parents of these children failed to realize this was a two-page instrument, and so did not complete the second page.

Externalizing Behaviors

Table 5–1 shows mean raw scores for externalizing behaviors obtained by each group. The authors of the CBCL reported a raw mean for their norma-

tive sample of 12.9, with a standard deviation of 7.7. That means that any raw score above 24 would indicate a child with a clinically significant number of negative externalizing behaviors. Table 5–1 shows that mean scores for all groups were well below this threshold. Statistical analyses revealed no significant differences for any of the comparisons: Children with hearing loss and those with normal hearing had similar scores; children with hearing loss scored similarly, regardless of whether they received sign support or not, and regardless of the age of ID of their hearing loss.

Internalizing Behaviors

Table 5–2 shows mean raw scores for internalizing behaviors obtained by each group. For this measure, the test authors reported a raw mean of 8.6, with a standard deviation of 6.2 for their normative sample. Clinical significance is suspected when scores exceed a raw score of 18. As with the externalizing scores, it is clear that means for all groups were well below that level. Again, no statistically significant differences were observed among groups.

In sum, we found no differences in the rate of problem behaviors observed for the children in this study. Generalizing to broader populations, it is appropriate to conclude that children with hearing loss are not at any greater risk than children with normal hearing of having behavioral problems that might be indicative of emerging personality difficulties. Regarding children with hearing loss, they are at no greater risk of behavior problems if their loss is not identified until the age of 1 or 2 years. Using signs with infants was not found to diminish the frequency of behaviors

Table 5–1. Mean raw scores for externalizing behaviors on the Child Behavior Checklist (CBCL), given at each test age, with standard deviations in parentheses and group numbers in italics.

Test Age (Months)	NH–s	NH+S	Early		Late	
			HL–s	HL+S	HL–s	HL+S
18	10.00 (6.04) *43*	9.86 (5.09) *28*	9.52 (7.93) *23*	5.31 (4.79) *13*	16.00 (9.90) *2*	*0*
24	8.72 (5.96) *32*	10.36 (7.30) *25*	10.28 (7.24) *29*	13.09 (10.25) *11*	11.40 (4.51) *5*	13.50 (7.78) *2*
30	10.56 (5.36) *25*	8.07 (5.08) *27*	11.41 (8.21) *37*	8.71 (9.82) *14*	10.50 (5.68) *12*	14.00 (6.68) *4*
36	9.13 (6.80) *31*	8.63 (5.83) *30*	10.18 (8.32) *34*	10.50 (10.61) *12*	9.71 (6.26) *14*	11.67 (6.80) *9*
42	9.22 (6.10) *27*	8.19 (5.00) *26*	10.87 (8.46) *38*	12.07 (10.87) *15*	9.30 (5.95) *23*	9.60 (7.79) *10*
48	8.73 (6.64) *26*	7.00 (6.63) *24*	10.88 (6.15) *33*	10.06 (9.43) *17*	8.08 (6.59) *26*	9.25 (6.52) *12*

arising from frustration, such as those of an aggressive nature. Based on this instrument, none of the children in this study appeared to be at risk for problem behaviors.

Cognitive Development

Measuring cognitive abilities in individuals with hearing loss is always tricky. Aside from actual test items that may be heavily dependent on language comprehension and expression, most tests require that some instruction be given. If a child has poor skills in the language of the person doing the testing, we cannot expect the child to understand those instructions as well as other children, and so performance may suffer for that reason alone. Fortunately, there is one cognitive assessment instrument that relies entirely on nonverbal communication for both instruction and administration: the Leiter International Performance Scale–Revised (LIPS-R; Roid & Miller, 2002), and it was used in

Table 5–2. Mean raw scores for internalizing behaviors on the Child Behavior Checklist (CBCL), given at each test age, with standard deviations in parentheses and group numbers in italics.

Test Age (Months)	NH–s	NH+S	Early		Late	
			HL–s	HL+S	HL–s	HL+S
18	4.84 (3.72) *43*	5.89 (5.10) *28*	5.09 (4.65) *23*	4.08 (4.21) *13*	11.50 (6.36) *2*	*0*
24	4.75 (3.51) *32*	5.64 (6.02) *25*	6.10 (4.97) *29*	7.00 (4.17) *11*	7.00 (3.46) *5*	6.00 (1.41) *2*
30	5.56 (3.54) *25*	5.67 (5.34) *27*	6.05 (4.13) *37*	5.43 (5.33) *14*	5.83 (2.79) *12*	7.00 (5.89) *4*
36	5.29 (3.17) *31*	6.33 (5.62) *30*	6.06 (5.59) *34*	7.67 (8.21) *12*	6.07 (2.43) *14*	5.67 (2.83) *9*
42	3.85 (2.58) *27*	5.81 (5.29) *26*	5.53 (4.93) *38*	7.13 (8.22) *15*	6.04 (4.14) *23*	5.50 (4.58) *10*
48	4.19 (2.83) *26*	5.04 (4.95) *24*	6.82 (5.72) *33*	6.88 (7.36) *17*	5.31 (3.89) *26*	3.58 (2.75) *12*

this study. Figure 5–1 illustrates the administration of this instrument. The LIPS-R consists of 20 subtests organized under two batteries: (1) Visualization and Reasoning and (2) Attention and Memory. For this study just three subtests from the Visualization and Reasoning Battery were selected for use.

The Figure Ground subtest was selected, and was believed to be least likely to produce significant differences in performance between children with normal hearing and those with hearing loss. This subtest taps into one's ability to recognize structure and detail in a visual display. As described in Chapter 3, Khan, Edwards, and Langdon (2005) used this instrument to measure cognitive abilities in preschool children with and without hearing loss, and reported finding the least variability across their three groups of children (NH, HL + CI, and HL – CI) on this subtest. It is completely visual in nature, and so likely requires no mediation by linguistic reasoning. Consequently, this subtest served as the strongest measure of whether there was any unintended

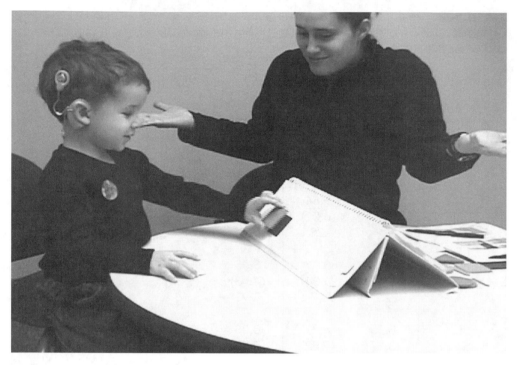

Figure 5–1. An examiner administers the Leiter International Performance Scales (LIPS-R) to a child.

variability across our groups in general cognitive abilities.

The Matching subtest was also selected for use in this study. This subtest requires participants to recognize similarities in objects, and to derive the relevant trait for matching those objects, such as size, color, or shape. Khan et al. found no significant differences among groups in their study, although children with normal hearing performed slightly better than either group of children with hearing loss (those with and without implants).

Finally, we selected the Classification subtest for use. In this subtest, participants must determine which trait forms the basis for grouping items together. Often, the relevant trait is abstract and not available from visual inspection. For example, being a fruit might be the basis of classification for a set of pic-

tures including a banana, grapes, and a pineapple; none of the specific exemplars of fruit bear a physical resemblance. Khan et al. found the strongest differences among groups of children on this task, and we thought it was the most likely to produce significant differences in our study because it is likely affected by linguistic reasoning.

The LIPS-R is designed for use with children as young as 2 years, although it is difficult to administer at very young ages. In the current study, we administered the three subtests selected for use at age 48 months only. Generally speaking, we wanted to restrict data collection to one session at each test age because some of the participants traveled a long distance to be tested. Consequently, it was important to preserve the time that was available for testing at each session to measures that were most likely to produce theoretically and clinically relevant data. We expected all participants in this study to be developing cognitive abilities in a typical fashion, with perhaps some minor differences on the Classification subtest. With all these considerations in mind it seemed most prudent to restrict the testing of cognitive abilities to one session only.

Three children became uncooperative during part of the LIPS-R testing: two with the Figure Ground subtest only, and one with both the Figure Ground and Classification subtests.

Figure Ground

Table 5–3 shows mean raw scores for the Figure Ground subtest. None of the statistical analyses revealed any significant differences among groups. In clin-

ical assessment it is generally the case that performance straying below the mean of a normative sample by more than one standard deviation is considered problematic. On this subtest, the test authors reported a raw mean of 10 for their normative sample of typically developing 48-month-olds, and one standard deviation below that mean was the raw score of 8. Means for all groups of children in this study were well above that mark.

Matching

Table 5–4 provides mean raw scores for the Matching subtest. Again, none of the statistical analyses revealed any significant differences among groups for this subtest. The test authors reported a raw mean score of 26 for their normative

Table 5–3. Mean raw scores for the Figure Ground subtest of the Leiter International Performance Scales–Revised (LIPS-R), with standard deviations in parentheses and group numbers in italics.

Test Age (Months)	NH–s	NH+S	Early		Late	
			HL–s	HL+S	HL–s	HL+S
48	12.42 (2.86) *26*	12.17 (3.41) *24*	10.55 (3.17) *31*	12.22 (2.41) *18*	11.16 (3.30) *25*	12.50 (3.09) *12*

Table 5–4. Mean raw scores for the Matching subtest of the Leiter International Performance Scales–Revised (LIPS-R), with standard deviations in parentheses and group numbers in italics.

Test Age (Months)	NH–s	NH+S	Early		Late	
			HL–s	HL+S	HL–s	HL+S
48	27.69 (3.00) *26*	27.13 (2.64) *24*	26.52 (4.18) *33*	26.50 (3.55) *18*	27.00 (3.72) *26*	28.00 (2.98) *12*

sample of 48-month-olds, with a raw score of 20 at one standard deviation below the mean. All groups in this study had means that were well above that criterion.

Classification

Table 5–5 shows mean raw scores for the Classification subtest. The FIRST ANOVA, done on scores for children with normal hearing and those in the early age-of-ID group, showed a significant main effect of hearing status, $F(1, 97) = 4.24$, $p = .042$. This result suggests that children with normal hearing performed slightly better than children with early-identified hearing loss. The main effect of signs was not significant in this analysis.

Next, analyses were performed to examine whether there were significant main effects of age of ID, signs, or type of prosthesis (implant or hearing aid) for children with hearing loss. No significant effects were found, and so we conclude that children with hearing loss all performed similarly. Consequently, the main conclusion is that children with normal hearing scored slightly better on this measure of classification than children with hearing loss.

For this subtest, the test authors reported a raw-score mean of 13.5 for 48-month-olds in their normative sample, and 10 was one standard deviation below that mean. So in spite of the slight difference between scores for children with normal hearing and those with hearing loss, means for all groups were well above the threshold for clinical concern.

It would be inappropriate to make too much of the significant effect of hearing status found for scores on the Classification subtest. Nonetheless, this was the only measure of cognitive development for which it was predicted that a difference between children with normal hearing and those with hearing loss might be found. Although the effect is small, the fact that one was found replicates findings of Khan et al. (2005). One difference between the two studies, however, was that children in this study with and without implants performed similarly, whereas Khan found that children with implants outscored children without implants. The small effect of hearing status on these scores may reflect differences in language abilities between children with normal hearing and those with hearing loss. If this is true, then the use of signs was not effective in compensating for the deficit.

Table 5–5. Mean raw scores for the Classification subtest of the Leiter International Performance Scales–Revised (LIPS-R), with standard deviations in parentheses and group numbers in italics.

Test Age (Months)	NH–s	NH+S	Early		Late	
			HL–s	HL+S	HL–s	HL+S
48	15.15 (2.29) *26*	15.04 (1.81) *24*	13.45 (4.17) *33*	14.28 (2.08) *18*	13.56 (2.96) *25*	13.83 (2.72) *12*

Adaptive Behavior

Closely related to the development of personality and social skills is the development of adaptive behavior. In its most technical sense, adaptive behavior refers to any behavior that allows an organism to adapt to its environment. In practice, instruments that evaluate adaptive behavior examine an individual's ability to live independently, socialize appropriately, communicate with others, and engage in both fine and gross motor activities. In this study, it was important to examine the development of independent living skills because intervention with young deaf children tends to be intensive. Parents are instructed to spend more time than usual communicating with their children, and so children have less time than usual to explore the world on their own. It is possible that this constrained independence could delay the development of daily living skills such as feeding and potty training. We wished to explore the possibility that the very procedures meant to help children with hearing loss (i.e., early identification and intervention) could have the unintended consequence of negatively impacting a child's ability to negotiate his environment independently.

To examine adaptive behavior in the children participating in this study, we selected the Scales of Independent Behavior–Revised (SIB-R; Bruininks, Woodcock, Weatherman, & Hill, 1996). The SIB-R is a measure of adaptive functioning that contains 14 subscales grouped into four clusters: Motor Skills (I), Social Interaction and Communication Skills (II), Personal Living Skills (III), and Community Living Skills (IV).

Additionally, the SIB-R assesses maladaptive behavior with eight subscales that group into three clusters: Internalized, Asocial, and Externalized. The SIB-R is administered in a structured interview to an adult with comprehensive knowledge of the child; in this study, that meant the parent. An example of test administration is shown in Figure 5–2. During the interview the examiner reads a statement that describes a task, and the parent must decide how frequently the child can perform that task by himself, with little or no help, and without being asked. A four-point scale is used to evaluate how frequently the child can do the task: *Never or rarely, even if asked (0); Does, but not well—or about ¼ of the time (1); Does fairly well—or about ¾ of the time (2);* or *Does very well—always or almost always (3).* For each subscale, a weighted sum of responses to these items is obtained. Cluster scores are derived by computing mean scores across the subscales that form the cluster. The SIB-R assesses the adaptive behavior of individuals from infancy to 80+ years, and so we could use it at every test age.

During testing we administered the complete SIB-R, but subsequently did not analyze the subscales that form the Community Living cluster because children in this study were not old enough to be expected to perform most of those behaviors, which include things such as punctuality and handling money. That left us with 10 subscales, fitting into three clusters.

In the Personal Living Skills cluster there are the five subscales of Eating and Meal Preparation, Toileting, Dressing, Personal Self-Care, and Domestic Skills. Examination of scores in this cluster allowed us to test the hypothesis that the enhanced parental attention received

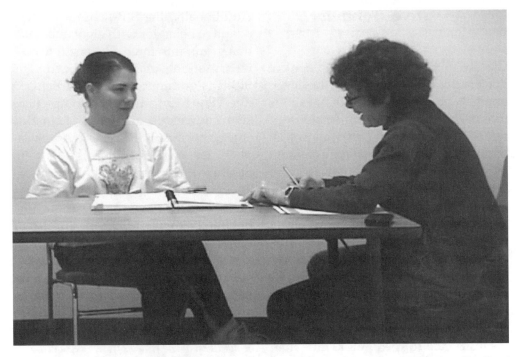

Figure 5–2. An examiner administers the Scales of Independent Behavior–Revised (SIB-R) to a parent.

by many children with hearing loss might slow down the acquisition of independent living skills.

In the Motor Skills cluster there are the subscales of Fine and Gross Motor Skills. Scores on subscales in this cluster would allow us to test the hypothesis that children with hearing loss have poorer fine and gross motor control than children with normal hearing.

In the Social Interaction and Communication Skills cluster there are the subscales of Social Interaction, Language Comprehension, and Language Expression. We particularly felt that the subscales of Language Comprehension and Language Expression would provide independent validation of our other language measures.

Data are missing for one child on the SIB-R because the examiner forgot to administer the instrument.

Personal Living Skills

For Personal Living Skills, we analyzed only cluster scores because there was no reason to suspect that the direction or magnitude of group differences, if found, would vary across the five subscales. Table 5–6 gives means and standard deviations of raw scores obtained for the Personal Living cluster. Values for each test age are shown separately. This table, as well as all others for this instrument, can be found at the chapter's end.

Figure 5–3 shows mean scores on the Personal Living cluster for all groups of children in this study. Here, as well as elsewhere, we chose not to attach error bars to symbols on the figures because they make it difficult to see differences among group means; readers are referred to the tables for standard deviations. Instead, we use dotted lines to

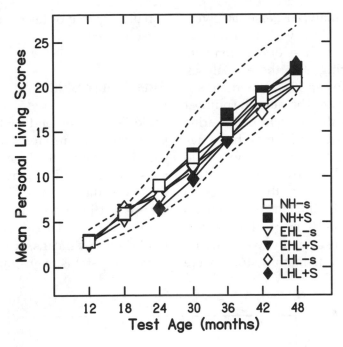

Figure 5–3. Mean raw scores for the Personal Living Skills cluster of the SIB-R for each group: NH–s (normal hearing, no signs); NH+S (normal hearing, signs); EHL–s (early-identified hearing loss, no signs); EHL+S (early-identified hearing loss, signs); LHL–s (late-identified hearing loss, no signs); and LHL+S (late-identified hearing loss, signs). Dotted lines show +/– one standard deviation from the mean, according to the normative data published by the test authors.

indicate one standard deviation above and below means for typically developing children according to data published by the test authors. These plus/minus one standard deviation values are generally considered to bound the range of "normal" scores. In particular, children are considered to be delayed in development if scores stray by more than one standard deviation below published means. Mean scores for the Personal Living cluster for all groups were well above this boundary.

The FIRST ANOVA failed to reveal significant main effects of either hearing status or signs. However, a third main effect was significant: In this and all subsequent analyses, test age is included as a factor. Here the effect of test age was highly significant, $F(1, 655) = 257.59$, $p < .001$, indicating only that children received higher scores as they got older. This will be true for all the measures reported from here on, in this and subsequent chapters. For this reason we will refrain from reporting statistical results for this main effect. However, we will report significant interactions between test age and other main effects because those interactions indicate that the rate of development differed significantly across groups.

Next, we analyzed Personal Living scores for children with hearing loss separately from those of children with normal hearing. For these analyses, only data between 30 and 48 months of age were analyzed because the number of children with late-identified hearing loss tested prior to 30 months of age was not large enough to allow a valid test. This will be true for all future analyses, as well. For these scores on the Personal Living cluster, no effects of age of ID, signs, or prostheses were observed. Consequently, we conclude that all children in this study were equally capable of taking care of their personal needs.

Fine Motor Skills

Table 5–7 (at the end of the chapter) gives mean scores for each group at each test time for the Fine Motor Skills subscale of the SIB-R, and Figure 5–4 illustrates these scores. Children in all groups performed similarly, and were within one standard deviation of the published raw means. No main effects of hearing status, signs, age of ID, or

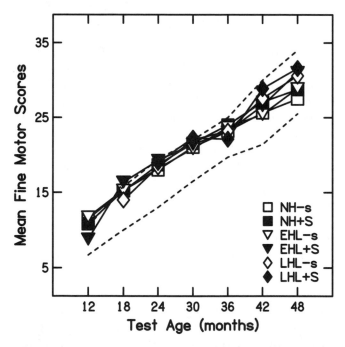

Figure 5–4. Mean raw scores for the Fine Motor Skills subscale of the SIB-R for each group: NH–s (normal hearing, no signs); NH+S (normal hearing, signs); EHL–s (early-identified hearing loss, no signs); EHL+S (early-identified hearing loss, signs); LHL–s (late-identified hearing loss, no signs); and LHL+S (late-identified hearing loss, signs). Dotted lines show +/– one standard deviation from the mean, according to the normative data published by the test authors.

auditory prosthesis were found for Fine Motor Skills.

Gross Motor Skills

Table 5–8 (at the end of the chapter) shows mean scores for each group at each test time for the Gross Motor Skills subscale of the SIB-R, and Figure 5–5 illustrates these scores. As with Fine Motor Skills, children in all groups performed similarly in terms of Gross Motor Skills, and were within one standard deviation of the published raw means.

No main effects of hearing status, signs, age of ID, or auditory prosthesis were found for Gross Motor Skills.

Social Interaction Skills

Table 5–9 (at the end of the chapter) presents mean scores for the Social Interaction subscale of the SIB-R, and Figure 5–6 illustrates these scores. Although there does not appear to be a great deal of difference among groups, the FIRST ANOVA revealed a significant main effect of hearing status, $F(1, 655)$

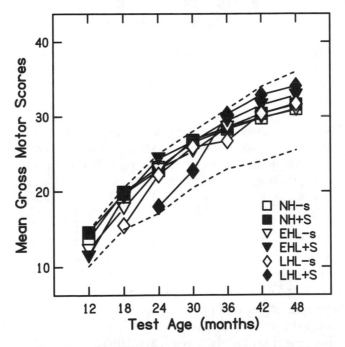

Figure 5–5. Mean raw scores for the Gross Motor Skills subscale of the SIB-R for each group: NH–s (normal hearing, no signs); NH+S (normal hearing, signs); EHL–s (early-identified hearing loss, no signs); EHL+S (early-identified hearing loss, signs); LHL–s (late-identified hearing loss, no signs); and LHL+S (late-identified hearing loss, signs). Dotted lines show +/– one standard deviation from the mean, according to the normative data published by the test authors.

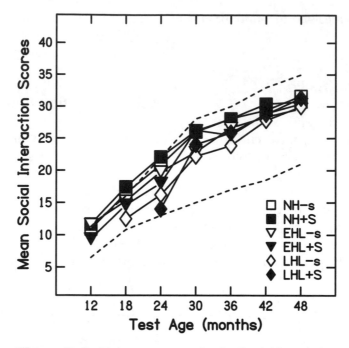

Figure 5–6. Mean raw scores for the Social Interaction subscale of the SIB-R for each group: NH–s (normal hearing, no signs); NH+S (normal hearing, signs); EHL–s (early-identified hearing loss, no signs); EHL+S (early-identified hearing loss, signs); LHL–s (late-identified hearing loss, no signs); and LHL+S (late-identified hearing loss, signs). Dotted lines show +/– one standard deviation from the mean, according to the normative data published by the test authors.

= 11.89, $p < .001$. The main effect of signs was not significant in that analysis. In the analyses done only on data from children with hearing loss, none of the main effects (age of ID, signs, and prosthesis) was found to be statistically significant. It is apparent from Figure 5–6 that means for all groups were within the boundaries of plus/minus one standard deviation from the means of the normative sample, shown by the dotted lines. Consequently, all that may be concluded about these scores is that children with normal hearing performed slightly better than children with hear-ing loss. This effect is particularly evi-dent during the toddler years (roughly 18–30 months), and diminishes as chil-dren get older.

Language Comprehension Skills

Table 5–10 (at the end of the chapter) shows mean scores for the Language Comprehension Skills subscale of the SIB-R. Figure 5–7 illustrates these scores for children with normal hearing and for children with early-identified hearing

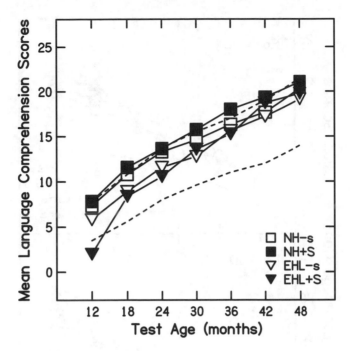

Figure 5-7. Mean raw scores for the Language Comprehension subscale of the SIB-R for children with normal hearing and early-identified hearing loss: NH−s (normal hearing, no signs); NH+S (normal hearing, signs); EHL−s (early-identified hearing loss, no signs); EHL+S (early-identified hearing loss, signs). Dotted lines show +/− one standard deviation from the mean, according to the normative data published by the test authors.

loss. Children with late-identified hearing loss are not included on this figure because with this measure we begin to see interesting differences among groups emerge.

The FIRST ANOVA revealed a significant main effect of hearing status, $F(1, 655) = 59.53, p < .001$. This difference is apparent on Figure 5–7, although it is again strongest during the toddler years; it appears to diminish as children get older. In spite of this significant main effect, however, it is evident that children in all groups performed well on this measure. Generally speaking, group means are close to one standard deviation above published means.

Figure 5–8 shows scores for children with early-identified and late-identified hearing loss separately. Means are given according to whether children used signs or not, and what kind of prosthesis they had. These means are plotted for test ages as young as 18 months, the youngest age at which we had late-identified children participate. Mean scores at these younger ages are displayed to illustrate continuity in the growth of these skills, but ANOVAs on data from children with hearing loss

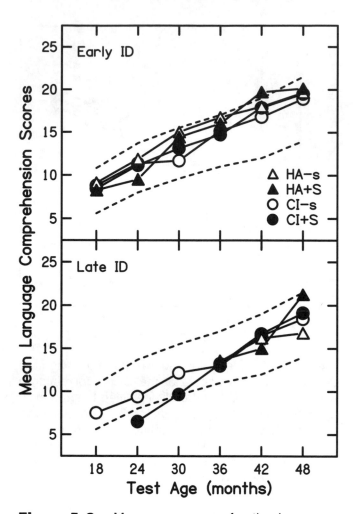

Figure 5–8. Mean raw scores for the Language Comprehension subscale of the SIB-R for children with early-identified (top) and late-identified (bottom) hearing loss: HA–s (hearing aids, no signs); HA+S (hearing aids, signs); CI–s (cochlear implants, no signs); and CI+S (cochlear implants, signs). Dotted lines show +/– one standard deviation from the mean, according to the normative data published by the test authors.

only were performed only on scores starting at 30 months of age.

When the SECOND ANOVA was performed only with children with hearing loss, a significant main effect of age of ID emerged, $F(1, 297) = 11.19$, $p = .001$. This finding indicates that those children identified with hearing loss at 1 or 2 years of age had poorer language comprehension than children whose hearing losses were identified before 6 months of age. To investigate further the differences in language comprehension of children with early- and late-identified hearing loss, a simple effects analysis was performed. Simple effects analysis, or SEA, is identical to standard ANOVAs, except that the error term used is the one obtained from all groups rather than just the subset being examined. This procedure is appropriate once it is determined that variances are similar across groups, and provides a slightly more sensitive test of the main effects for each group. In this SEA, the effects of signs and prosthesis (implant or hearing aids) were examined separately for children with early- and late-identified hearing loss, using the error term obtained from all children with hearing loss. Scores obtained from 30 to 48 months of age were used. All that was found was a significant effect of prosthesis for children with early-identified hearing loss, $F(1, 281) = 6.57$, $p = .011$. [When an ANOVA is performed on children with early-identified hearing loss using the error term obtained with only these children, we find a similar result for the prosthesis effect, $F(1, 187) = 6.59$, $p = .011$, so clearly SEA provides similar information.] Figure 5–8 illustrates this prosthesis effect in the top panel: Children who wore hearing aids scored slightly higher than children who had implants, although the effect appears to diminish as the children get older.

In sum, it was found that children with normal hearing had slightly better language comprehension than children with hearing loss. Children whose hearing losses were identified before 6 months of age had better language comprehension than those whose losses were identified after 12 months of age, and of the children with hearing loss identified before 6 months of age, those who wore hearing aids had slightly higher scores than those who had cochlear implants. Figure 5–7 and Figure 5–8 show that these main effects were small, and that mean scores for all groups were better than one standard

deviation below the means of the normative sample. The lack of evidence for a developmental delay in children with hearing loss is likely due to the fact that this instrument only generally assesses an individual's ability to understand what is said. A typical item for a young child is *Points to familiar pictures in a book on request*. This instrument does not explicitly examine an individual's comprehension of syntactic and grammatical devices. That sort of assessment was obtained with the Auditory Comprehension task, to be discussed in Chapter 6.

Language Expression Skills

Although it may be possible to understand others without having strong underlying language abilities, those abilities are taxed more strongly during expression. Therefore, the Language Expression subscale of the SIB-R is the first measure to be reported here that significantly tapped into children's language processes.

Table 5–11 (at the end of the chapter) shows mean raw scores for the Language Expression subscale for each group. Figure 5–9 shows these scores for children with normal hearing and for those with early-identified hearing loss.

A clear gap can be seen on Figure 5–9 between the developmental trajectories of children with normal hearing and those with hearing loss. For the first time, we see scores for the children with hearing loss at or below one standard deviation below the mean of the published normative data. This effect appeared in the FIRST ANOVA as a significant main effect of hearing status, $F(1, 655) = 82.60$, $p < .001$: Children with early-identified hearing loss had poorer

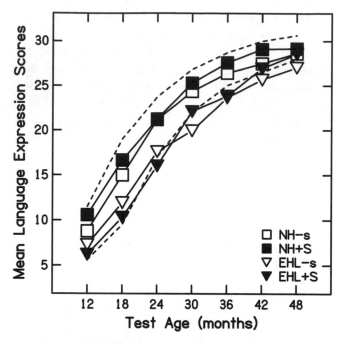

Figure 5–9. Mean raw scores for the Language Expression subscale of the SIB-R for children with normal hearing and those with early-identified hearing loss: NH–s (normal hearing, no signs); NH+S (normal hearing, signs); EHL–s (early-identified hearing loss, no signs); EHL+S (early-identified hearing loss, signs). Dotted lines show +/– one standard deviation from the mean, according to the normative data published by the test authors.

language expression than children with normal hearing.

The FIRST ANOVA also showed a significant main effect of signs, $F(1, 655) = 5.70, p = .017$. A SEA was performed to trace the source of that effect: The main effect of signs was tested separately for children with normal hearing and for those with (early-identified) hearing loss. Results showed a significant main effect of signs only for children with normal hearing, $F(1, 655) = 10.11, p = .002$. In looking at Table 5–11 it is clear that children receiving sign support scored an average of one point higher across all test ages than children not receiving that sign support. However,

means for both groups of children were within plus/minus one standard deviation of the published normative means.

The SECOND ANOVA showed significant main effects of both age of ID, $F(1, 297) = 33.18, p < .001$, and of signs, $F(1, 297) = 4.36, p = .038$. In addition, there was a significant Age of ID × Signs interaction, $F(1, 297) = 16.97, p < .001$, which prompted a SEA examining scores for signing and nonsigning children separately. The purpose of that SEA was to test for a significant main effect of age of ID for each signing group separately. In fact, a significant age-of-ID effect was found only for children who received sign support, $F(1, 297) = 34.46$,

$p < .001$: Of the children with hearing loss who used signs, those who were identified early had the highest scores on the Language Expression measure. Among children who did not receive sign support, there was no difference in scores based on when the hearing loss was identified.

Figure 5–10 illustrates the Language Expression scores for children with early- and late-identified hearing loss separately. Here children were grouped according to whether or not they used signs, and according to whether they had hearing aids or a cochlear implant. A SEA was done with the main effects

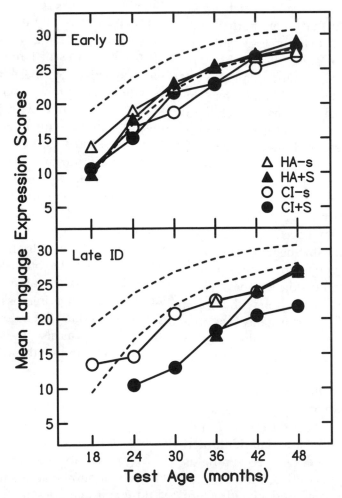

Figure 5–10. Mean raw scores for the Language Expression subscale of the SIB-R for children with early-identified (top) and late-identified (bottom) hearing loss: HA–s (hearing aids, no signs); HA+S (hearing aids, signs); CI–s (cochlear implants, no signs); and CI+S (cochlear implants, signs). Dotted lines show +/– one standard deviation from the mean, according to the normative data published by the test authors.

of signs, prosthesis, and test age looking at scores for early- and late-identified children separately. For children with early-identified hearing loss, only the main effect of prosthesis was significant, $F(1, 297) = 7.78$, $p = .006$: Children who wore hearing aids for the duration of the study had better Language Expression scores than children who received cochlear implants, although children with implants appear to catch up by the end of the study. For children with late-identified hearing loss, only the main effect of signs was significant, $F(1, 297) = 6.44$, $p = .012$: Children not receiving sign support had better Language Expression scores than children who used signs. This effect is apparent at all test ages for those children who received implants. Signers who wore hearing aids caught up by the end of the study, although the Prosthesis × Signs interaction term was not significant.

With this Language Expression subscale of the SIB-R we begin to see highly significant trends across our groups. Children with hearing loss performed more poorly than children with normal hearing, and that performance was poor enough that it would meet the criterion of being clinically significant for many of these children: For more than half of the children with hearing loss, scores were more than one standard deviation below the published means. With this subscale we find that late-identified deaf children were not performing as well as early-identified children, but only if they used signs. For children not using signs, there was no additional decrement in performance associated with late identification. Finally, there was a small decrement in performance among the children with early-identified losses associated with wearing a cochlear implant.

Chapter Summary

We learn from this chapter that children with hearing loss are not at any greater risk for behavioral, personality, or social problems than are children with normal hearing. No effects, either positive or negative, were uncovered for the use of signs or for differences in auditory prostheses. However, we found significant and potentially important differences among these groups of children on the measures of language acquisition provided by these instruments: Language comprehension scores were poorer for children with hearing loss than for those with normal hearing, although scores for all children were generally within the range considered to be normal. Where we saw differences that appear clinically significant was on the SIB-R Language Expression subscale. Children with hearing loss were generally more than one standard deviation below the published mean for this subscale, and signing children with late-identified hearing loss were generally two standard deviations below the mean. There was also an effect of prosthesis for children with early-identified hearing loss, such that those children with hearing aids performed better than the children with cochlear implants. These trends will be examined more closely in the following chapters.

Cognitive abilities were generally found to be similar across the groups of children participating in this study. The only effect of having a hearing loss was found for the Classification subtest of the LIPS-R, and it seems reasonable to suspect that this may be explained by potential differences in underlying language abilities. The following chapters explore those abilities.

Table 5–6. Mean raw scores for the Personal Living Skills cluster of the Scales of Independent Behavior–Revised (SIB-R), given at each test age, with standard deviations in parentheses and group numbers in italics.

Test Age (Months)	NH–s	NH+S	Early		Late	
			HL–s	HL+S	HL–s	HL+S
12	2.86 (1.16) *29*	3.00 (1.54) *12*	2.73 (0.90) *11*	2.40 (0.55) *5*	*0*	*0*
18	5.95 (2.37) *43*	5.86 (1.76) *28*	5.13 (1.62) *24*	6.31 (2.69) *13*	6.50 (0.71) *2*	*0*
24	9.03 (3.03) *32*	9.04 (2.81) *25*	8.07 (2.45) *30*	8.18 (2.23) *11*	7.80 (1.30) *5*	6.50 (0.71) *2*
30	12.12 (4.34) *25*	12.48 (4.12) *27*	10.65 (3.43) *37*	11.07 (2.40) *14*	11.25 (3.44) *12*	9.75 (0.96) *4*
36	15.03 (5.22) *31*	16.90 (4.15) *30*	14.14 (4.43) *35*	15.25 (4.47) *12*	14.00 (3.91) *15*	14.00 (5.77) *9*
42	18.74 (4.49) *27*	19.35 (4.21) *26*	18.00 (5.01) *38*	19.40 (4.56) *15*	17.13 (4.21) *23*	18.67 (6.54) *9*
48	20.65 (3.82) *26*	22.08 (3.46) *25*	20.32 (4.88) *34*	21.28 (4.34) *18*	20.19 (3.89) *26*	22.50 (5.57) *12*

Table 5–7. Mean raw scores for the Fine Motor subscale of the Scales of Independent Behavior–Revised (SIB-R), given at each test age, with standard deviations in parentheses and group numbers in italics.

Test Age (Months)	NH–s	NH+S	Early		Late	
			HL–s	HL+S	HL–s	HL+S
12	11.48 (2.82) *29*	10.83 (3.64) *12*	11.73 (3.80) *11*	8.80 (1.64) *5*	*0*	*0*
18	15.28 (3.31) *43*	15.21 (2.56) *28*	15.29 (2.68) *24*	16.38 (2.60) *13*	14.00 (0.00) *2*	*0*
24	18.00 (3.11) *32*	18.68 (2.51) *25*	18.20 (2.86) *30*	19.27 (1.42) *11*	18.40 (1.95) *5*	19.00 (2.83) *2*
30	21.04 (3.09) *25*	21.56 (4.40) *27*	20.84 (3.72) *37*	21.43 (2.47) *14*	22.00 (3.25) *12*	22.25 (5.85) *4*
36	23.16 (3.69) *31*	24.00 (4.46) *30*	23.71 (2.83) *35*	23.08 (2.15) *12*	23.20 (3.47) *15*	22.11 (3.76) *9*
42	25.63 (4.74) *27*	27.08 (5.26) *26*	25.42 (3.30) *38*	26.60 (4.56) *15*	27.57 (4.52) *23*	28.89 (5.51) *9*
48	27.50 (6.10) *26*	28.76 (4.53) *25*	28.91 (4.93) *34*	31.06 (5.09) *18*	30.58 (4.97) *26*	31.58 (7.09) *12*

Table 5–8. Mean raw scores for the Gross Motor subscale of the Scales of Independent Behavior–Revised (SIB-R), given at each test age, with standard deviations in parentheses and group numbers in italics.

Test Age (Months)	NH–s	NH+S	Early		Late	
			HL–s	HL+S	HL–s	HL+S
12	13.72 (3.57) *29*	14.58 (2.61) *12*	12.27 (3.10) *11*	11.40 (3.97) *5*	*0*	*0*
18	19.91 (4.02) *43*	19.71 (2.80) *28*	17.79 (3.86) *24*	19.23 (3.44) *13*	15.50 (3.54) *2*	*0*
24	23.19 (4.61) *32*	22.80 (3.65) *25*	22.97 (4.61) *30*	24.36 (2.34) *11*	22.20 (1.79) *5*	18.00 (1.41) *2*
30	26.52 (4.40) *25*	26.81 (5.31) *27*	25.35 (4.44) *37*	26.64 (5.60) *14*	25.92 (5.32) *12*	22.75 (4.35) *4*
36	28.32 (4.74) *31*	28.57 (4.92) *30*	28.57 (4.68) *35*	29.42 (3.32) *12*	26.73 (5.02) *15*	30.33 (4.53) *9*
42	29.78 (4.13) *27*	30.38 (3.81) *26*	29.84 (4.40) *38*	31.53 (2.50) *15*	30.39 (5.06) *23*	32.89 (3.59) *9*
48	31.00 (4.04) *26*	31.60 (4.02) *25*	30.88 (4.30) *34*	32.83 (3.75) *18*	31.73 (4.51) *26*	34.08 (4.36) *12*

Table 5–9. Mean raw scores for the Social Interaction subscale of the Scales of Independent Behavior–Revised (SIB-R), given at each test age, with standard deviations in parentheses and group numbers in italics.

Test Age (Months)	NH–s	NH+S	Early		Late	
			HL–s	HL+S	HL–s	HL+S
12	10.90 (2.08) *29*	11.67 (1.72) *12*	11.64 (3.56) *11*	9.40 (2.30) *5*	*0*	*0*
18	16.42 (4.72) *43*	17.43 (3.77) *28*	15.25 (5.25) *24*	14.62 (4.96) *13*	12.50 (6.36) *2*	*0*
24	20.84 (4.89) *32*	22.08 (4.10) *25*	19.77 (6.04) *30*	18.00 (4.00) *11*	16.20 (2.86) *5*	14.00 (2.83) *2*
30	25.96 (5.73) *25*	26.11 (5.39) *27*	22.81 (6.86) *37*	26.21 (6.38) *14*	22.17 (5.80) *12*	24.00 (6.48) *4*
36	28.10 (6.40) *31*	28.10 (5.16) *30*	26.66 (7.19) *35*	25.50 (6.79) *12*	23.87 (6.53) *15*	25.89 (8.92) *9*
42	29.44 (5.06) *27*	30.42 (4.48) *26*	28.37 (6.38) *38*	28.93 (6.15) *15*	27.83 (5.03) *23*	28.78 (6.85) *9*
48	31.65 (5.39) *26*	30.76 (5.02) *25*	29.68 (6.11) *34*	30.44 (5.36) *18*	30.00 (4.81) *26*	31.33 (7.43) *12*

Table 5–10. Mean raw scores for the Language Comprehension subscale of the Scales of Independent Behavior–Revised (SIB-R), given at each test age, with standard deviations in parentheses and group numbers in italics.

Test Age (Months)	NH–s	NH+S	Early		Late	
			HL–s	HL+S	HL–s	HL+S
12	7.31 (2.39) *29*	7.83 (1.75) *12*	5.82 (2.68) *11*	2.00 (3.08) *5*	*0*	*0*
18	10.79 (2.19) *43*	11.57 (1.73) *28*	8.92 (2.96) *24*	8.38 (4.93) *13*	7.50 (0.71) *2*	*0*
24	13.28 (1.71) *32*	13.64 (1.73) *25*	11.57 (3.06) *30*	10.55 (4.37) *11*	9.40 (3.71) *5*	6.50 (7.78) *2*
30	14.60 (2.20) *25*	15.74 (2.25) *27*	12.76 (3.75) *37*	13.57 (3.92) *14*	12.00 (2.76) *12*	9.75 (4.19) *4*
36	16.32 (3.03) *31*	18.00 (2.94) *30*	15.63 (3.81) *35*	15.25 (3.41) *12*	13.13 (2.92) *15*	13.44 (4.33) *9*
42	17.67 (3.14) *27*	19.35 (2.77) *26*	17.21 (3.46) *38*	18.73 (4.45) *15*	16.43 (2.37) *23*	16.33 (4.90) *9*
48	20.35 (3.30) *26*	21.08 (2.94) *25*	19.15 (3.46) *34*	19.78 (2.78) *18*	18.12 (3.43) *26*	19.83 (4.71) *12*

Table 5–11. Mean raw scores for the Language Expression subscale of the Scales of Independent Behavior–Revised (SIB-R), given at each test age, with standard deviations in parentheses and group numbers in italics.

Test Age (Months)	NH–s	NH+S	Early		Late	
			HL–s	HL+S	HL–s	HL+S
12	8.79 (3.44) *29*	10.58 (4.46) *12*	7.27 (3.32) *11*	6.20 (0.84) *5*	*0*	*0*
18	14.98 (4.66) *43*	16.64 (5.00) *28*	11.92 (5.12) *24*	10.31 (5.63) *13*	13.50 (2.12) *2*	*0*
24	21.16 (3.69) *32*	21.24 (4.95) *25*	17.60 (5.57) *30*	16.00 (6.48) *11*	14.60 (6.07) *5*	10.50 (10.61) *2*
30	24.32 (3.41) *25*	25.26 (2.44) *27*	19.92 (5.82) *37*	22.07 (3.20) *14*	20.58 (3.80) *12*	13.75 (5.56) *4*
36	26.39 (2.91) *31*	27.57 (2.36) *30*	23.63 (4.16) *35*	23.83 (3.10) *12*	22.60 (2.87) *15*	17.89 (6.58) *9*
42	27.48 (1.78) *27*	29.08 (1.26) *26*	25.66 (3.87) *38*	26.93 (2.63) *15*	23.87 (2.90) *23*	21.22 (7.21) *9*
48	28.62 (1.83) *26*	29.16 (2.44) *25*	27.03 (3.59) *34*	28.56 (1.89) *18*	26.88 (3.19) *26*	23.42 (6.80) *12*

References

Achenbach, T. M. (1992). *Manual for the Child Behavior Checklist/2–3 and 1992 profile.* Burlington, VT: University of Vermont, Department of Psychiatry.

Achenbach, T. M., & Rescorla, L. A. (2000). *Manual for the ASEBA preschool forms and profiles.* Burlington, VT: University of Vermont, Research Center for Children, Youth, & Families.

Bruininks, R. H., Woodcock, R. W., Weatherman, R. F., & Hill, B. K. (1996). *Scales of Independent Behavior–Revised.* Itasca, IL: Riverside.

Khan, S., Edwards, L., & Langdon, D. (2005). The cognition and behaviour of children with cochlear implants, children with hearing aids and their hearing peers: A comparison. *Audiology & Neurotology, 10,* 117–126.

Roid, G. H., & Miller, L. J. (2002). *Leiter International Performance Scale–Revised (LIPS-R).* Wood Dale, IL: Stoelting.

6

Basic Language Measures: Comprehension, Vocabulary, and Intelligibility

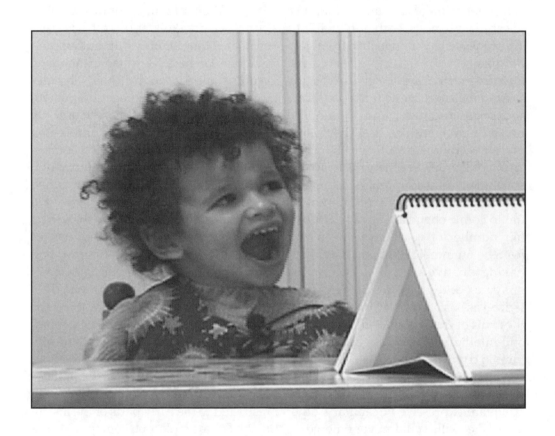

In the last chapter we uncovered some evidence of language delay for children with hearing loss using their parents' responses to commercially available developmental inventories. Those instruments are not designed to investigate language acquisition independently of other aspects of development, and so may not be as sensitive to variability among our groups of children as instruments specifically designed to examine language might be. This chapter reports data from four measures that examined three basic language abilities: auditory comprehension of language, expressive vocabulary, and speech intelligibility. These measures were obtained from standardized, commercially available test instruments that are designed explicitly to examine language acquisition. All are simple to administer and so are used routinely in clinical practice. The abilities measured by these tools are characterized as basic because they are, relatively speaking, easily acquired. As Chapter 2 discussed, it is possible for an individual to comprehend a language, know a fair number of vocabulary items, and even be an intelligible speaker without having a native speaker's appreciation of syntax and grammar. Being characterized as basic, however, does not make the skills of comprehension, vocabulary, and intelligibility any less important to human communication than syntax and grammar: In fact, without being able to understand others and possessing an adequate expressive vocabulary, other language skills could never emerge.

Auditory Comprehension of Spoken Language

A child with hearing loss must be able to understand what others say if that child is going to participate in mainstream, hearing society. For this study we were interested specifically in how well children with hearing loss could understand spoken language. We selected the Auditory Comprehension portion of the Preschool Language Scales 4 (PLS-4; Zimmerman, Steiner, & Pond, 2002) as our measure of this construct. The PLS-4 is a commercially available, standardized assessment tool generally used to examine the development of language comprehension and expression in children between birth and 7 years of age. The first edition of this test was published in 1969, and so it has been evaluated thoroughly by the authors and other researchers interested in language acquisition. Although it has subscales that evaluate both language comprehension and expression, we chose to use only the subscale that examines comprehension. The Language Expression component would have provided information largely redundant with that obtained from numerous other measures used in this study. The time available for testing these children was constrained, and we wanted to use the testing time we had wisely by carving it up so that all aspects of development could be examined.

Data collected by the authors of the PLS-4 reveal that the Auditory Comprehension subscale has excellent reliability. We had some concerns about the validity of a few test items, but those items were few in number and were restricted to the early parts of the instrument. For example, one item was *Mouths objects*. We questioned how validly such an item measures a child's ability to understand language, but these few examples did not detract from our general enthusiasm for the instrument.

Overall, the items on the Auditory Comprehension subscale index a child's ability to understand specific components of communication and language. The items are organized in a hierarchical order, going from those we would expect a child to understand at the youngest ages to those we would expect the child to understand later in development. For example, an early item is *Reacts to sounds other than voices in the environment*. A late item is *Understands the "-er" ending to be "one who . . . "* Figure 6–1 illustrates test administration.

On this project all data collection for the auditory comprehension task was done with exactly the same materials. We generally used the materials provided by the publisher or recommended by the test authors, with one exception: For the item *Discriminates one sound from another*, it is recommended that the sound of car keys rattling be compared to the sound of paper crinkling. We would not expect children with hear-

ing loss to hear these sounds very well, if at all. Therefore, we designed and built small metal boxes that had two sound generators inside: one that made a steady 500-Hz tone, and one with an interrupted tone. The box was equipped with a switch so that the sounds could be changed once the child habituated to the first one presented. For all test items, examiners were trained to give each child two opportunities, and only two, to demonstrate a response before moving to the next item. Testing was stopped after three consecutive failures on the child's part to respond.

Data are missing for one child on this task because the child was extremely uncooperative, and so could not be tested. Table 6–1 shows mean scores for the auditory comprehension task for each group. This table, as well as several others in this chapter, can be found at the chapter's end. Figure 6–2 plots

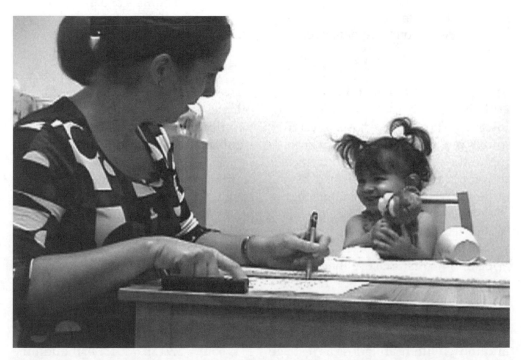

Figure 6–1. An examiner administering the Auditory Comprehension task to a child.

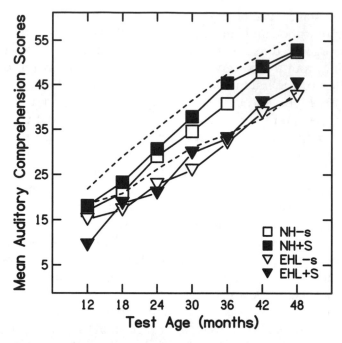

Figure 6–2. Mean scores on the Auditory Comprehension task for children with normal hearing and those with early-identified hearing loss: NH–s (normal hearing, no signs); NH+S (normal hearing, signs); EHL–s (early-identified hearing loss, no signs); EHL+S (early-identified hearing loss, signs). Dotted lines show +/– one standard deviation from the mean, according to the normative data published by the test authors.

means for children with normal hearing and those with early-identified hearing loss. The dotted lines show plus/minus one standard deviation according to the normative data for typically developing children published by the authors. It is apparent in this figure that children with normal hearing had higher scores than children with early-identified hearing loss. A trend that appears for this measure that was not present for the language measures reported in the last chapter is that there is an increasingly larger gap in scores for the children with normal hearing and those with hearing loss as test age increases. The FIRST ANOVA performed on these scores supported these two descriptions of the results: There was a significant main effect of hearing status, $F(1, 654) = 201.01$, $p < .001$, as well as a significant Hearing Status × Test Age interaction, $F(6, 654) = 2.43$, $p = .025$. It is apparent from Figure 6–2 that children with early-identified hearing loss performed more poorly than children with normal hearing, and the magnitude of this difference is greater at older test ages.

There was also a significant main effect of signs in this FIRST ANOVA, $F(1, 654) = 5.91$, $p = .015$. Although the

Hearing Status × Sign interaction was not significant, we wanted to examine this sign effect more closely. Therefore, a SEA was performed looking at the sign effect for children with normal hearing and those with early-identified hearing loss separately. Only children with normal hearing showed a significant effect of signs when examined this way, $F(1, 654) = 10.28$, $p < .001$. The small difference between children who used signs and those who did not is apparent on Figure 6–2. Across all test ages, it was a difference of two points: Means for the NH–s and NH+S groups were 34.7 and 36.8, respectively. The effect appears to be strongest at 30 and 36 months, which is curious because parents of children with normal hearing who used signs reported that they stopped doing so by 24 months of age. This sign effect disappears by 48 months of age.

Figure 6–3 illustrates scores on the auditory comprehension task for children with hearing loss only. The dotted lines are the same plus/minus one standard deviation from the mean raw scores reported by the test authors for their normative sample of typically developing children. The SECOND ANOVA performed on these data, with scores from children with normal hearing excluded, revealed a significant main effect of age of ID, $F(1, 297) = 15.99$, $p < .001$. Although the main effect of signs was not significant, the Age of ID × Signs interaction was $F(1, 297) = 13.14$, $p < .001$. To investigate further, a SEA was performed, examining scores separately for children who used signs and those who did not. A significant age-of-ID effect was found only for signing children, $F(1, 297) = 20.61$, $p < .001$: Signing children whose hearing loss was identified early had better scores than signing

children whose losses were identified late. Among children who did not use signs, there was no age-of-ID effect.

Next, a SEA was done examining scores for early- and late-identified children separately with signs, prosthesis, and test age as main effects. For children with early-identified hearing loss, the main effect of prosthesis was significant, $F(1, 297) = 12.11$, $p < .001$, but not the main effect of signs; for the late-identified children, the sign effect was significant, $F(1, 297) = 6.64$, $p = .011$, but not the prosthesis effect. These effects are apparent in Figure 6–3: On the top panel we see that scores for children with hearing aids were higher than those for children who received implants. On the bottom panel we see that scores for children who did not use signs were higher than those for children who did use signs.

This auditory comprehension task tapped into children's abilities to respond to communicative acts in general, such as by acknowledging that something was said by a communication partner. That aspect of the instrument was similar to the Language Comprehension subscale of the SIB-R discussed in Chapter 5. However, this Auditory Comprehension subscale from the PLS-4 also examined children's abilities to respond specifically to lexical, syntactic, and grammatical devices. The nature and direction of effects were similar to those obtained for the Language Comprehension subscale reported in Chapter 5, but the magnitude of these effects was greater. Children with hearing loss, even when it was identified before 6 months of age, failed to understand language constructions as well as children with normal hearing. Children with late-identified hearing loss

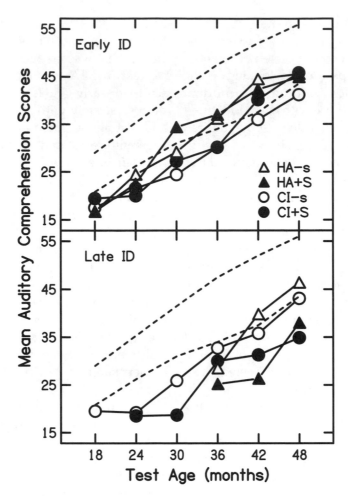

Figure 6–3. Mean scores on the Auditory Comprehension task for children with hearing loss only: HA–s (hearing aids, no signs); HA+S (hearing aids, signs); CI–s (cochlear implants, no signs); and CI+S (cochlear implants, signs). Dotted lines show +/– one standard deviation from the mean, according to the normative data published by the test authors.

performed more poorly than children whose losses were identified early, but only if they used signs. For children not using signs, there was no decrement in performance for the late-identified children compared to the early-identified children. Finally, of the children whose losses were identified early, those with implants had poorer scores than those who wore hearing aids.

How the Independent Measures Correlated with Auditory Comprehension Scores

This measure of auditory comprehension of language revealed some important differences in abilities among groups. Other than the main effects examined in our ANOVAs, we wanted to see what might account for variability in the scores. To do that, we used Auditory Comprehension scores obtained at the 48-month test session: Because those scores represented the culmination of 4 years of language learning, we thought they would be most sensitive to these effects. For children with hearing loss, we examined the effects of BE-PTA, ID-Age (the continuous variable), mean number of monthly intervention sessions (both before 36 months of age and between 36 and 48 months of age), and SES. None of these independent variables correlated significantly with Auditory Comprehension scores. That was true even when we computed these correlation coefficients for children with hearing aids and cochlear implants separately, and for children with early- and late-identified hearing loss separately.

For children with normal hearing, we computed the correlation coefficient between Auditory Comprehension scores and SES, and found it to be significant: $r(51) = .50$, $p < .001$. By squaring this correlation coefficient, we can estimate that 25% of the variance in scores was explained by SES: Children with normal hearing who came from families with lower SES had poorer Auditory Comprehension scores. Generally speaking, correlation coefficients between .3 and .5 indicate moderate relations between two variables. Any coefficient greater than .5 indicates a fairly strong relation, especially when it comes to explaining the sources of a human behavior as complex as language. We had the same range of SES scores among children with hearing loss as among children with normal hearing, yet did not find a significant correlation for the children with hearing loss. Two reasons come to mind for why this might be. First, it may be the case that scores were sufficiently depressed as a result of

having a hearing loss that SES imposed no additional decrement on performance for these children. It may also be the case that the intervention provided to children with hearing loss helped to ameliorate the effects of low SES just as it ameliorates the effects of hearing loss. We have no way of separating these two possibilities, and in fact suspect that both explanations contribute to our failure to find a SES effect on these scores for children with hearing loss.

Results of a Longitudinal and Repeated-Measures Analysis

Some readers might worry that results from this study could be compromised either because the samples of children in this study were not strictly longitudinal or because too many children were tested repeatedly, and so learning effects could have arisen. Believing the first of these potential concerns to be most prevalent, we compared results of children who were in the study for most sessions to the results of all participants. We used data from the 100 children with normal hearing or early-identified hearing loss who participated in at least four of these test sessions. Children with late-identified hearing loss were excluded from this analysis because there were not enough of them who were in four or more test sessions: In most cases, they had already missed several test sessions by the time their hearing loss was identified. Figure 6–4 shows results for children who participated in four or more test sessions on the bottom panel, with data from all children with normal hearing and early-identified hearing loss on the top. The developmental patterns across groups are clearly the same in both displays. This finding

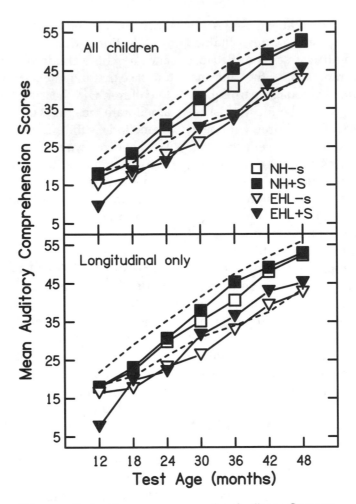

Figure 6–4. Mean scores on the Auditory Comprehension task for children who participated in four or more test sessions (bottom panel) compared to scores for all participants (top panel): NH–s (normal hearing, no signs); NH+S (normal hearing, signs); EHL–s (early-identified hearing loss, no signs); EHL+S (early-identified hearing loss, signs). Dotted lines show +/– one standard deviation from the mean, according to the normative data published by the test authors.

reassures us that we were accurately capturing representative performance for the children in these groups.

A concern regarding data analysis might similarly exist. Statistically astute readers will have noticed by now that test age is being treated as a between-

subjects factor. That follows from the fact that not all children were tested at each test age. Nonetheless, it could raise concern that the conclusions being reached may be different from what they would be if this was a strictly longitudinal design. To evaluate the veracity of that concern, we performed ANOVAs on data for those 100 children with normal hearing or with early-identified hearing loss who participated in at least four of the six sessions between 18 and 48 months of age. Data from the 12-month test session were excluded from these analyses because that test age had the fewest participants. We performed these ANOVAs using both a repeated-measures and between-subjects design. Table 6–2 presents statistical results for these analyses, as well as those for analyses of all children with normal hearing and early-identified hearing loss, regardless of how many sessions they participated in. Clearly, outcomes were similar for all analyses, and this was true for all other dependent measures in the study, as well. All indications were that there were no underlying differences between those children who participated in most test sessions and those who did not. We were obtaining representative measures of performance for the populations of children we were studying.

Expressive Vocabulary

There is perhaps no single measure of language development that is used in research with deaf children as commonly as expressive vocabulary. This construct indexes how many separate words a child is able to produce, spontaneously and with correct reference. With young children, estimates of expressive vocabulary are generally obtained from word lists that the parent completes. These measures are easy to obtain and are reliable. Although our ultimate interest on this project was in measures

of complex language abilities, we felt it was important to have an indication of expressive vocabulary for the children in this study as well. Measures of receptive vocabulary are also frequently used in studies of child language, but our own experiences indicate that these measures can be so strongly influenced by a child's SES that other effects are difficult to estimate (Nittrouer, 1996; Nittrouer & Burton, 2005). Therefore, we did not explicitly measure receptive vocabulary.

To the extent possible, instruments used in this study were selected so that they could serve as measures over the entire age range from 12 to 48 months. However, at the time we were designing this study, there was no one measure of expressive vocabulary that allowed us to do that. Measures of children's early expressive vocabularies are usually word lists given to the parents to evaluate. With these instruments, parents are asked to recall from experience the words that their children can say. That is what was done on this project for the youngest ages. As soon as children were old enough, which was at age 36 months, we began to assess expressive vocabulary directly, eliciting words from the child, rather than relying on parents' memories.

For this project, we used the Language Development Survey (LDS; Achenbach & Rescorla, 2000) with children between the ages of 12 and 30 months. The test authors have shown that the LDS correlates well with direct measures of children's expressive vocabularies. The LDS consists of 310 words. Parents were asked to circle the words that their children say spontaneously, rather than just through imitation. They could count words their children do not pronounce correctly, according to the adult form,

Table 6–2. ANOVA results for Auditory Comprehension scores performed on data from participants who were in four or more test sessions (longitudinal), done as a repeated-measures design and as a between-groups design, and on data from all participants with normal hearing and early-identified hearing loss between 18 and 48 months. Numerator degrees of freedom were 1 in all cases; denominator degrees of freedom are provided (df). MS is the Mean Square for between-groups variance estimates.

	df	Hearing Status			Signs			Hearing Status × Signs		
		MS	F	p	MS	F	p	MS	F	p
Longitudinal										
Repeated Measures	96	6973.02	63.01	<.001	657.09	5.94	.017	19.78	0.18	.673
Between Groups	576	6973.02	223.95	<.001	657.09	21.10	<.001	19.78	0.64	.426
All participants										
Between Groups	601	8903.09	215.07	<.001	502.85	12.15	.001	18.59	0.45	.503

as long as those words were consistently pronounced in the same form. In addition to counting the number of words that each child was able to say, we provided a column in which parents were asked to check the item if their child had only a signed version of the vocabulary item. In this way, we could estimate the total size of a child's productive vocabulary, both spoken and signed.

Beginning at 36 months of age, we administered the Expressive One-Word Picture Vocabulary Test (EOWPVT; Brownell, 2000). In this task, the child is shown a picture and is expected to provide the vocabulary item that names that picture. We modified procedures from the standard by giving all instructions nonverbally, through mime. It was felt that children who had spoken language supplemented with signs might be inappropriately hampered in their abilities to participate if instructions were only provided in spoken form. We also removed all pictures representing supraordinate category labels, such as *appliances* and *clothing*. Users of American Sign Language are less likely to use supraordinate category labels than speakers of English, and so children receiving sign support might have less exposure to those lexical items. Again, we did not want to bias results against those children with strong sign support to their spoken language input.

Language Development Survey (LDS)

Three parents failed to complete the second page of this two-page form at one test session each, and so data are missing for those children. Table 6–3 (at the end of the chapter) shows mean raw scores for the numbers of spoken words, and Figure 6–5 plots these values for children with normal hearing and those with early-identified hearing loss. One impression that is immediately apparent in the table is how large the variability is for this measure. In fact, we did not plot lines indicating plus/minus one standard deviation from the test authors' data because the variability for the normative sample was similarly large. The impressions gathered from Figure 6–5 are that children with normal hearing have more spoken words in their vocabularies than children with early-identified hearing loss, and that the magnitude of the difference in scores between children with normal hearing and those with early-identified hearing loss increases as children get older. This trend resembles that found for the auditory comprehension of language.

The FIRST ANOVA revealed a significant effect of hearing status, $F(1, 347) = 33.5, p < .001$, and a significant Hearing Status × Test Age interaction, $F(1, 347) = 6.27, p < .001$. Thus, statistical support was obtained for the observations that children with hearing loss had fewer words in their spoken vocabularies than children with normal hearing, and that the gap increased as children got older.

The SECOND ANOVA was not performed on the numbers of spoken words that children with hearing loss had. For other measures, these analyses are done on results from 30 to 48 months of age, but only results for 30 months were available for LDS spoken words. And variability was so high for this measure as to render a statistical analysis pointless. Nonetheless, Table 6–3 shows the pattern of results at 30 months that has

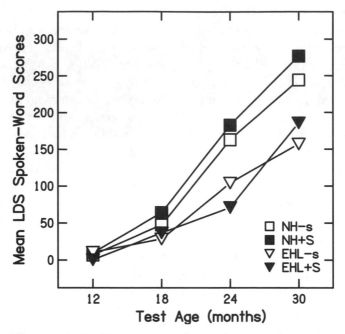

Figure 6–5. Mean scores for spoken words on the Language Development Survey (LDS) for children with normal hearing and those with early-identified hearing loss: NH–s (normal hearing, no signs); NH+S (normal hearing, signs); EHL–s (early-identified hearing loss, no signs); EHL+S (early-identified hearing loss, signs).

been seen for other language measures reported thus far: Children with early-identified hearing loss, regardless of whether they used signs or not, and nonsigning children with late-identified hearing loss had similar numbers of spoken words reported by their parents. Signing children with late-identified hearing loss had far fewer.

Table 6–4 shows the numbers of words for which children had only signed versions. No statistical analyses were performed on these numbers because they were so small. We collected this information in the belief that children who were receiving sign input might be learning some words in their signed forms before they knew how to say them. If so, it might be the case that the sums of words these children knew in the spoken and signed forms would equal or surpass the numbers of words that children in nonsigning programs knew in the spoken form. That is indeed the case for signing children with early-identified hearing loss at both 24 and 30 months: For example, at 24 months these children had a mean of 126.82 items in their expressive vocabularies (70.91 spoken and 55.91 signed), which is more than the 103.93 items that nonsigning children with early-identified hearing loss had as spoken vocabulary items. However, this was not the case for signing children with late-identified hearing loss. So, the late-identified chil-

Table 6–4. Mean number of words on the Language Development Survey (LDS) for which children had only signed versions, obtained at each test age, with standard deviations in parentheses and group numbers in italics.

Test Age (Months)	NH–s	NH+S	Early		Late	
			HL–s	HL+S	HL–s	HL+S
12	2.21 (8.21) *29*	7.17 (10.29) *12*	1.27 (2.97) *11*	7.80 (3.70) *5*	*0*	*0*
18	2.33 (4.43) *43*	18.00 (21.50) *28*	2.67 (5.90) *24*	20.75 (18.42) *12*	0.00 (0.00) *2*	*0*
24	1.19 (5.39) *31*	7.88 (19.15) *24*	0.80 (2.67) *30*	55.91 (40.10) *11*	0.00 (0.00) *5*	15.50 (19.09) *2*
30	0.08 (0.28) *25*	0.00 (0.00) *27*	0.11 (0.46) *37*	17.79 (27.73) *14*	0.00 (0.00) *12*	5.75 (8.26) *4*

dren who were receiving sign support had fewer spoken items in their expressive vocabularies than other children, and these deficits were not compensated for by their signed vocabularies.

Expressive One-Word Picture Vocabulary Test (EOWPVT)

Five children were uncooperative for this task at one test age, and so data are missing for them at those ages. Our first concern in analyzing these data was in how similarly the LDS and EOWPVT measure children's expressive vocabularies. To examine that question, we computed a correlation coefficient between LDS scores from the 30-month test session and EOWPVT scores from the 36-month session for children who

participated at both ages: A strong correlation was observed, $r(100) = .72, p < .001$. Consequently, we conclude that both measures examine the same underlying construct.

Table 6–5 (at the end of the chapter) shows means for the numbers of items children in each group were able to provide lexical labels for on the EOWPVT. Figure 6–6 displays these results for children with normal hearing and with early-identified hearing loss. The dotted lines show plus/minus one standard deviation according to the normative data for typically developing children published by the authors. Unlike results for the LDS, the separation between children with normal hearing and those with early-identified hearing loss remains consistent in magnitude for the EOWPVT across the 1 year that scores

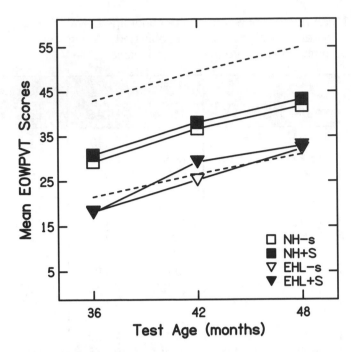

Figure 6–6. Mean scores on the Expressive One-Word Picture Vocabulary Test (EOWPVT) for children with normal hearing and those with early-identified hearing loss: NH–s (normal hearing, no signs); NH+S (normal hearing, signs); EHL–s (early-identified hearing loss, no signs); EHL+S (early-identified hearing loss, signs). Dotted lines show +/– one standard deviation from the mean, according to the normative data published by the test authors.

are available. This trend was supported by the FIRST ANOVA: Only the main effect of hearing status was significant, $F(1, 302) = 79.22, p < .001$.

Figure 6–7 shows mean scores from the EOWPVT for children with early- and late-identified hearing loss. The dotted lines are the same plus/minus one standard deviation from the mean raw scores shown in Figure 6–6. For children with early-identified hearing loss, whose scores are shown in the top panel, it appears that children who wore hearing aids for the entire study scored better than children who received im-

plants. For children with late-identified hearing loss, it is clear that the children who were not in signing programs scored better than children in programs that used signs.

In order to examine the factors influencing scores on the EOWPVT, the SECOND ANOVA was performed on scores for children with hearing loss only, with age of ID, signs, and test age as the main effects. The main effects of both age of ID and signs were significant: for age of ID, $F(1, 231) = 10.06, p = .002$; for signs, $F(1, 231) = 5.20, p = .024$. In addition, the Age of ID × Signs inter-

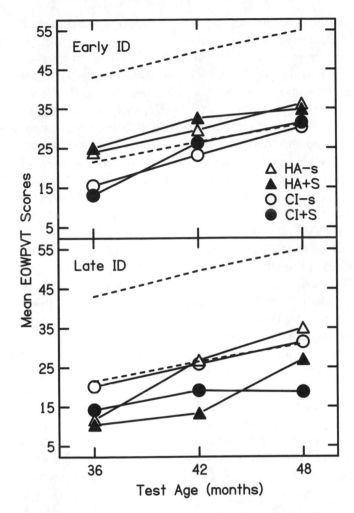

Figure 6–7. Mean scores on the Expressive One-Word Picture Vocabulary Test (EOWPVT) for children with hearing loss only: early-identified children on the top panel; late-identified children on the bottom panel. Means are plotted separately as a function of type of prosthesis and sign use. *HA–s* = hearing aid users, nonsigners; *HA+S* = hearing aid users, signers; *CI–s* = cochlear implant users, nonsigners; *CI+S* = cochlear implant users, signers. Dotted lines show +/− one standard deviation from the mean, according to the normative data published by the test authors.

action was significant, $F(1, 231) = 10.80$, $p = .001$, prompting further investigation. A SEA was performed, examining scores separately for children who used signs and for those who did not. A significant age-of-ID effect was found only for signing children, $F(1, 231) = 15.40$, $p < .001$: Children who did not use signs performed similarly, regardless of age of ID. Among children who used signs, however, those whose hearing loss was identified late had lower EOWPVT scores than those with early-identified hearing loss.

Next, a SEA was done examining scores for early- and late-identified children separately with signs, prosthesis, and test age as main effects. For children with early-identified hearing loss, the main effect of prosthesis was significant, $F(1, 219) = 13.65$, $p < .001$, but not the main effect of signs. For the late-identified children, the sign effect was significant, $F(1, 219) = 10.15$, $p = .002$, but not the prosthesis effect. These effects are apparent in Figure 6–7: On the top panel we see that scores for children with hearing aids were higher than those for children who received implants. On the bottom panel we see that scores for children who did not use signs were higher than those for children who did use signs. This is precisely the pattern observed for scores on the Auditory Comprehension task.

How the Independent Measures Correlated with Expressive Vocabulary Scores

As with our measure of auditory comprehension, we were interested in how well these measures of expressive vocabulary correlated with the independent measures. Looking first at scores on the LDS, obtained at the 30-month test session, we found that no significant portion of the variance was explained by SES, for either children with NH or those with HL. However, unlike the correlational analysis done for Auditory Comprehension scores, a significant portion of the variance in LDS scores was found to be explained by factors related to children's hearing loss, for the children with hearing loss. Significant correlations were found for LDS scores at 30 months and BE-PTA, $r(67) = -.27$, $p = .026$, and ID-Age, $r(67) = -.26$, $p = .033$. But although these correlations are significant, they indicate that these factors explain only a little of the variance in LDS scores (6 to 7%). The amount of time that children spent with intervention specialists did not explain any variance in LDS scores.

Correlations computed for EOW-PVT scores obtained at the 48-month test session revealed trends more like those found for Auditory Comprehension. For children with hearing loss, BE-PTA, ID-Age, and mean number of monthly intervention sessions all failed to correlate significantly with EOWPVT scores. On the other hand, SES was found to explain some of the variance for both children with normal hearing, $r(51) = .27$, $p = .055$, and those with hearing loss, $r(90) = .22$, $p = .036$. Again, however, these amounts are not great.

Speech Intelligibility

We were concerned with how well children in this study could generally be understood by others, or how intelligible they were. Speech intelligibility is a construct of interest to speech scientists and clinicians from a number of subspecialties. It is used to evaluate the productive capacities of adults who have neurogenic disorders, or those who are second-language learners of English. Such measures are also commonly used with children with developmental apraxia or phonological processing problems. Many methods have been described for indexing speech intelligibility. In some tasks, listeners are presented with a sample of connected speech, and are asked to estimate what percentage of the speaker's sample is intelligible. Although these methods enjoy a high degree of validity, it is very difficult to ensure reliability (Schiavetti, Metz, & Sitler, 1981).

One of the first tests of speech intelligibility developed for deaf children was a sentence identification task, devised by Marjorie Magner at the Clarke School for the Deaf (1972). In this task, children are asked to read a series of sentences. Typically, tape recordings are made of these samples, and listeners subsequently transcribe what they hear when listening to the tapes. Clearly, this task could not be used with children too young to read, as the children were in the current study. In addition, on that task listeners are supported in their recognition of speech samples by having sentence context. We wanted to investigate listeners' abilities to understand these children, independent of contextual support. Therefore, we selected an intelligibility measure that consisted of single words, which the child imitated after the examiner.

The Children's Speech Intelligibility Measure (CSIM; Wilcox & Morris, 1999) was used in this project starting when children were 36 months of age. On this task, children repeat 50 words, one at a time, after the examiner. The instrument consists of 200 such word lists that are constructed from a master list of 600 words. Most words are single syllable, but some have two syllables. These words were recorded onto the same digital videotape used to record the parent-child interactions. The samples were recorded at a 48-kHz sampling rate with 16-bit digitization. Once

the tape got to the central facility, the CSIM portion was downloaded to a hard drive, and the child's word productions were separated into their own audio files. Listeners unfamiliar with the speech of deaf speakers came to the laboratory and listened to these samples. The task of the listener was to select the word that was produced from a set of 12 phonetically similar choices. Each listener heard only three lists so that no listener would have the opportunity to become skilled at recognizing the speech of deaf children. Two naïve listeners scored the samples from each child. Here we used the mean score from the two listeners for each child, and report these scores as the percentage of words the listeners identified correctly when produced by the child. The correlation coefficient between first and second listeners was computed, and showed excellent agreement, $r(358) = .94$.

This is the task for which there is the most missing data. A total of 41 CSIM tests were missed at the 36-month test age, either because examiners did not administer it or because children refused to repeat the test words. These missing tests are evenly distributed across groups. Twenty-one tests are missing across the 42- and 48-month test ages, largely because children were uncooperative.

Table 6–6 (at the end of the chapter) shows mean percent correct scores for the CSIM. Figure 6–8 displays these results for children with normal hearing and for those with early-identified hearing loss. Here we plotted the plus/minus one standard deviation boundaries according to our own sample of children with normal hearing. It is evident from Figure 6–8 that children with early-identified hearing loss were less intelligible in their speech production than were children with normal hearing,

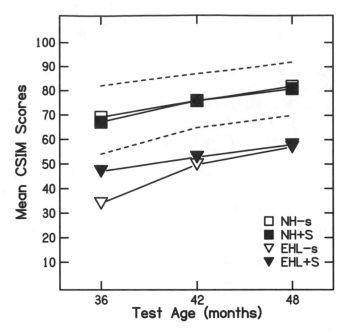

Figure 6–8. Mean scores on the Children's Speech Intelligibility Measure (CSIM) for children with normal hearing and those with early-identified hearing loss: NH–s (normal hearing, no signs); NH+S (normal hearing, signs); EHL–s (early-identified hearing loss, no signs); EHL+S (early-identified hearing loss, signs). Dotted lines show +/− one standard deviation from the mean, according to data from children with normal hearing in this study.

and the FIRST ANOVA supported that observation: The main effect of hearing status was significant, $F(1, 257) = 167.75, p < .001$.

Figure 6–9 plots CSIM scores for children with hearing loss only. The SECOND ANOVA performed on these scores showed a significant main effect of age of ID, $F(1, 194) = 12.70, p < .001$, as well as a significant Age of ID × Signs interaction, $F(1, 194) = 14.91, p < .001$. As with other measures, a SEA was performed, examining scores separately for children who used signs and those who did not to determine if both groups of children showed an effect of age of ID. As with other measures, a significant

age-of-ID effect was found only for signing children, $F(1, 194) = 20.75, p < .001$: Signing children whose losses were identified late performed more poorly than those with early-identified hearing loss. Children who did not use signs performed similarly, regardless of age of ID.

Next, a SEA was done examining scores for early- and late-identified children separately with signs, prosthesis, and test age as main effects. For children with early-identified hearing loss, no main effects or interactions were found (other than the main effect of test age, of course). The lack of a prosthesis effect for the CSIM differs from findings for other language-related measures

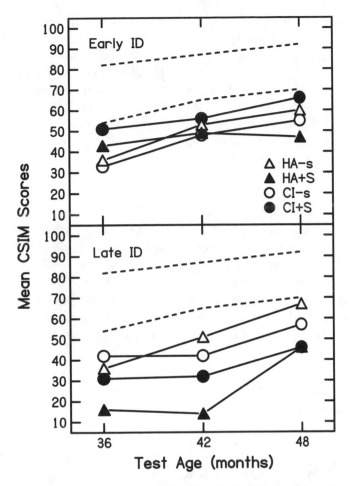

Figure 6–9. Mean scores on the Children's Speech Intelligibility Measure (CSIM) for children with hearing loss only: early-identified children on the top panel; late-identified children on the bottom panel. Means are plotted separately as a function of type of prosthesis and sign use. *HA–s* = hearing aid users, nonsigners; *HA+S* = hearing aid users, signers; *CI–s* = cochlear implant users, nonsigners; *CI+S* = cochlear implant users, signers. Dotted lines show +/– one standard deviation from the mean, according to data from children with normal hearing in this study.

involving children with early-identified hearing loss. For the late-identified children, the sign effect was significant, $F(1, 182) = 16.32$, $p < .001$, as has been the case for other language-related measures.

In general, children with hearing loss were quite unintelligible, with listeners able to understand less than half of the words these children said. In considering this finding, it is important to bear in mind that listeners were hearing these words without linguistic context, and without visual cues from watching the child speak.

How the Independent Measures Correlated with Speech Intelligibility

As with measures of auditory comprehension and expressive vocabulary, we wished to see if the independent variables explained significant portions of the variance in this measure of speech intelligibility. The same correlational analyses were performed as for the other measures, but in this case, no significant outcomes were obtained. Of particular importance, we found no evidence that the severity of a child's hearing loss explained any variance in the child's ability to produce intelligible speech. Again, factors other than these independent variables must explain that ability.

Using Cohen's *d* to Select Assessment Measures

The statistical analyses that have been reported so far indicate which measures show significant differences between (or among) groups, but provide no way of gauging the magnitude of those differences. Differences between group means must be evaluated according to how much variability there is in scores within the groups: The question we are always asking when we perform analyses of variance is whether the variability among groups is greater than what we would expect based on how much variability tends to be found among individual participants. Thus, if we want an estimate of the size of those group differences we must use our within-groups variance estimate as our ruler. Specifically, the difference between the means of any two groups can be normalized according to the standard devi-

ation pooled across those two groups using Cohen's *d* (Cohen, 1960). Generally speaking, any value of greater than 0.8 represents a large difference between two groups. For example, if we compute Cohen's *d* on CSIM scores at 48 months for children with normal hearing and those with hearing loss, we obtain a value of 1.64, representing a rather large effect of hearing status on this measure.

One problem consistently faced by clinicians involves how to select measures that can serve as sensitive indices of language acquisition in deaf children. One contributing factor to that selection may actually be how sensitive measures are to differences between children with normal hearing and those with hearing loss. If a measure demonstrates a large effect between these two groups, it should be better at evaluating whether a score for an individual child is closer to those of children with normal hearing or to those of other children with hearing loss than measures that do not vary greatly between the two groups of children. This follows from the fact that the range of scores between the two endpoints is wider. In effect, we have a longer ruler, and so can examine the spread of scores more accurately.

Of course, various measures will differ in how sensitive they are to group differences as children mature. For some measures, there is likely to be little difference in scores obtained for children with normal hearing and those with hearing loss at young ages because it indexes a skill that children do not acquire until they are older. We saw that with the LDS: At 12 months of age, even typically developing children produce few words. Consequently, we would not expect measures of expressive vocabulary to be sensitive to how well a child is progressing in language development at very young ages. In the chapters to come we will see that some measures lose their sensitivity because there are upper limits on performance, and all children eventually hit those limits, even if development is slow.

We have already seen that the measure of speech intelligibility used here was sensitive to differences between children with normal hearing and those with hearing loss, at least at 48 months. Effect sizes, using Cohen's *d*, were computed

for the other two measures discussed in this chapter, as well: auditory comprehension and expressive vocabulary.

Cohen's *d*s were computed at each test age from 12 to 48 months, using scores and standard deviations from children with normal hearing and children with early-identified hearing loss, collapsed across signers and nonsigners. These values are shown on Figure 6–10, along with values for CSIM at 36 to 48 months of age. The dashed line at 0.8 separates the space into values that

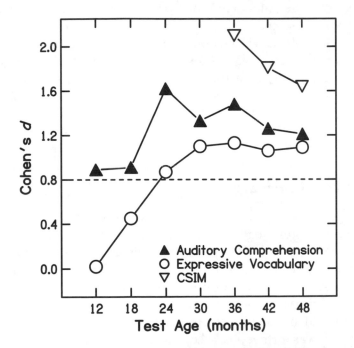

Figure 6–10. Cohen's *d*s for each test age for the auditory comprehension task and for expressive vocabulary measures. From 12 to 30 months these values for expressive vocabulary were derived from the LDS; from 36 to 48 months the values were derived from the EOWPVT. Cohen's *d*s are shown for CSIM scores from 36 to 48 months. Cohen's *d*s were computed for mean scores from children with normal hearing and those with early-identified hearing loss, across nonsigners and signers. The dashed line at 0.8 separates the space into values that represent large effects (above the line) from those that show moderate or weak effects (below the line).

represent large effects (above the line) from those that represent moderate or weak effects (below the line). This figure reveals that the Auditory Comprehension subscale of the PLS-4 provides a sensitive indicator of how well children understand spoken language across the ages tested here. Similarly, the EOWPVT was a sensitive indicator of differences in expressive vocabulary starting at 36 months of age. The LDS, on the other hand, was not a very sensitive measure, at least not until 24 months of age. The effect of hearing status was large for CSIM. Consequently, the Auditory Comprehension subscale of the PLS-4, the EOWPVT, and the CSIM can all be used with confidence to assess progress for children with hearing loss, at least when administered as we have. Expressive vocabulary at young ages does not offer a very sensitive index of that progress.

Chapter Summary

In this chapter, we found that the children with hearing loss lagged behind their peers with normal hearing on three measures of basic language development: auditory comprehension, expressive vocabulary, and intelligibility. Generally speaking, it was further observed that these skills were not affected by whether children used signs or not—at least not for children with normal hearing or with early-identified hearing loss. The only exception to this trend involved auditory comprehension, for which children with normal hearing showed slightly better scores than their nonsigning peers. For children with late-identified hearing loss, however, the use of signs was associated with a strong decrement in performance on all measures. This difference in the sign effect based on age of ID also meant that there was a difference in the effect of age of ID across signing groups: For nonsigning children with hearing loss, it did not matter whether their losses were identified before 6 months of age or at 2 years of age; these nonsigning deaf children performed similarly. For children who used signs, however, there was a consistent effect of age of ID such that those signing children identified with hearing loss at 1 or 2 years of age were poorer in these language abilities than signing children identified before 6 months of age. It may be that we have uncovered a piece of evidence for the notion of critical periods. Although perhaps not as rigidly formed as the concepts described in Chapter 1, it may be that the ability to acquire language capacities diminishes after the 1st year, such that interfering effects are not well tolerated by the system. Signing generally had no effect on language learning for children with normal hearing or with early-identified hearing loss: It neither facilitated nor interfered with that learning. But for children identified later, the effect of using signs on these basic language abilities was clearly one of an inhibitory nature.

Table 6–1. Mean raw scores on the Auditory Comprehension subscale of the Preschool Language Scales–4 (PLS–4), given at each test age, with standard deviations in parentheses and group numbers in italics.

Test Age (Months)	NH–s	NH+S	Early		Late	
			HL–s	HL+S	HL–s	HL+S
12	17.00 (3.77) *29*	18.08 (3.70) *12*	15.09 (3.73) *11*	9.40 (5.94) *5*	*0*	*0*
18	20.91 (5.23) *43*	23.29 (4.50) *28*	17.17 (4.14) *24*	18.62 (3.95) *13*	19.50 (0.71) *2*	*0*
24	29.06 (3.83) *32*	30.72 (4.33) *25*	22.83 (5.11) *30*	20.91 (4.97) *11*	19.20 (3.03) *5*	18.50 (4.95) *2*
30	34.60 (6.07) *25*	37.85 (5.64) *27*	26.00 (7.72) *36*	29.79 (7.56) *14*	25.75 (5.88) *12*	20.00 (2.94) *4*
36	40.81 (5.99) *31*	45.47 (4.61) *30*	32.06 (8.31) *35*	33.00 (9.52) *12*	31.60 (6.90) *15*	27.33 (6.63) *9*
42	47.96 (5.00) *27*	49.27 (5.03) *26*	38.87 (8.97) *38*	41.13 (8.75) *15*	36.65 (9.73) *23*	29.80 (10.81) *10*
48	52.50 (5.36) *26*	53.00 (4.24) *25*	42.59 (10.02) *34*	45.39 (8.82) *18*	43.73 (8.59) *26*	35.92 (12.80) *12*

Table 6–3. Mean number of spoken words on the Language Development Survey (LDS), obtained at each test age, with standard deviations in parentheses and group numbers in italics.

Test Age (Months)	NH–s	NH+S	Early		Late	
			HL–s	HL+S	HL–s	HL+S
12	6.86 (7.35) *29*	9.75 (6.17) *12*	10.64 (25.28) *11*	0.40 (0.55) *5*	*0*	*0*
18	47.58 (37.85) *43*	64.04 (58.79) *28*	28.54 (49.24) *24*	36.83 (65.85) *12*	46.00 (8.49) *2*	*0*
24	162.39 (80.76) *31*	182.25 (98.01) *24*	103.93 (84.97) *30*	70.91 (86.53) *11*	54.60 (58.17) *5*	34.00 (48.08) *2*
30	244.08 (79.25) *25*	276.70 (48.88) *27*	157.08 (104.56) *37*	185.79 (103.19) *14*	122.25 (69.34) *12*	38.75 (29.64) *4*

Table 6–5. Mean raw scores for the Expressive One-Word Picture Vocabulary Test (EOWPVT), given at each test age, with standard deviations in parentheses and group numbers in italics.

Test Age (Months)	NH–s	NH+S	Early		Late	
			HL–s	HL+S	HL–s	HL+S
36	29.30 (8.96) *30*	30.87 (9.25) *30*	18.24 (10.93) *34*	18.08 (14.46) *12*	17.93 (8.00) *15*	12.11 (8.88) *9*
42	36.59 (8.59) *27*	38.00 (9.22) *26*	25.22 (11.30) *37*	29.20 (12.32) *15*	26.10 (7.39) *21*	17.40 (11.80) *10*
48	41.73 (6.86) *26*	43.24 (9.74) *25*	32.18 (10.81) *34*	32.89 (8.76) *18*	32.12 (7.86) *26*	21.50 (13.40) *12*

Table 6–6. Mean proportion of words recognized correctly by naïve listeners on the Children's Speech Intelligibility Measure (CSIM), given at each test age, with standard deviations in parentheses and group numbers in italics.

Test Age (Months)	NH–s	NH+S	Early		Late	
			HL–s	HL+S	HL–s	HL+S
36	.69 (.14) *23*	.67 (.15) *21*	.34 (.14) *24*	.47 (.19) *6*	.40 (.11) *9*	.23 (.16) *8*
42	.76 (.12) *26*	.76 (.10) *25*	.50 (.18) *33*	.53 (.13) *13*	.44 (.18) *18*	.27 (.22) *10*
48	.81 (.11) *25*	.81 (.12) *24*	.57 (.17) *32*	.58 (.19) *17*	.59 (.16) *25*	.46 (.25) *11*

References

Achenbach, T. M., & Rescorla, L. A. (2000). *Manual for the ASEBA preschool forms and profiles.* Burlington, VT: University of Vermont, Research Center for Children, Youth, & Families.

Brownell, R. (Ed.). (2000). *Expressive One-Word Picture Vocabulary Test (EOWPVT)* (3rd ed.). Novato, CA: Academic Therapy.

Cohen, J. A. (1960). A coefficient of agreement for nominal scales. *Educational and Psychological Measurement, 20,* 37–46.

Magner, M. E. (1972). *A Speech Intelligibility Test for Deaf Children.* Northampton, MA: Clarke School for the Deaf.

Nittrouer, S. (1996). The relation between speech perception and phonemic awareness: Evidence from low-SES children and children with chronic OM. *Journal of Speech and Hearing Research, 39,* 1059–1070.

Nittrouer, S., & Burton, L. T. (2005). The role of early language experience in the development of speech perception and phonological processing abilities: Evidence from 5-year-olds with histories of otitis media with effusion and low socioeconomic status. *Journal of Communication Disorders, 38,* 29–63.

Schiavetti, N., Metz, D. E., & Sitler, R. W. (1981). Construct validity of direct magnitude estimation and interval scaling of speech intelligibility: Evidence from a study of the hearing impaired. *Journal of Speech and Hearing Research, 24,* 441–445.

Wilcox, K., & Morris, S. (1999). *Children's Speech Intelligibility Measure.* San Antonio, TX: The Psychological Corporation.

Zimmerman, I. L., Steiner, V. G., & Pond, R. E. (2002). *Preschool Language Scale* (4th ed.). San Antonio, TX: The Psychological Corporation.

7

Language in the Real World: What We Learn from Natural Samples

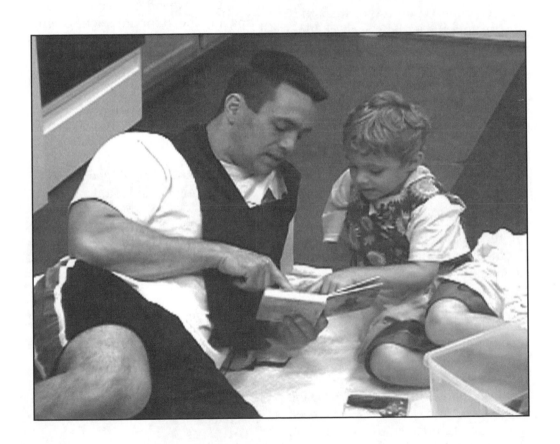

The most debilitating consequence of childhood hearing loss is that it disrupts language acquisition. Severely impaired language can isolate deaf children from family members. It can interfere with normal social relationships outside of the family, as well. It constrains children's abilities to succeed academically and so eventually follow desired career paths. These are the problems that pioneers in deaf education, such as Thomas Gallaudet and Alexander Graham Bell, hoped to solve, and the problems that we continue to struggle with today.

The primary purpose of this study was to investigate how well children with hearing loss are using language, spontaneously and in natural settings. The measures reported in Chapter 6 are important and help us address that purpose. But those measures were derived from clinical assessment tools, and so do not provide a picture of how children use language in natural settings. We really wanted to know how children with hearing loss who have been recipients of current technology are functioning when they are out and about in everyday settings, trying to negotiate their world using language. That meant that samples of children's language had to be collected in contexts as natural as could be obtained within an experimental paradigm.

Fortunately, procedures for obtaining natural language samples from a child, and subsequently categorizing the child's communicative acts, have been developed through studies of children with normal hearing (e.g., Coggins, Olswang, & Guthrie, 1987; Eisenberg, Fersko, & Lundgren, 2001; Wetherby, Cain, Yonclas, & Walker, 1988). In one experimental paradigm, a child and parent are videotaped interacting in as natural a setting as possible. Subse-

quently, experimenters review the tapes and categorize the individual communication acts according to function and form. We drew on these methods to develop a standard procedure for collecting and analyzing samples of children's language, modifying techniques as needed to ensure high levels of validity and reliability.

Sampling

In this study, we videotaped one parent sitting on the floor interacting with her child. Although the decision about which parent would participate in this activity was left up to the family, more than 95% of the time it was the mother. Toys available to the parent and child were consistent at all test sites, and were the following:

1. A felt board with felt people comprising a family and various pets
2. A set of small, plastic people comprising a family
3. A cell phone
4. A Teddy bear
5. A toy truck
6. The largely wordless book *Good Night Gorilla* by Peggy Rathmann (1994)
7. A set of see-through plastic blocks with little toys in the middle (peek-a-blocks)
8. A plastic tea set

When these materials were given to the parent, the instructions that accompanied them were that they (the parent and child) should play exactly as they do at home; they were not told explicitly that the recording being made with these toys would be used for evaluating the child's language. In general, parents knew that their children's language would be evaluated at the test sessions in which parent and child were participating, but these were long sessions. Several parts of each session were videotaped. The portion of each videotape used for deriving these measures of children's communicative attempts was just one part of the general videotaping procedures that occurred. So, although parents knew of the overall goals of the test procedures, they usually were unable to match specific test segments to specific dependent measures.

The dyad was videotaped for 21 minutes. Each videotape was made with a high-quality video camera. An FM transmitter and receiver were used in combination with the camera to ensure optimal audio signals. All recordings were made using a 48-kHz sampling rate with 16-bit resolution. To keep the FM transmitter in place the child wore a small vest with a pocket designed to hold the transmitter on the back.

Once a videotaped sample of a parent-child interaction arrived at the central site, 20 minutes of the sample (starting after the first minute) was transferred from the videotape to a DVD. A time code with 10-second observation intervals followed by 2-second scoring intervals was embedded in the visual display starting after the first minute, so there were 100 scoring intervals in all (5 per minute × 20 minutes; Figure 7–1). A visual code on-screen helped staff members keep track of scoring. For example, the code *8-2-O* indicated that it was the 8th minute of scoring, the second interval of the 8th minute, and that

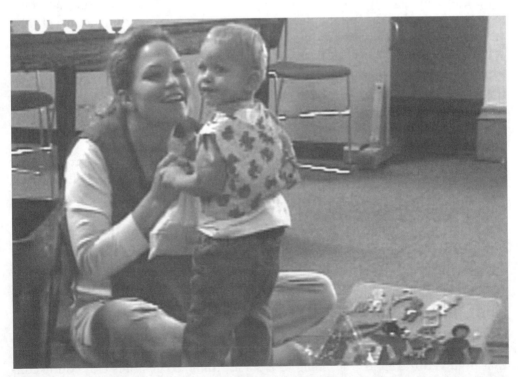

Figure 7–1. Parent and child playing during the videotaping of a natural language sample.

it was an observation interval, rather than a scoring interval. An *S* in the third position indicated scoring intervals. Different tones accompanied the ends of the observation intervals and the ends of the scoring intervals to serve as auditory cues as to what state the task was in.

Scoring

Two scorers independently watched each videotaped sample. Their responsibilities were to decide if the child communicated during each observation interval, and if so, how. They recorded their responses on paper forms during the scoring intervals. Each communicative act was coded for its function and for its form. Appendix B shows the decision tree that scorers used in evaluating these videotapes. The first decision that needed to be made was whether or not a behavior really fit the criterion of being communication. Not all sounds or manual acts emanating from a child are meant to communicate something to one's self or the communication partner. It was also necessary to have a consistent way of defining what constituted a discrete act. Separate communicative acts were generally discernible because they alternated with parental utterances. When they did not, separate acts were defined as those with at least 3 seconds of silence between one another.

There were 13 categories of communicative function that fell into three broader categories: (a) communicative acts that were *initiated* by the child and directed towards the parent; (b) acts that involved the child *responding* to a communication act initiated by the parent; and (c) acts that involved the child

talking to himself, babbling, talking to an object, pretending to talk to someone on the cell phone, or having dolls or toy animals talk to one another; these acts were *nondirected*. Appendix C lists the 13 categories of communicative functions under those three broad headings.

In terms of form, the scorer needed to evaluate whether the communication act involved a real word, a nonword vocalization, or a manual gesture only. The decision as to whether a spoken communication act should be scored as a real-word utterance or as a vocalization was tricky, and so was based on several considerations. First, an observed communication act was unambiguously recognized as a vocalization if it was a completely open, nonresonant production. Similarly, if the production was clearly a reduplicated or variegated babble, it was recorded as a vocalization. The majority of vocalizations met these descriptions. Ambiguity between real words and vocalizations arose for some of the more phonologically complex productions: The question became whether these were complex vocalizations or poor renditions of real words. In these cases, factors considered in deciding whether to score an utterance as including real words or vocalizations only were whether it was a phonetically consistent form with a clear referent through an entire recording session (if it was, it was recorded as a real word), and/or if the parent responded to the production with an obvious understanding that resulted in a definite action (if so, it was recorded as a real word). If there was even one real word in an utterance, it was coded as "real word."

Manual gestures included both signs and ritualized gestures that young children tend to use, such as reaching their hands out for an object that they want and alternately opening and closing their fingers. If a manual gesture accompanied an utterance consisting of real words or vocalizations, it was not scored as a gesture. A communicative act had to be completely nonvocal to be coded as "manual." The primary focus of this study was on the acquisition of spoken language, and so we were primarily interested in scoring vocal productions.

In summary, the procedure was that the scorer would observe a 10-second interval, and then pause the DVD. The decisions to be made were:

1. Did a communication act occur?
2. If so, was it directed to the parent or not?
3. If it was directed, was it initiated by the child or was the child responding to something the parent said?
4. What was the function of the act, according to the 13 categories provided?
5. What was the form of the communication act? Was it a vocalization, a real word (or string of words), or a manual gesture?

After the paper scoring was complete, two other individuals entered the recorded data for each scorer into the database independently. A software utility compared entered data between the two individuals responsible for entering data for one scorer on an interval-by-interval basis. At this point, if a discrepancy was found in data entry for a single scorer it was corrected by going back to the paper form to see what that scorer had written. This routine ensured that data were entered according to how they had been recorded on paper.

Reliability between the two scorers was checked for each participant. *Occur-*

rence reliability was used in this study and was computed on an interval-by-interval basis. Occurrence reliability differs from *agreement* reliability, with the latter more typically used. The difference in these techniques is that occurrence reliability evaluates reliability only when one or the other scorer judges that a behavior occurred, whereas agreement reliability includes intervals in which both scorers agreed that the behavior did not occur. Figure 7–2 illustrates all possible combinations of scoring across the two scorers. Using the cell descriptions from Figure 7–2, the general formula for scoring agreement reliability is:

$$R = (A + D) / (A + B + C + D)$$

That formula inflates reliability scores when behaviors are not frequently occurring (Kent & Foster, 1977). The formula for occurrence reliability, used here, is:

$$R = A / (A + B + C)$$

The difference between these methods is apparent if one considers a result in

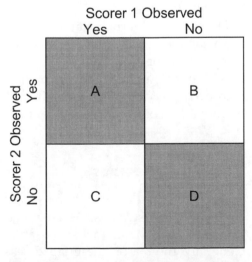

Figure 7–2. Grid used for computation of inter-rater reliability during scoring of unstructured language samples.

which the proportion of responses falling into each of cells A, B, and C is .05, and the proportion of responses falling into D is .85. Using the first formula, a reliability coefficient of .90 would be obtained; using the second formula, a reliability coefficient of .33 would be obtained. Thus, occurrence reliability is the more rigorous of the two, and that is what we used.

For each videotape scored, reliability between the two scorers was checked. If reliability for the 39 possible combinations of function/form codes was less than 60%, that videotape was viewed by all laboratory staff. Discussion of the troublesome communication acts helped to establish and maintain standards for scoring. Any videotape falling below the 60% reliability criterion was rescored by two independent scorers after group discussion. This process of discussing how to score tapes was particularly useful when videotapes for a specific test age were initially being scored, because children's communicative styles changed as they got older. New issues arose with the scoring of each new test age.

For statistical purposes in this study, the mean raw number of each behavior recorded by the two scorers was used. However, the numbers of occurrences recorded by each scorer rarely differed by more than one observation, if at all.

Results

Across all test sessions, 22 language samples were found to be unusable. Generally, the reason these taped sessions could not be scored was that they were not a full 21 minutes long, but other problems included finding a bad audio track (because the FM transmitter was not set up properly) or a poor video recording (because the taping was done in front of a window or the lens cap was left on).

Total Communication Acts

Mean reliability across all participants at all test ages for whether a communication act occurred or not was 93.7%. This is quite good, and so was considered acceptable.

Table 7–1 shows the mean numbers of total communication acts for each group at each test age. In this chapter, all tables are provided at the end. Figure 7–3 illustrates these results for the six groups of children with hearing loss. In this and all subsequent figures our own data are used to mark plus/minus one standard deviation (*SD*) from means for children with normal hearing. The FIRST ANOVA performed on these data showed that there was a significant effect of hearing status, $F(1, 635)$ = 46.13, $p < .001$. Children with normal hearing attempted to communicate more often than children with early-identified hearing loss, but the difference was not great: Across all test ages and both signing conditions, mean number of communication attempts was 123.6 (*SD* = 45.3) for children with normal hearing, and 114.3 (*SD* = 41.3) for children with early-identified hearing loss. (Means for children with late-identified hearing loss cannot be compared to means across test ages for the other groups because they were only tested at older ages, and so results are weighted to higher scores.) No statistically significant differences were found in analyses

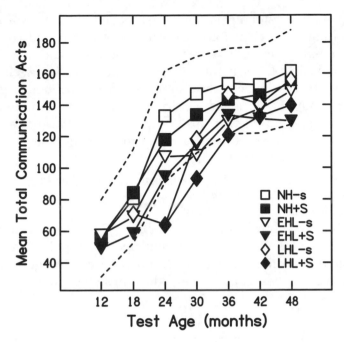

Figure 7–3. Mean numbers of total communication acts for each group at each test age for children with normal hearing and children with early-identified hearing loss: NH–s (normal hearing, no signs); NH+S (normal hearing, signs); EHL–s (early-identified hearing loss, no signs); EHL+S (early-identified hearing loss, signs); LHL–s (late-identified hearing loss, no signs); and LHL+S (late-identified hearing loss, signs). In this and all subsequent figures in this chapter, dotted lines show +/– one standard deviation from the mean, according to data from children with normal hearing in this study.

of the numbers of total communication acts done on data only from children with hearing loss. Thus, we may conclude that children in all groups defined by hearing loss attempted to communicate equally often.

Because of this slight difference in overall numbers of communicative acts between children with normal hearing and with hearing loss, we considered using proportions of each type of act to total numbers of acts in statistical analyses of function and form. However, it quickly became apparent that

using proportions did not change any outcomes, and so doing so only needlessly complicated the reporting of these data. Consequently, we report outcomes of statistical analyses performed on raw numbers.

Communicative Functions

Examining the functions that communication served for these children separately from the forms of the communication acts was an important goal of this work. We understood from the start that finding a deficit in one or the other area, but not in both, would explain a great deal about the nature of the deficit faced by children with hearing loss, and about how to intervene. Were we studying children with disorders from the autism spectrum, for example, we might expect the children to show significant deficits in the area of communicative function; the form of their communication attempts might be accurate, though slightly delayed for their ages.

To examine the functions that communication served for these children we first looked at the three supraordinate categories of initiated communication acts, responses, and nondirected communication acts. Mean reliability across all test ages and both signing conditions was 77.7% for judging in which supraordinate category an act fit. This was considered to be good agreement.

Communication Initiated by the Child

Table 7–2 shows mean numbers of initiated communication acts for each group at each test age, and Figure 7–4 illustrates these numbers for the six

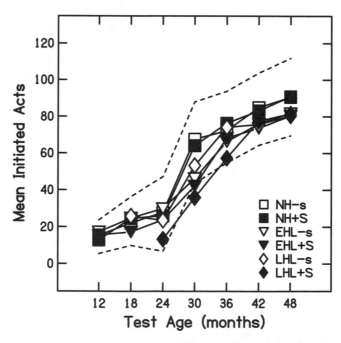

Figure 7–4. Mean numbers of initiated communication acts for each group at each test age for children with normal hearing and children with early-identified hearing loss: NH–s (normal hearing, no signs); NH+S (normal hearing, signs); EHL–s (early-identified hearing loss, no signs); EHL+S (early-identified hearing loss, signs); LHL–s (late-identified hearing loss, no signs); and LHL+S (late-identified hearing loss, signs).

groups of children. These results look similar to those for total communication acts: Children with hearing loss initiated communication only slightly less often than did children with normal hearing. Outcomes of the statistical analyses were similar to those for total communication acts, as well: For the FIRST ANOVA, there was a significant main effect of hearing status, $F(1, 635) = 16.11$, $p < .001$, but nothing else. Again, there were no differences found in the numbers of initiated communication acts for children with hearing loss depending on age of ID or sign use. It may appear from Figure 7–4 that signing children with late-identified hearing loss were initiating communication less often than other children, but that is primarily seen for young ages. It will be recalled that statistical analyses involving only children with hearing loss are done on data from 30 to 48 months of age. Certainly by 3 years of age it is clear that children in all groups were trying to initiate communication with their parents to similar extents.

Children's Responses

Table 7–3 shows mean numbers of responses for each group at each test age, and Figure 7–5 illustrates these numbers for children with normal hearing

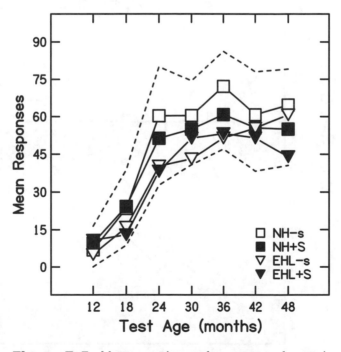

Figure 7–5. Mean numbers of responses for each group at each test age for children with normal hearing and children with early-identified hearing loss: NH–s (normal hearing, no signs); NH+S (normal hearing, signs); EHL–s (early-identified hearing loss, no signs); EHL+S (early-identified hearing loss, signs).

and with early-identified hearing loss. The FIRST ANOVA revealed a significant effect of hearing status, $F(1, 635) = 31.69, p < .001$, which mirrors what was found for the numbers of initiated communication acts. No other differences were found for these children.

These sorts of communication acts showed differences among the children with hearing loss. Figure 7–6 shows the numbers of communication acts categorized as responses for children with early- and late-identified hearing loss separately, coded according to whether the children use signs or not and what kind of prosthesis they wore. To start with, the SECOND ANOVA uncovered a significant main effect of signs, $F(1, 291) = 8.75, p = .003$, as well as a significant Age of ID × Signs interaction, $F(1, 291) = 3.98, p = .047$. A SEA was done examining scores for early- and late-identified

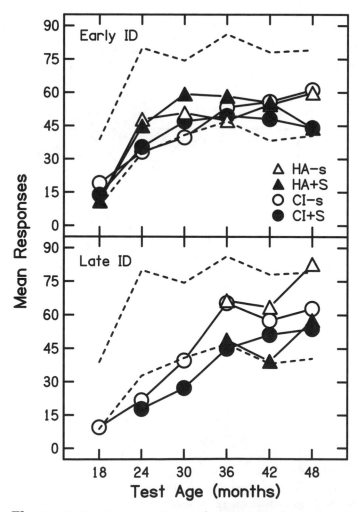

Figure 7–6. Mean numbers of responses for children with hearing loss only: HA–s (hearing aids, no signs); HA+S (hearing aids, signs); CI–s (cochlear implants, no signs); and CI+S (cochlear implants, signs).

children separately with signs, prosthesis, and test age as main effects. (Results of analyses looking at the age-of-ID effect separately for signing and non-signing children will no longer be reported. It should be apparent by now that those analyses provide the same information that is provided when we examine the sign effect for early- and late-identified children separately.) In this analysis, the only effect that was significant was the main effect of signs for the late-identified children with hearing loss, $F(1, 275) = 9.47, p = .002$. As was found for language measures reported in Chapter 6, children with late-identified hearing loss who used signs were generally performing more poorly than the other children with hearing loss. Here it was found that they responded to their parents less often than did other children with hearing loss. This difference is apparent in Figure 7–6.

Nondirected Communication

Table 7–4 shows mean numbers of non-directed communication acts for each group at each test age, and Figure 7–7 illustrates these numbers. The most interesting aspect of these numbers is the precipitous nature with which these behaviors decline across test ages. Before conducting this study we had expected

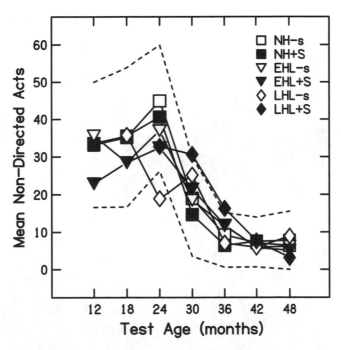

Figure 7–7. Mean numbers of nondirected communication acts for each group at each test age for children with normal hearing and children with early-identified hearing loss: NH–s (normal hearing, no signs); NH+S (normal hearing, signs); EHL–s (early-identified hearing loss, no signs); EHL+S (early-identified hearing loss, signs); LHL–s (late-identified hearing loss, no signs); and LHL+S (late-identified hearing loss, signs).

that there might have been more pretend play at older test ages, especially for children with normal hearing, but that was not found to be the case. Perhaps having a communication partner present in the form of a parent diminished the amount of pretend play exhibited by the children; perhaps there would have been more pretend play if the partner had been another child or if the child had been playing alone. Those are questions left for future studies to examine. Here we find that the numbers of nondirected communication acts were similar across all groups. No significant effects, other than test age, were observed in the statistical analyses.

Linguistic Form

The forms of children's communication acts were examined next: Did these acts consist of real words, vocalizations only, or manual gestures only?

Manual-Only Communication

The numbers of communication acts consisting of only manual gestures were analyzed. Table 7–5 shows numbers of manual-only communication acts for each group at each test age, and Figure 7–8 illustrates these numbers for children with normal hearing and with early-identified hearing loss.

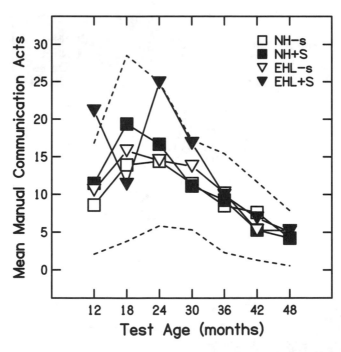

Figure 7–8. Mean numbers of manual-only communication acts for each group at each test age for children with normal hearing and children with early-identified hearing loss: NH–s (normal hearing, no signs); NH+S (normal hearing, signs); EHL–s (early-identified hearing loss, no signs); EHL+S (early-identified hearing loss, signs).

Over roughly the first half of all test sessions it is apparent that signing children produced more communication acts that consisted of manual gestures only. However, this trend is highly confounded by the large dip in manual-only communication acts observed for signing children with early-identified hearing loss at 18 months of age. On first consideration, this appears to be a spurious point in the developmental trajectory, but that data point at 18 months represents results of 13 children, and variability was not large for that group at that test age. We considered possible explanations for that dip, but in the end were never able to explain it.

Whatever the explanation, the dip in the numbers of manual-only communication acts observed at 18 months for signing children with early-identified hearing loss complicated statistical analyses. Table 7–5 shows that signing children with normal hearing consistently produced more manual-only communication acts than nonsigning children with normal hearing up to 24 months of age; after that the numbers are similar for the two groups. For children with early-identified hearing loss, this discrepancy between signing and nonsigning children exists through 30 months, except for the dip at 18 months. Because of these differences at the early test ages, a significant effect of signs was observed in the FIRST ANOVA, $F(1, 635) = 9.59$, $p = .002$, for children with normal hearing and those with early-identified hearing loss. There was no Hearing Status × Signs interaction. This outcome was not surprising: Children whose parents signed to them produced more manual gestures. Additionally, there were significant two-way interactions and the three-way interaction of Hearing Status

× Signs × Test Age was significant, but these interactions undoubtedly reflect the 18-month dip for the signing children with early-identified hearing loss.

Figure 7–9 shows the mean numbers of manual-only communication acts for all children with hearing loss. This figure illustrates the finding that the late-identified children who used signs did not show a particularly great number of communication acts consisting only of manual gestures. Consequently, the emerging pattern of results showing that signing children with late-identified hearing loss are behind other children, even those with hearing loss, on all measures of spoken language development cannot be attributed to their using signs more than other children: They were not signing without vocalizing any more often than other children were gesturing without vocalizing.

In the SECOND ANOVA, there was a significant main effect of signs, $F(1, 291) = 5.30$, $p = .022$, and this result reflects similar trends for early- and late-identified children: Those in the signing groups used slightly more manual-only gestures, particularly at the younger test ages. These differences were small, however. In fact, when a SEA was done on the numbers of manual-only communication acts for early- and late-identified children separately with signs, prosthesis, and test age as main effects, the effect of signs was not significant for either group.

In summary, we found that children whose parents signed to them communicated more frequently through the use of manual gestures only, albeit not by much. In addition, we found that children whose parents signed to them as infants decreased their use of manual communication as they got older. We

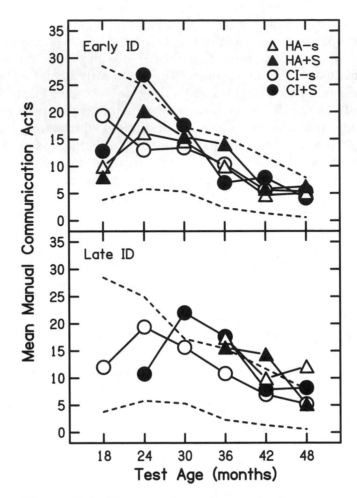

Figure 7–9. Mean numbers of manual-only communication acts for children with hearing loss only: HA–s (hearing aids, no signs); HA+S (hearing aids, signs); CI–s (cochlear implants, no signs); and CI+S (cochlear implants, signs).

saw in Chapter 4 that many of these hearing parents gradually diminished their own use of signs with their children, and here we see that children's use of manual communication independent of spoken language similarly diminished. It may simply be that in homes where spoken language is the customary means of communication there is not sufficient environmental support for manual communication for its use to continue once a child starts being able to use spoken language to any degree at all.

Real-Word Utterances

The second kind of linguistic form examined was the numbers of communication acts involving real words. Table 7–6 shows the mean numbers of communication acts that contained real words for each group at each test age. Figure 7–10 illustrates these numbers for children with normal hearing and with early-identified hearing loss. Here we see the same pattern of results found in Chapter 6 for the language-related measures of auditory comprehension, expressive vocabulary, and speech intelligibility: Children with early-identified hearing loss trail their peers with normal hearing in the acquisition of this skill, and there is little difference within these groups depending on whether children were signing or not. The FIRST ANOVA revealed only a significant main effect of hearing status, $F(1, 635) = 97.39$, $p < .001$. The Hearing Status × Test Age interaction was also significant,

$F(1, 635) = 4.54$, $p < .001$, indicating that developmental trajectories were different for children with normal hearing and for those with early-identified hearing loss. In particular, the numbers of real-word communication acts appears to plateau for children with normal hearing after roughly 36 months of age. This trend likely indicates that there is an upper limit to the number of times a person can say something within a 20-minute period. In addition to limits imposed purely by sampling time, that number may be constrained by the fact that children's productions were getting longer as children get older and acquired better syntactic skills. This effect will be examined in Chapter 8.

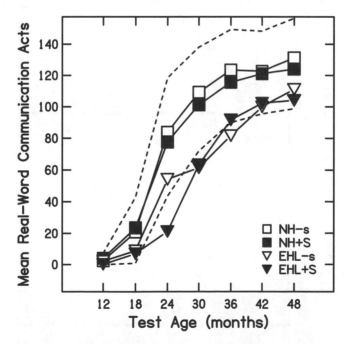

Figure 7–10. Mean numbers of real-word communication acts for each group at each test age for children with normal hearing and children with early-identified hearing loss: NH–s (normal hearing, no signs); NH+S (normal hearing, signs); EHL–s (early-identified hearing loss, no signs); EHL+S (early-identified hearing loss, signs).

Figure 7–11 displays the mean numbers of real-word utterances for children with early- and late-identified hearing loss separately, as a function of whether they used signs and the type of prosthesis they used. Again, trends similar to those reported in Chapter 6 are evident: There is little difference among children with early-identified hearing loss, but there appears to be a very strong effect of using signs for children with late-identified hearing loss. The

SECOND ANOVA, done on numbers from children with hearing loss only, showed two significant main effects: age of ID, $F(1, 291) = 11.55$, $p = .001$, and signs, $F(1, 291) = 21.09$, $p < .001$. The Age of ID × Signs interaction was also significant, $F(1, 291) = 24.73$, $p < .001$. A SEA done on the numbers of real-word utterances for early- and late-identified children separately with signs, prosthesis, and test age as main effects revealed a significant effect of signs for late-identified

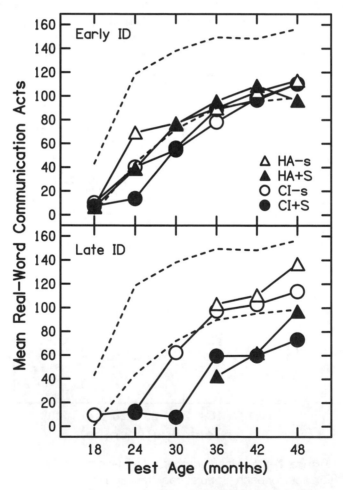

Figure 7–11. Mean numbers of real-word communication acts for children with hearing loss only: HA–s (hearing aids, no signs); HA+S (hearing aids, signs); CI–s (cochlear implants, no signs); and CI+S (cochlear implants, signs).

children, $F(1, 275) = 22.49, p < .001$. There were no other significant main effects or interactions for either group.

In summary, children's use of real words to communicate their wants, needs, and ideas increased dramatically from 12 to 48 months of age. At 12 months none of these children were using real words in natural communication settings. For children with normal hearing, real-word productions increased precipitously over the next 2 years, reaching a plateau at roughly 36 months of age. Children with hearing loss were slower in their growth of real-word communication acts: All children with early-identified hearing loss and those with late-identified hearing loss who did not use signs followed a trajectory that had the means for their groups at just one standard deviation below the mean for children with normal hearing. Children with late-identified hearing loss who used signs were much slower in their acquisition of real-word communications.

Vocalizations

The third and last linguistic form examined with these language samples was nonword vocalizations. Table 7–7 shows the mean numbers of communication acts that consisted only of vocalizations for each group at each test age. Figure 7–12 illustrates these numbers for children with normal hearing and those with early-identified hearing loss.

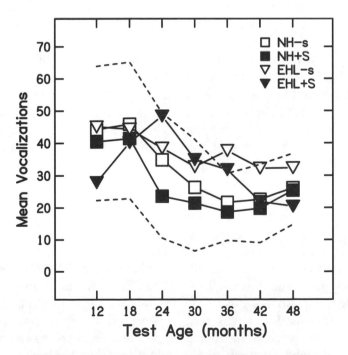

Figure 7–12. Mean numbers of vocalizations for each group at each test age for children with normal hearing and children with early-identified hearing loss: NH–s (normal hearing, no signs); NH+S (normal hearing, signs); EHL–s (early-identified hearing loss, no signs); EHL+S (early-identified hearing loss, signs).

Here, for the first time, we see a trend that differs from what has been reported so far. Here we see that children with hearing loss were producing more of this kind of communication than were children with normal hearing, at least during many of the test sessions. For children with normal hearing, the numbers of nonword vocalizations decreased after 18 months of age, but that was not so for children with hearing loss. For this measure the FIRST ANOVA revealed a significant effect of hearing status, $F(1, 635) = 11.13$, $p = .001$, as well as a significant Hearing Status × Test Age interaction, $F(1, 635) = 3.14$, $p = .005$. Children with early-identified hearing loss produced more pure vocalizations than children with normal hearing, and the pattern of change over test sessions was different for these two groups of children: The decline in vocalizations occurred earlier and was more precipitous for children with normal hearing.

This FIRST ANOVA also produced one result that was unexpected: There was a significant main effect of signs, $F(1, 635) = 9.03$, $p = .003$. The Hearing Status × Signs interaction was not significant. Regardless of whether children had normal hearing or hearing loss, those who used signs were producing fewer vocalizations than those who did not. This effect is consistent across test ages for children with normal hearing, but apparent only at older ages for children with early-identified hearing loss. We are unable to explain this effect. One explanation we considered was that children who do not learn signs during these early years may be more likely to communicate wants and needs with nonword vocalizations. Children who know even a few signs, on the other hand, can use those signs to make those wants and needs known. However, the numbers of manual-only communication acts do not support that hypothesis: Signing children did not use manual-only gestures much more frequently than nonsigning children during the 20-minute language sample. All we can think is that it may have involved more global learning: Perhaps signing children just never developed a communication strategy of using vocalizations because they had those signs available to them.

Figure 7–13 shows mean numbers of communication acts consisting only of nonword vocalizations for children with early- and late-identified hearing loss separately. It is apparent for children with early-identified hearing loss that those who received cochlear implants produced more pure vocalizations than children who wore hearing aids for much of the study. For children with late-identified hearing loss we find an outcome that contradicts what was observed for children with normal hearing and early-identified hearing loss: There is a strong trend for signing children to communicate with vocalizations only. The SECOND ANOVA, done on data from children with hearing loss only, resulted in two significant main effects: age of ID, $F(1, 291) = 28.14$, $p < .001$, and signs, $F(1, 291) = 8.30$, $p = .004$. The Age of ID × Signs interaction was also significant, $F(1, 291) = 26.45$, $p < .001$. The SEA performed on these vocalizations for children with early- and late-identified hearing loss, using signs, prosthesis, and test age as main effects, identified the source of this interaction: A significant sign effect was found for the late-identified children only, $F(1, 275) = 16.35$, $p < .001$. No other significant effects or interactions were found for this

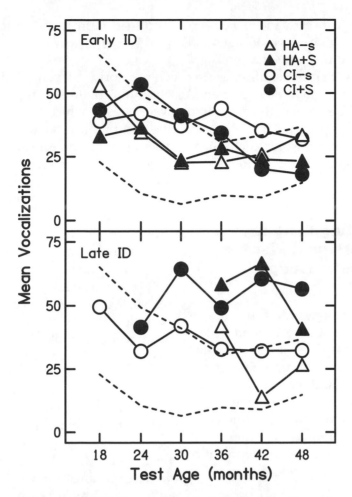

Figure 7–13. Mean numbers of vocalizations for children with hearing loss only: HA–s (hearing aids, no signs); HA+S (hearing aids, signs); CI–s (cochlear implants, no signs); and CI+S (cochlear implants, signs).

group. For children with early-identified hearing loss, the main effect of signs was not significant, suggesting that the main effect found in the FIRST ANOVA may have been largely driven by a sign effect for children with normal hearing. However, the prosthesis effect was significant in this SEA, $F(1, 275) = 4.54$, $p = .034$. Of the children whose hearing loss was identified early, those who received cochlear implants communi-cated with pure vocalizations longer through their toddler years than did the children who continued to use hearing aids only.

In summary, this measure of pure vocalizations showed trends that were mirror images of all other language-related measures reported thus far: Children with normal hearing decreased the numbers of this kind of production sooner than did children with hearing loss. Children with early-identified hearing loss, both those who used signs and those who did not, as well as nonsigning children with late-identified hearing loss, showed similar developmental trajectories. The late-identified children who used signs persisted in their use of high numbers of nonword vocalizations through the entire study period.

Putting Language Functions under the Microscope

Chapter 8 examines the form of children's communication in more detail. That chapter is devoted to examining communication acts consisting of real words or vocalizations. In this section, the nature of communicative functions is examined more closely in the belief that why children are communicating may tell us about the development of communicative capacities in general.

Nondirected Communication, under the Microscope

Earlier in this chapter we found that communication generally served the same functions for children with normal hearing and for those with hearing loss. Looking first at the numbers of nondirected communication acts used by children, we found no differences: The numbers of nondirected communication acts were few at all test ages and similar across all groups. Therefore, the individual acts comprising the supraordinate category of nondirected communication were not examined further.

Initiated Communication, under the Microscope

The majority of communication acts observed in these language samples were ones in which the child initiated the communication with the parent. There were some differences between children with normal hearing and those with hearing loss, but these differences were not great: The mean numbers of initiated communication acts for all groups of children with hearing loss were well within one standard deviation of the numbers found for children with normal hearing. That finding is reassuring; we would have expected a very different result for children with autism, for example. Instead, we find that these children with hearing loss were trying to communicate with their parents every bit as much as were their peers with normal hearing.

Because the majority of communication acts observed in this study were ones initiated by the child, however, we were curious as to whether children differed with regard to the specific kind of initiated communication. Therefore, we looked at the numbers of each kind of act listed under Child-Initiated Communications in Appendix C: requests for objects, requests for actions, rejections/protests, directed comments, inquiries, and routines. When these individual acts were examined, it was found that the categories of requests for actions, directed comments, and inquiries accounted for 84% of all initiated communication acts across all test ages. Only these three kinds of initiated communication were ever observed more than five times in a single recording session.

Table 7–8, Table 7–9, and Table 7–10 show mean numbers of each of these kinds of initiated communication: directed comments, requests for action, and inquiries. Figure 7–14, Figure 7–15, and Figure 7–16 illustrate these results. In these figures, means for all six groups are shown on the same plot. Quite clearly, directed comments (Figure 7–14) accounted for the greatest proportion of all initiated communication, at all test ages. Between 60 and 75% of all communication initiated by children consisted of a child commenting to his parent about an activity the pair was doing together, or an object they were looking at jointly. And quite clearly, there is very little difference in the numbers of directed comments across the six groups of children: Chil-

dren with normal hearing produced a few more directed comments than children with hearing loss, but that was the only effect found. In the FIRST ANOVA, the main effect of hearing status was significant, $F(1, 635) = 12.98$, $p < .001$.

Requests for action (Figure 7–15) reveal just one pattern found in previously reported measures: Signing children with late-identified hearing loss produced the fewest of this kind of communication act. In the SEA, late-identified signers were found to produce fewer requests for action than late-identified nonsigners, $F(1, 275) = 15.96$, $p < .001$. No differences among other groups were observed.

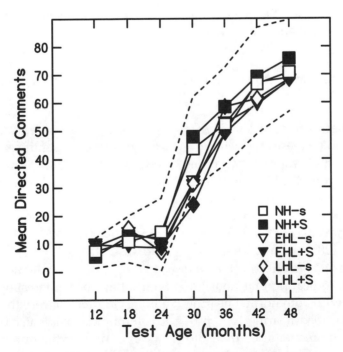

Figure 7–14. Mean numbers of directed comments for each group at each test age: NH–s (normal hearing, no signs); NH+S (normal hearing, signs); EHL–s (early-identified hearing loss, no signs); EHL+S (early-identified hearing loss, signs); LHL–s (late-identified hearing loss, no signs); and LHL+S (late-identified hearing loss, signs).

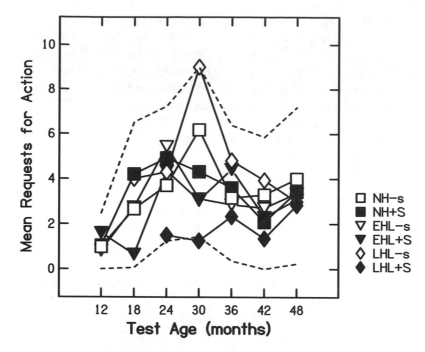

Figure 7–15. Mean numbers of requests for action for each group at each test age: NH–s (normal hearing, no signs); NH+S (normal hearing, signs); EHL–s (early-identified hearing loss, no signs); EHL+S (early-identified hearing loss, signs); LHL–s (late-identified hearing loss, no signs); and LHL+S (late-identified hearing loss, signs).

The numbers of inquiries (Figure 7–16) produced by these children show a closer pattern of results to what has been found before. Children with normal hearing produced the most inquiries. In the FIRST ANOVA there was a significant main effect of hearing status, $F(1, 635) = 32.28$, $p < .001$. There was also a significant sign effect, $F(1, 635) = 5.10$, $p = .024$, indicating that nonsigning children, with both normal hearing and early-identified hearing loss, produced a few more inquiries than did signing children. Children in three of the four hearing loss groups (early-identified signers and nonsigners alike and late-identified nonsigners) were comparable in the numbers of inquiries they used. Signing children with late-identified hearing loss asked the fewest questions of their parents, indicated by the finding of a significant difference between late-identified signers and non-signers, $F(1, 275) = 3.75$, $p = .054$.

Responses, under the Microscope

Some of the most interesting differences among children concern their responses to communication initiated by the parent.

We found that the numbers of times that children simply acknowledged something their parents said were consistent across groups: Between 60 and 90% of all responses were simple acknowledgments, and this number was similar for all groups. This kind of communication act, of acknowledging that a communica-

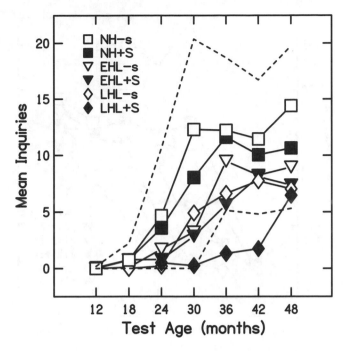

Figure 7–16. Mean numbers of inquiries for each group at each test age: NH–s (normal hearing, no signs); NH+S (normal hearing, signs); EHL–s (early-identified hearing loss, no signs); EHL+S (early-identified hearing loss, signs); LHL–s (late-identified hearing loss, no signs); and LHL+S (late-identified hearing loss, signs).

tion partner has said something, is basic, and so it won't be discussed further.

Answers, on the other hand, require the speaker to understand what the communication partner said, and generate an appropriate response. Table 7–11 shows the mean numbers of answers across each test age, for each group, and Figure 7–17 illustrates these numbers for all groups. Here we see the pattern found in many other language measures: Children with normal hearing produced the most answers: In the FIRST ANOVA there was a significant main effect of hearing status, $F(1, 635) = 35.07, p < .001$. Children in three of the four hearing loss groups (early-identified signers and nonsigners, and late-identified nonsigners) were comparable in the numbers of an-

swers they produced, but they produced fewer than children with normal hearing. Signing children with late-identified hearing loss were least likely to provide an answer to their parents. In the SEA for children with late-identified hearing loss, there was a significant sign effect, $F(1, 275) = 7.19, p = .008$.

Finally, the number of times children imitated their parents' communication acts was examined. In Chapter 2 it was explained that imitations are important language learning devices at the early stages of acquisition, but eventually children need to begin generating their own language. It is not absolutely necessary to understand what the communication partner said in order to imitate it. Table 7–12 shows the mean numbers

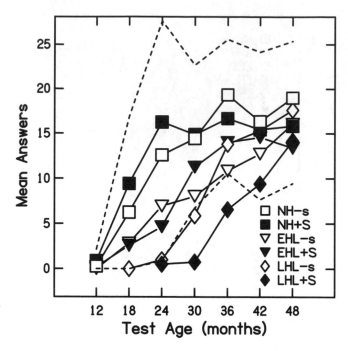

Figure 7–17. Mean numbers of answers for each group at each test age: NH–s (normal hearing, no signs); NH+S (normal hearing, signs); EHL–s (early-identified hearing loss, no signs); EHL+S (early-identified hearing loss, signs); LHL–s (late-identified hearing loss, no signs); and LHL+S (late-identified hearing loss, signs).

of imitations children produced across each test age, and Figure 7–18 illustrates these numbers for all groups. There are clear curvilinear functions in these numbers, and the age at which these functions reach a maximum differs across groups: Children with normal hearing reach that maximum first, followed by children with hearing loss who were identified early, and lastly by children with late-identified hearing loss.

One effect involving imitation was particularly intriguing: It appears as if there is a signing effect for children with normal hearing. In fact, the FIRST ANOVA supports this observation. There was a main effect of signs, $F(1, 635) = 8.57$, $p = .004$, and the SEA done on data from children with normal hearing and those with early-identified hearing loss separately revealed a significant sign effect only for children with normal hearing, $F(1, 635) = 6.19$, $p = .013$. Among children with normal hearing, those who used signs imitated their parents' vocal productions less often than did children who did not use signs.

One other finding is intriguing, and potentially very informative: Nonsigning children with late-identified hearing loss have the highest peak. It appears as if they engaged in a great deal of imitation shortly after having their hearing loss identified. This behavior may have had a facilitative effect that helped them catch up in their language learning to children with hearing loss that was identified early.

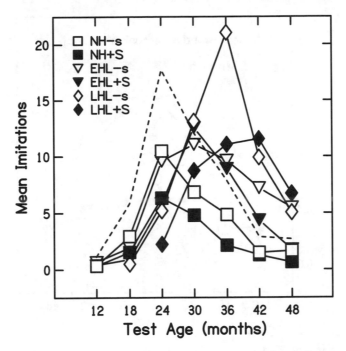

Figure 7–18. Mean numbers of imitations for each group at each test age: NH–s (normal hearing, no signs); NH+S (normal hearing, signs); EHL–s (early-identified hearing loss, no signs); EHL+S (early-identified hearing loss, signs); LHL–s (late-identified hearing loss, no signs); and LHL+S (late-identified hearing loss, signs).

Effect Sizes

Cohen's *d* was computed for four measures that showed significant effects of hearing loss: numbers of real-word utterances, vocalizations, answers, and imitations. Figure 7–19 shows these values for each test age. The numbers of real-word communication acts show the strongest effects, with the largest of those effects occurring at 30 months, a trend that matches the fact that there is an S-shape to this developmental trajectory. Children in all groups produced few real-word utterances at the earliest test ages, and children with normal hearing reached a plateau starting at 36 months. Consequently, children

with hearing loss were able to close the gap after that. Cohen's *d* for answers shows a similar trend because there was an S-shape to the developmental trajectory for these communication acts, as well. Cohen's *d* for imitations shows that this metric becomes more sensitive to differences between children with normal hearing and those with hearing loss as they get older. Overall effect sizes were not particularly large for vocalizations. However, this measure is interesting because it is one behavior of only two (the other being imitations) that occurs in higher numbers for children with hearing loss than for children with normal hearing. In addition, vocalizations can take on many forms. Differences in those forms might inform us about

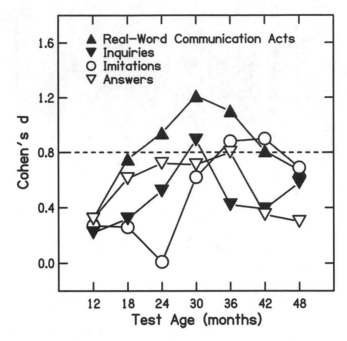

Figure 7–19. Cohen's *d*s for each test age for numbers of real-word communication acts, inquiries, imitations, and answers. Cohen's *d*s were computed for mean scores from children with normal hearing and those with early-identified hearing loss, across nonsigners and signers.

language acquisition in children with hearing loss, and how that acquisition differs from acquisition for children with normal hearing. More will be said on this in Chapter 8.

Correlations with Independent Variables

One sensitive measure derived from these natural language samples was the number of communication acts consisting of real words. This measure is used in subsequent chapters to explore more specific trends regarding these children. Precisely because it is used as a metric of language advancement, we wanted to

examine the extent to which variability in this measure was explained by independent variables. Therefore, we computed correlation coefficients between numbers of real-word utterances and SES for children with normal hearing. For children with hearing loss, we computed these correlation coefficients between numbers of real-word utterances and SES, BE-PTA, ID-age, and numbers of intervention visits, both before and after 36 months of age. These correlations were computed for real-word scores at 30 months of age, when this measure was most sensitive to differences between children with normal hearing and with hearing loss, and at 48 months of age, the last test age in this study. None of these independent variables was found to explain even a modest amount of variance in the numbers of real-word communication acts that children in this study produced, at either test age. For example, r for real-word utterances and BE-PTA was −.155 at 30 months of age and −.076 at 48 months of age. Apparently, factors unrelated to the degree of hearing loss a child has, his SES, or the age at which his hearing loss was identified can explain how well that child learns to use real words in communication. In subsequent chapters, we examine factors that might explain this variability.

Longitudinal Results

The number of communicative acts consisting of real words was another measure (in addition to auditory comprehension) that we submitted to careful scrutiny to ensure that the outcomes we were obtaining with our samples were not somehow different from what we might have obtained if we had insisted on including data only from participants who were in every test session. Figure 7–20 shows the numbers of

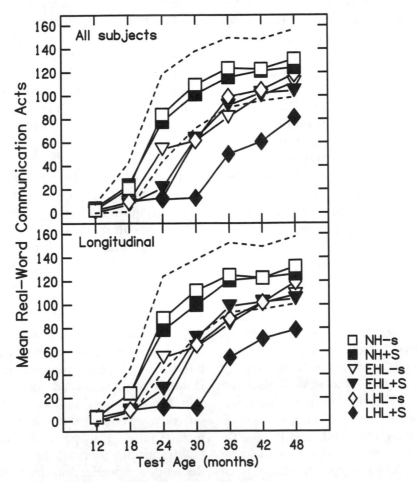

Figure 7–20. Mean numbers of real-word communication acts for all children participating in this study (*top*), and for only those who participated in at least four test sessions (*bottom*).

real-word communication acts for all participants and just for those children who participated in four or more test sessions. Developmental trajectories are strikingly similar, and so we conclude that these outcomes were not affected by allowing participants to miss test sessions if they needed to.

Chapter Summary

This chapter has explored the characteristics of the language that children in this study produced in natural settings. The function and form of that language were examined. Generally speaking, communication served the same functions for all children: those with normal hearing and those with hearing loss; those whose parents signed to them, and those whose parents never did. Apparently, the drive to communicate was similar for all these children.

There were slight differences observed, however, when specific communicative functions were examined. Simply requesting an object, directing a parent's attention to an object or event, or acknowledging that the parent had communicated something were actions that all children performed with the same frequency. However, acts that required more linguistic sophistication and necessitated that a spoken utterance be generated in a more thoughtful manner, such as answers, were observed less frequently for children with hearing loss. Of those children, these sorts of acts were observed least frequently for those with late-identified hearing loss who used signs. The category of imitated communication acts showed perhaps the most interesting differences across groups: Children in all groups displayed growth in the numbers of imitations over the early test sessions, with a subsequent decline over the later sessions. What differed across groups was the age at which these numbers reached a maximum: Those children who were acquiring language at a faster rate, according to other language measures, produced their maximum number of imitations at younger ages. After that, language production became more generative. Among children with normal hearing, signing children generally imitated less than nonsigning children.

The forms of these linguistic functions were also examined. Although signing children, both those with normal hearing and those with hearing loss, produced more manual gestures unaccompanied by vocal production, the difference was not large. Communication consisting of real-word utterances showed what has come to be predictable patterns: Children with hearing loss used real-word utterances less frequently in their communications than did children with normal hearing, with the late-identified, signing children showing the fewest real-word utterances. This trend is important because quite obviously a child cannot develop syntax and grammar until he has mastered the task of using real words in communicative attempts. By contrast, the numbers of communicative acts consisting of pure vocalizations showed the inverse pattern: The highest numbers of vocalizations were observed for the late-identified, signing children, and the fewest were observed for children with normal hearing. In particular, signing children with normal hearing produced pure vocalizations least often of all groups.

By now, several trends are starting to emerge consistently in the data generated by this study—some of them good, and some not so good. The first trend that should be noted is that children with hearing loss, even those with only moderate losses that were identified early in life, are generally not keeping up with their peers with normal hearing in language acquisition. Is this the best we can hope for, that children with hearing loss will be, on average, one standard deviation below their normal-hearing peers? Or is there more we can be doing? By examining language outcomes in more detail in the chapters that follow, we find evidence to help answer these questions.

Regarding type of prosthesis, children who receive implants are showing performance close to that of their peers who use hearing aids. This is indeed one of the good findings to come out of this study because the children who received implants had poorer unaided BE-PTAs than children who used hearing aids. Complementary to that finding, we have found no evidence that unaided auditory sensitivity explains language outcomes for these children. If a child has a hearing loss that is significant enough to interfere with language acquisition at all, factors unrelated to the degree of that loss explain language learning. Subsequent chapters will help uncover what those other factors might be.

Finally, no evidence has been provided to support the use of signs with infants, either those with normal hearing or those with hearing loss. The best that can be said of the practice of supporting language input to young children with signs is that it does not appear to have deleterious effects—unless a child has a late-identified hearing loss.

Table 7–1. Mean total communication acts for each group at each test age. Standard deviations are in parentheses, and group numbers are in italics.

Test Age (Months)	NH–s	NH+S	Early		Late	
			HL–s	HL+S	HL–s	HL+S
12	55.30 (23.68) *28*	55.96 (27.04) *12*	57.82 (13.55) *11*	49.20 (23.85) *5*	*0*	*0*
18	80.66 (31.13) *40*	84.30 (27.45) *28*	69.12 (32.05) *21*	58.58 (34.67) *13*	71.00 (19.80) *2*	*0*
24	132.98 (34.49) *32*	117.90 (35.46) *25*	107.09 (38.52) *27*	94.40 (24.14) *10*	64.10 (30.70) *5*	63.75 (22.27) *2*
30	146.98 (32.42) *25*	133.70 (28.24) *27*	107.88 (39.67) *36*	114.96 (27.05) *14*	118.59 (38.73) *11*	93.25 (24.17) *4*
36	153.58 (26.90) *31*	143.50 (27.27) *29*	129.47 (32.85) *33*	133.25 (26.25) *12*	146.73 (40.32) *15*	120.72 (27.30) *9*
42	152.79 (26.26) *26*	146.14 (29.29) *25*	137.38 (27.26) *37*	131.03 (19.91) *15*	140.43 (32.40) *23*	132.75 (29.29) *10*
48	161.60 (32.42) *25*	153.64 (28.08) *25*	148.68 (31.07) *33*	129.56 (18.06) *18*	156.16 (31.53) *25*	139.79 (30.67) *12*

Table 7–2. Mean numbers of initiated communication acts for each group at each test age. Standard deviations are in parentheses, and group numbers are in italics.

Test Age (Months)	NH–s	NH+S	Early		Late	
			HL–s	HL+S	HL–s	HL+S
12	15.29 (8.50) *28*	12.79 (10.62) *12*	17.18 (10.33) *11*	15.50 (6.72) *5*	*0*	*0*
18	22.06 (12.41) *40*	24.54 (14.44) *28*	24.76 (18.05) *21*	17.19 (11.07) *13*	25.75 (6.72) *2*	*0*
24	27.75 (20.80) *32*	25.94 (19.85) *25*	29.85 (20.23) *27*	23.75 (10.56) *10*	23.50 (13.80) *5*	13.25 (6.01) *2*
30	67.60 (22.98) *25*	64.07 (21.71) *27*	46.22 (23.91) *36*	42.14 (20.45) *14*	53.23 (23.51) *11*	35.88 (15.45) *4*
36	72.27 (15.88) *31*	76.29 (22.95) *29*	66.32 (21.82) *33*	68.25 (14.57) *12*	74.10 (23.86) *15*	57.28 (14.91) *9*
42	84.94 (20.31) *26*	83.14 (19.50) *25*	76.05 (23.56) *37*	73.67 (19.72) *15*	75.70 (24.16) *23*	77.50 (20.61) *10*
48	90.60 (24.29) *25*	90.90 (17.98) *25*	81.77 (23.03) *33*	80.42 (17.74) *18*	80.46 (23.54) *25*	81.54 (17.32) *12*

Table 7–3. Mean numbers of responses for each group at each test age. Standard deviations are in parentheses, and group numbers are in italics.

Test Age (Months)	NH−s	NH+S	Early		Late	
			HL−s	HL+S	HL−s	HL+S
12	6.84 (7.44) *28*	9.63 (11.34) *12*	5.00 (3.35) *11*	10.80 (13.04) *5*	*0*	*0*
18	23.46 (15.33) *40*	24.25 (14.96) *28*	15.93 (17.98) *21*	12.92 (11.80) *13*	9.50 (2.12) *2*	*0*
24	60.30 (22.27) *32*	51.34 (24.78) *25*	40.26 (21.66) *27*	38.25 (15.17) *10*	21.70 (20.47) *5*	17.75 (8.13) *2*
30	60.40 (18.39) *25*	54.98 (14.99) *27*	43.14 (24.71) *36*	51.36 (12.63) *14*	40.23 (19.68) *11*	26.75 (6.09) *4*
36	72.10 (20.94) *31*	60.78 (16.44) *29*	51.48 (20.13) *33*	53.17 (18.69) *12*	65.60 (24.98) *15*	47.17 (15.29) *9*
42	60.73 (18.26) *26*	55.48 (21.48) *25*	55.39 (18.36) *37*	51.53 (14.78) *15*	58.83 (22.94) *23*	47.65 (24.25) *10*
48	64.64 (20.06) *25*	55.00 (17.53) *25*	60.74 (19.51) *33*	44.03 (10.47) *18*	66.82 (24.78) *25*	55.13 (21.80) *12*

Table 7–4. Mean numbers of nondirected communication acts for each group at each test age. Standard deviations are in parentheses, and group numbers are in italics.

Test Age (Months)	NH–s	NH+S	Early		Late	
			HL–s	HL+S	HL–s	HL+S
12	33.18 (17.16) *28*	33.54 (16.24) *12*	35.64 (13.59) *11*	22.90 (6.70) *5*	*0*	*0*
18	35.14 (17.90) *40*	35.52 (19.84) *28*	28.43 (17.62) *21*	28.46 (25.17) *13*	35.75 (10.96) *2*	*0*
24	44.94 (13.44) *32*	40.62 (20.47) *25*	36.98 (14.71) *27*	32.40 (22.50) *10*	18.90 (10.97) *5*	32.75 (8.13) *2*
30	18.98 (14.14) *25*	14.65 (12.23) *27*	18.51 (12.76) *36*	21.46 (15.08) *14*	25.14 (18.97) *11*	30.63 (38.01) *4*
36	9.21 (8.05) *31*	6.43 (6.20) *29*	11.67 (9.63) *33*	11.83 (6.85) *12*	7.03 (5.51) *15*	16.28 (20.19) *9*
42	7.12 (6.26) *26*	7.52 (7.16) *25*	5.93 (7.39) *37*	5.83 (4.67) *15*	5.91 (7.23) *23*	7.60 (13.30) *10*
48	6.36 (7.53) *25*	7.74 (9.47) *25*	6.17 (8.71) *33*	5.11 (4.63) *18*	8.88 (10.81) *25*	3.13 (2.56) *12*

Table 7–5. Mean numbers of manual-only communication acts for each group at each test age. Standard deviations are in parentheses, and group numbers are in italics.

Test Age (Months)	NH–s	NH+S	Early		Late	
			HL–s	HL+S	HL–s	HL+S
12	8.59 (6.43) *28*	11.46 (9.21) *12*	10.55 (5.83) *11*	21.10 (16.13) *5*	*0*	*0*
18	13.91 (11.78) *40*	19.36 (12.66) *28*	15.79 (13.42) *21*	11.35 (8.12) *13*	12.00 (1.41) *2*	*0*
24	14.39 (7.02) *32*	16.66 (12.10) *25*	14.50 (8.73) *27*	24.85 (9.68) *10*	19.40 (12.71) *5*	10.75 (0.35) *2*
30	11.44 (6.44) *25*	11.11 (5.59) *27*	13.74 (7.45) *36*	16.79 (8.88) *14*	14.86 (8.49) *11*	20.00 (6.68) *4*
36	8.50 (6.02) *31*	9.24 (7.18) *29*	10.20 (6.16) *33*	9.88 (7.49) *12*	12.57 (8.55) *15*	16.50 (9.01) *9*
42	7.62 (5.42) *26*	5.30 (4.75) *25*	5.26 (4.11) *37*	6.90 (3.44) *15*	7.59 (5.72) *23*	9.80 (6.85) *10*
48	4.22 (3.32) *25*	4.22 (4.02) *25*	5.23 (4.24) *33*	5.06 (3.62) *18*	6.58 (8.84) *25*	7.17 (3.24) *12*

Table 7–6. Mean numbers of real-word communication acts for each group at each test age. Standard deviations are in parentheses, and group numbers are in italics.

Test Age (Months)	NH–s	NH+S	Early		Late	
			HL–s	HL+S	HL–s	HL+S
12	2.46 (3.48) *28*	4.04 (5.74) *12*	2.18 (5.08) *11*	0.20 (0.45) *5*	*0*	*0*
18	20.90 (21.27) *40*	23.52 (21.01) *28*	8.98 (16.70) *21*	7.04 (12.70) *13*	9.50 (2.12) *2*	*0*
24	83.80 (34.24) *32*	77.66 (41.61) *25*	54.19 (38.45) *27*	21.20 (29.94) *10*	12.70 (17.82) *5*	11.50 (16.26) *2*
30	109.24 (37.45) *25*	101.19 (28.51) *27*	61.47 (39.23) *36*	63.32 (34.99) *14*	61.64 (39.50) *11*	12.75 (14.36) *4*
36	123.44 (28.56) *31*	115.64 (30.91) *29*	81.65 (37.59) *33*	91.63 (23.38) *12*	98.97 (39.40) *15*	49.94 (33.05) *9*
42	122.62 (26.51) *26*	121.08 (26.86) *25*	99.93 (27.88) *37*	102.27 (21.80) *15*	104.65 (34.91) *23*	60.55 (45.57) *10*
48	131.24 (30.53) *25*	124.06 (27.28) *25*	111.15 (31.28) *33*	104.11 (20.87) *18*	118.44 (34.80) *25*	81.29 (53.13) *12*

Table 7–7. Mean numbers of vocalizations for each group at each test age. Standard deviations are in parentheses, and group numbers are in italics.

Test Age (Months)	NH–s	NH+S	Early		Late	
			HL–s	HL+S	HL–s	HL+S
12	44.25 (20.57) *28*	40.46 (21.92) *12*	45.09 (14.94) *11*	27.90 (10.18) *5*	*0*	*0*
18	45.85 (21.55) *40*	41.43 (20.58) *28*	44.36 (23.08) *21*	40.19 (26.39) *13*	49.50 (19.09) *2*	*0*
24	34.80 (21.65) *32*	23.58 (14.08) *25*	38.41 (21.97) *27*	48.35 (25.59) *10*	32.00 (10.61) *5*	41.50 (6.36) *2*
30	26.30 (20.32) *25*	21.41 (13.97) *27*	32.67 (22.06) *36*	34.86 (26.37) *14*	42.09 (20.51) *11*	60.50 (38.41) *4*
36	21.65 (10.11) *31*	18.62 (10.68) *29*	37.62 (24.37) *33*	31.75 (16.27) *12*	35.20 (18.98) *15*	54.28 (28.51) *9*
42	22.56 (13.33) *26*	19.76 (10.90) *25*	32.19 (20.14) *37*	21.87 (12.09) *15*	28.20 (18.84) *23*	62.40 (30.72) *10*
48	26.14 (10.99) *25*	25.36 (11.24) *25*	32.30 (19.92) *33*	20.39 (8.80) *18*	31.14 (13.76) *25*	51.33 (30.02) *12*

Table 7–8. Mean numbers of directed comments for each group at each test age. Standard deviations are in parentheses, and group numbers are in italics.

Test Age (Months)	NH–s	NH+S	Early		Late	
			HL–s	HL+S	HL–s	HL+S
12	7.32 (6.00) *28*	5.46 (3.21) *12*	9.05 (3.45) *11*	9.80 (5.08) *5*	*0*	*0*
18	10.80 (8.66) *40*	12.80 (7.84) *28*	13.79 (12.10) *21*	9.00 (7.61) *13*	15.50 (4.95) *2*	*0*
24	14.17 (13.01) *32*	12.14 (12.92) *25*	11.35 (9.08) *27*	8.60 (3.83) *10*	7.10 (6.17) *5*	8.75 (5.30) *2*
30	43.66 (16.72) *25*	47.87 (15.71) *27*	31.92 (19.53) *36*	30.61 (17.42) *14*	31.23 (15.06) *11*	23.88 (10.43) *4*
36	52.26 (12.52) *31*	58.48 (20.98) *29*	49.11 (17.56) *33*	52.67 (11.17) *12*	58.50 (24.71) *15*	49.39 (16.42) *9*
42	66.60 (19.16) *26*	69.20 (19.03) *25*	59.88 (18.69) *37*	59.17 (19.04) *15*	61.30 (20.91) *23*	67.20 (18.60) *10*
48	70.76 (17.88) *25*	75.68 (14.61) *25*	67.62 (20.21) *33*	67.92 (15.95) *18*	68.34 (20.43) *25*	68.83 (12.40) *12*

Table 7–9. Mean numbers of requests for action for each group at each test age. Standard deviations are in parentheses, and group numbers are in italics.

Test Age (Months)	NH–s	NH+S	Early		Late	
			HL–s	HL+S	HL–s	HL+S
12	0.98 (1.44) *28*	1.04 (1.60) *12*	0.82 (1.78) *11*	1.60 (2.43) *5*	*0*	*0*
18	2.66 (2.53) *40*	4.20 (3.90) *28*	2.74 (2.85) *21*	0.65 (0.85) *13*	4.00 (1.41) *2*	*0*
24	3.70 (2.72) *32*	4.92 (3.26) *25*	5.44 (5.30) *27*	4.35 (2.98) *10*	4.30 (4.69) *5*	1.50 (2.12) *2*
30	6.18 (3.78) *25*	4.31 (3.61) *27*	3.11 (3.08) *36*	3.04 (1.74) *14*	9.00 (4.59) *11*	1.25 (0.50) *4*
36	3.15 (3.05) *31*	3.60 (2.99) *29*	2.85 (2.31) *33*	4.42 (5.56) *12*	4.80 (3.29) *15*	2.33 (4.06) *9*
42	3.29 (3.91) *26*	2.08 (2.03) *25*	2.70 (3.02) *37*	2.30 (1.51) *15*	3.93 (3.68) *23*	1.35 (1.42) *10*
48	4.00 (3.45) *25*	3.42 (3.56) *25*	3.36 (3.05) *33*	3.08 (2.12) *18*	2.98 (2.19) *25*	2.83 (3.07) *12*

Table 7–10. Mean numbers of inquiries for each group at each test age. Standard deviations are in parentheses, and group numbers are in italics.

Test Age (Months)	NH–s	NH+S	Early		Late	
			HL–s	HL+S	HL–s	HL+S
12	0.00 (0.00) *28*	0.08 (0.29) *12*	0.00 (0.00) *11*	0.00 (0.00) *5*	*0*	*0*
18	0.74 (1.61) *40*	0.77 (1.30) *28*	0.10 (0.30) *21*	0.77 (1.48) *13*	*2*	*0*
24	4.67 (7.70) *32*	3.58 (4.39) *25*	1.72 (4.37) *27*	0.80 (1.32) *10*	0.20 (0.45) *5*	0.50 (0.71) *2*
30	12.28 (12.35) *25*	8.04 (7.59) *27*	3.24 (4.34) *36*	2.86 (3.51) *14*	4.91 (8.08) *11*	0.25 (0.50) *4*
36	12.21 (7.37) *31*	11.60 (6.20) *29*	9.48 (10.45) *33*	5.63 (4.73) *12*	6.63 (5.35) *15*	1.33 (2.60) *9*
42	11.44 (5.63) *26*	10.04 (6.31) *25*	8.23 (8.18) *37*	8.10 (4.24) *15*	7.74 (5.42) *23*	1.75 (2.23) *10*
48	14.40 (8.64) *25*	10.64 (4.95) *25*	8.95 (7.34) *33*	7.36 (6.16) *18*	7.02 (5.75) *25*	6.46 (8.66) *12*

Table 7–11. Mean number of answers for each group at each test age. Standard deviations are in parentheses, and group numbers are in italics.

| Test Age (Months) | NH–s | NH+S | Early | | Late | |
			HL–s	HL+S	HL–s	HL+S
12	0.27 (1.00) *28*	0.88 (2.73) *12*	0.00 (0.00) *11*	0.20 (0.45) *5*	*0*	*0*
18	6.25 (7.99) *40*	9.43 (10.84) *28*	2.83 (6.95) *21*	2.58 (4.62) *13*	0.00 (0.00) *2*	*0*
24	12.64 (10.65) *32*	16.32 (16.22) *25*	6.94 (8.91) *27*	4.65 (4.71) *10*	1.00 (1.73) *5*	0.50 (0.71) *2*
30	14.48 (8.32) *25*	14.93 (7.83) *27*	8.04 (8.20) *36*	11.29 (7.75) *14*	5.86 (6.61) *11*	0.75 (1.50) *4*
36	19.37 (7.67) *31*	16.71 (7.22) *29*	10.85 (8.35) *33*	14.04 (8.38) *12*	13.83 (7.82) *15*	6.56 (5.90) *9*
42	16.35 (7.72) *26*	15.44 (8.91) *25*	12.74 (6.34) *37*	14.57 (7.66) *15*	15.33 (9.82) *23*	9.40 (9.06) *10*
48	18.98 (7.32) *25*	15.82 (8.41) *25*	16.06 (7.83) *33*	13.39 (6.51) *18*	17.60 (9.98) *25*	14.17 (11.67) *12*

Table 7–12. Mean number of imitations for each group at each test age. Standard deviations are in parentheses, and group numbers are in italics.

Test Age (Months)	NH–s	NH+S	Early		Late	
			HL–s	HL+S	HL–s	HL+S
12	0.34 (0.88) *28*	0.33 (0.65) *12*	0.68 (1.15) *11*	0.40 (0.89) *5*	*0*	*0*
18	2.95 (3.64) *40*	1.55 (3.05) *28*	1.95 (3.28) *21*	0.92 (1.02) *13*	0.50 (0.71) *2*	*0*
24	10.48 (8.65) *32*	6.32 (9.21) *25*	9.59 (8.36) *27*	5.85 (5.01) *10*	5.20 (6.73) *5*	2.25 (3.18) *2*
30	6.84 (6.51) *25*	4.80 (6.03) *27*	11.07 (12.63) *36*	12.57 (8.12) *14*	13.14 (9.04) *11*	8.75 (7.53) *4*
36	4.85 (5.31) *31*	2.14 (2.22) *29*	9.65 (9.07) *33*	8.92 (7.12) *12*	21.07 (21.85) *15*	11.06 (4.81) *9*
42	1.50 (1.63) *26*	1.28 (1.39) *25*	7.20 (8.68) *37*	4.37 (3.83) *15*	9.91 (12.14) *23*	11.55 (9.84) *10*
48	1.66 (1.96) *25*	0.64 (0.74) *25*	5.48 (6.96) *33*	1.78 (2.42) *18*	5.06 (5.93) *25*	6.71 (5.40) *12*

References

Coggins, T. E., Olswang, L. B., & Guthrie, J. (1987). Assessing communicative intents in young children: Low structured observation or elicitation tasks? *Journal of Speech and Hearing Disorders, 52,* 44–49.

Eisenberg, S. L., Fersko, T. M., & Lundgren, C. (2001). The use of MLU for identifying language impairment in preschool children: A review. *American Journal of Speech-Language Pathology, 10,* 323–342.

Kent, R. N., & Foster, S. L. (1977). Direct observational procedures: Methodological issues in naturalistic setting. In A. R. Ciminero, K. S. Calhoun, & H. E. Adams (Eds.), *Handbook of behavioral assessment* (pp. 279–328). Toronto, Canada: John Wiley & Sons.

Rathmann, P. (1994). *Good night gorilla.* New York: G. P. Putnam's Sons.

Wetherby, A. M., Cain, D. H., Yonclas, D. G., & Walker, V. G. (1988). Analysis of intentional communication of normal children from the prelinguistic to the multiword stage. *Journal of Speech and Hearing Research, 31,* 240–252.

Real-World Language: Developing Native Competencies

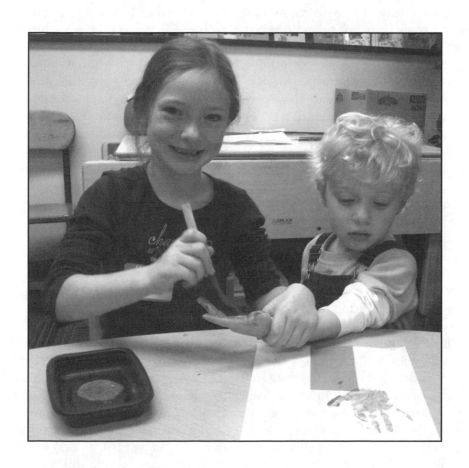

Language is a complex behavior. As users of our native language, we are completely comfortable structuring our utterances in ways that are highly specific only to the language we learned as young children. For example, we inflect verbs to mark whether the action is happening at the moment, or happened in the past (e.g., *walk/walks* vs. *walked*). We signal whether the action was ongoing in the past, or completed at some past time (*was/were walking* vs. *walked*). We can even indicate if the action was merely intended (*were going to walk*). And we can even do all this with verbs that require irregular forms when inflected (*kept, came*). With inflections we indicate the number of people performing the action (*he walks, they walk*). In some languages, even the gender of those people is signaled. To make our productions more efficient and comprehensible, we substitute short, consistent nouns (pronouns) for proper nouns. We even omit words or phrases entirely under some circumstances to make communication more efficient. Performing all of these linguistic maneuvers requires great sophistication and a high level of familiarity with one's native language.

Thus far, we have examined the language abilities of children, both with and without hearing loss, using measures that index general levels of language proficiency. Some of these measures are ones that are commercially available and used routinely in clinical assessment. Nonetheless, the argument could be made that the measures described in earlier chapters are not sensitive to the level of linguistic sophistication that specifies native-like abilities. In the first part of this chapter, results of more detailed kinds of analysis than those used in earlier chapters are provided.

Here we examine how well these children were mastering the nuances of their native language, which was English for all children.

In the second section of this chapter, we take on a different challenge. We have thus far presented a picture of overall language development showing that sensorineural hearing loss has detrimental effects, although those effects appear rather mild. At the same time, we learned in Chapter 5 that all of these children display normal nonverbal intelligence. In Chapter 7 we found that they all were trying to communicate with those around them with roughly the same frequency, for all the same reasons. What do children with normal intelligence who want to communicate do when their language abilities are not keeping up with their cognitive and pragmatic development? As one way to examine that question we looked at children's nonword vocalizations. Perhaps there would be differences in these productions that mark this discrepancy in development.

Syntactic and Grammatical Competency

Procedures for analyzing early syntax and grammar are fairly well standardized, with a software utility named the Systematic Analysis of Language Transcripts (or SALT) most commonly used. According to these procedures a written transcript of a set of spoken utterances from a child is entered into a computer file. The SALT software counts the numbers of various linguistic devices that research into child language development has ascertained are predictive of language ability, and computes several relevant metrics. Of course, the validity of the picture of language development provided by these procedures is only as valid as the language sample used. If young children are recorded reciting nursery rhymes, for example, outcomes will not be indicative of their natural language because such rhymes consist of preexisting verses. Similarly, if older children are recorded reading text, analyses of those samples will be unrepresentative of their natural language. It is critical that a sample be obtained that represents what a child typically produces in a natural setting. The language samples reported in Chapter 7 were deemed appropriate for this purpose.

Those language samples were 20 minutes in length. It will be recalled that each minute was divided into five intervals, with 10 seconds used for observing and 2 seconds used for scoring. In all, there were 100 intervals per sample, each of which had been scored according to language function and form. Our procedures provided us with a particularly objective manner of selecting utterances for further analysis. Typically in the procedures used in SALT, experimenters listen to the language sample as they are selecting which utterances to include in the analysis. Even if only unwittingly, that can lead to some bias in the selection of utterances to be analyzed. In this study the selection of utterances was handled without knowledge of the content of those utterances. First, we completed the analyses reported in Chapter 7 for all children at a particular test age. That provided us with records of where in the language samples utterances occurred that could be used to complete the syntactic/grammatical analyses reported in this chap-

ter. Laboratory staff used those score sheets to identify communicative acts containing real words, and those acts were marked for later transcription. In this way, staff members did not know the content of the utterances they would be transcribing beforehand.

Even at that questions arose regarding how to pick the utterances to be transcribed. As a general rule, SALT needs to be performed on a minimum of 50 utterances in order to ensure that a valid and reliable picture of each child's language production is obtained. Most children with hearing loss in this study produced far fewer than 50 real-word communication acts before 36 months of age. Therefore SALT could be used only on language samples obtained at 36 to 48 months. Samples were used from all children with hearing loss tested at each of the ages 36, 42 and 48 months. However, because these sorts of analyses are extremely labor-intensive, we restricted analysis to just 40 children with normal hearing at each of those test ages: 20 who used signs and 20 who did not. These children were randomly selected at each age.

Just as validity and reliability would be threatened by using too few utterances from children with hearing loss, so would validity and reliability be threatened by using too short of a time sample from children with normal hearing. Some children with normal hearing produced as many as eight or nine real-word utterances during some single minute intervals by 48 months of age. That would give us a 50-utterance sample with as little as 6 minutes of videotape. Such a short time frame restricts the range of activities that would be represented in the sample. Consequently, we implemented the additional restriction that at least 8 minutes of language sample had to be included in the transcriptions used.

In sum, exact procedures for obtaining these transcripts were as follows: A laboratory staff member went through each score sheet from the language analyses reported in Chapter 7. She began at the start of the 5th minute, and marked each communication act that consisted of a real-word utterance. If 50 utterances could not be found by the end of the score sheet, she went to the beginning to try to obtain a 50-utterance sample. At least 8 minutes (forty intervals) of the language sample had to be included. These procedures produced sets of transcripts that included 50 utterances on average, although there was some variability in exact numbers. To deal with this variability we normalized all measures that were counts of linguistic devices to a 50-utterance sample using the formula:

$$\text{Count}_{\text{normalized}} = (50/\text{Number of Utterances}) * \text{Count}$$

where *Number of Utterances* was the number actually obtained from any given participant, and *Count* was the number of linguistic devices obtained from those samples. This method provided a very precise comparison of counts across groups, although we found that results did not differ much at all from those obtained without the correction: Counts changed by very little, and statistical outcomes were identical with and without the normalization. This fact assures us of the robustness of the methods.

To obtain a language transcript of these utterances, one staff member watched the videotape and transcribed each utterance, according to SALT conventions. Subsequently, a second staff member watched the same videotape and checked the veracity of the transcription. If the two transcribers disagreed about some utterances in the sample, they viewed the videotape together and arrived at an agreement. If they were unable to reach an agreement by themselves, a third staff member was asked to serve as the referee. These transcripts were then entered into a file, and Systematic Analysis of Language Transcripts, Version 9 (SALT; Miller & Chapman, 2006) was used to analyze those transcripts.

The SALT software makes a number of different counts and calculations of linguistic measures. We selected five that were deemed most appropriate for the stage of language development at which most children in this study were. These were the following:

■ *Total words:* Just as the term suggests, the total number of words produced by the child across the 50 utterances was computed.
■ *Number of different words (NDW):* The number of unique words used by the child was computed, and is reported. Although we had measures of the size of children's expressive lexicons from the LDS and EOWPVT, discussed in Chapter 6, this SALT measure was an indication of how well children could productively use the words within their lexicons during the course of conversation.
■ *Mean length of utterance (MLU):* This metric was the average length of a child's utterances, in morphemes. It serves as an index of how well children are able to combine words.

■ *One-word utterances:* The number of utterances consisting of just one word is generally complementary to MLU, such that as MLU increases the number of one-word utterances decreases. Nonetheless, the number of one-word utterances can serve as an important metric of language advance, and so we included it.

■ *Pronouns:* The number of pronouns produced across the 50-utterance sample was counted. SALT provides counts of eight different kinds of pronouns. However, for these children we found that roughly 60% of all pronouns were personal pronouns (e.g., *she* and *he*) and another 20% were demonstrative pronouns (e.g., *this* and *that*). These percentages were similar across all three ages at which analyses were performed, and across all six groups of children. Consequently, we analyzed the sum of pronouns, across all kinds, for this report.

Although not reported in detail, we also examined the number of conjunctions used by children. Means for children with normal hearing and those with hearing loss are shown on Table 8–1. Also shown are the numbers of occurrences of the word *and* as a conjunction.

Children with hearing loss used fewer conjunctions overall than children with normal hearing, but higher proportions of these conjunctions were the word *and*. This conjunction is among the first to appear in language development. The finding that it accounted for a higher proportion of conjunctions used by children with hearing loss than by children with normal hearing is consistent with all other findings showing that these children with hearing loss were generally delayed in learning to use language. Children with normal hearing used a wider variety of conjunctions, with more that typically appear at later stages of development. Ultimately, we decided that reporting on the frequency of conjunction use added nothing to our understanding of children's language development that we could not derive from other measures. For that reason, nothing more will be said of conjunction use by these children.

Results of SALT

Figures 8–1 through 8–4 show mean numbers of total words, NDW, MLU, and pronouns for each of the six groups of children in this study. Tables 8–2 through 8–5, at the end of the chapter,

Table 8–1. Mean number of conjunctions per language sample, occurrences of the conjunction *and*, and ratios of *and*/total conjunctions, across the three test ages of 36, 42, and 48 months for children with normal hearing and those with hearing loss.

	Total Conjunctions	*and* Conjunctions	*and*/Total
Normal Hearing	8.2	5.7	.70
Hearing Loss	2.3	1.9	.81

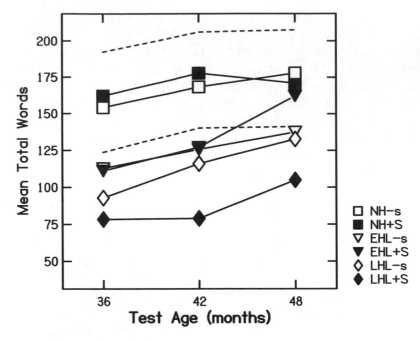

Figure 8–1. Mean numbers of total words derived from SALT for each group at each test age for six groups of children: NH–s (normal hearing, no signs); NH+S (normal hearing, signs); EHL–s (early-identified hearing loss, no signs); EHL+S (early-identified hearing loss, signs); LHL–s (late-identified hearing loss, no signs); and LHL+S (late-identified hearing loss, signs). The dotted lines show +/– one standard deviation from the mean, according to data from children with normal hearing in this study.

also provide this information. In Figure 8–1 we see a pattern that has been found for almost all of the language measures previously reported: Children with early-identified hearing loss had outcomes that were poorer than those of children with normal hearing, regardless of whether they used signs or not. What is different for these results from those reported in earlier chapters is the magnitude of those differences. Here we find that children with hearing loss were generally performing more than one standard deviation below the means of children with normal hearing. Children with late-identified hearing

loss performed similarly to those early-identified children, if they were not using signs. Those late-identified children who were using signs were performing even more poorly, sometimes more than two standard deviations below the means of children with normal hearing. Figure 8–2, 8–3, and 8–4, for NDW, MLU, and number of pronouns, all show patterns similar to those described above.

The same series of statistical analyses was conducted on data from these SALT results as were done on data reported in earlier chapters, and outcomes were similar. Because of that

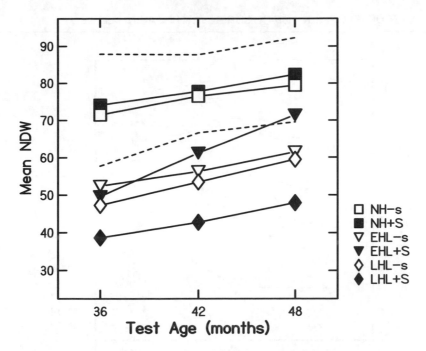

Figure 8–2. Mean numbers of different words (NDW) derived from SALT for each group at each test age for six groups of children. See legend for Figure 8–1 for details.

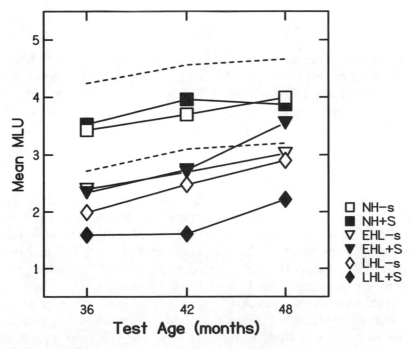

Figure 8–3. Means for mean length of utterances (MLU) derived from SALT for each group at each test age for six groups of children. See legend for Figure 8–1 for details.

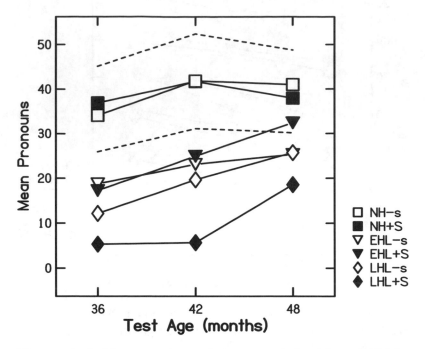

Figure 8–4. Mean numbers of pronouns derived from SALT for each group at each test age for six groups of children. See legend for Figure 8–1 for details.

redundancy the tedious details of the statistical outcomes will be forgone in favor of a summary. The FIRST ANOVA showed that children with normal hearing and those with early-identified hearing loss performed differently from each other: $p < .001$ for all four measures of total words, NDW, MLU, and pronouns. In the SECOND ANOVA, the main effect of age of ID was significant, $p < .001$ for all measures, as was the Age of ID × Signs interaction, $p \leq .003$ for all. When SEA was performed on outcomes for early-identified and late-identified children separately, results for children with early-identified hearing loss consistently demonstrated a significant effect of prosthesis, $.008 \leq p \leq .034$, indicating that children with hearing aids performed slightly better than children with cochlear implants. Results for children with late-identified hearing loss consistently showed a significant sign effect, $p \leq .003$, indicating that those children who used signs performed more poorly than those who did not. In sum, the same trends were obtained for these measures of language development as for measures reported earlier, except that there was a stronger effect of hearing loss for three of the four measures: NDW, MLU, and numbers of pronouns.

Even at that, there are more profound differences between the language of children with hearing loss and the language of children with normal hearing by the 4th year of life than has been revealed thus far. For example, we just learned that children with normal hearing produced a greater number of different words than did children with hearing loss, but the difference runs deeper still. By examining the kinds of words that these children used, we obtain a clearer picture of how they were communicating. Over these three test sessions (36 to 48 months of age), 64% of words produced by children with hearing loss were nouns. That contrasts with the fact that nouns accounted for just 39% of the words produced by children with normal hearing. By contrast, verbs accounted for only 33% of the different words used by children with hearing loss, but 44% for children with normal hearing. These differences suggest that children with hearing loss were more likely to label objects when communicating, whereas children with normal hearing were more often producing sentences with noun-verb structures.

Roger Brown, who developed the metric of MLU (1973), used it to classify children's language development into stages. We can apply the same criteria that he used to the MLU measures we obtained, shown on Table 8–4. In doing so we learn that children with normal hearing generally reached Brown's Stage V by 42 months of age, which fits nicely with what was found for typically developing children by Brown. Children with early-identified hearing loss in this study generally reached Stage IV, but not until 48 months of age. Brown reported that the typical age for reaching this stage was roughly 36 months of age, and so these children were close to a year behind in language development. Nonsigning children with late-identified hearing loss would be classified as Stage III at 48 months of age, which put them a full year or more behind in development. Signing children with late-identified hearing loss were even further behind, never progressing past Stage II by the end of this study. That meant that these children were 2 full years behind in language development. Thus, we find that children with hearing loss were generally quite delayed in the form of the language they were producing. In contrast to some earlier findings, we find that this delay is slightly greater for late-identified children, regardless of whether they used signs or not. However, the greatest delay is again observed for those late-identified children who used signs.

Figure 8–5 shows mean numbers of one-word utterances computed from SALT, and these data are also in Table 8–6 at the end of the chapter. In this case, we see that children with hearing loss produced more of this type of utterance than did children with normal hearing. We also see that signing children with late-identified hearing loss produced many more one-word utterances than did other children with hearing loss: Roughly 60% of all utterances consisted of only one word for these children. The FIRST ANOVA revealed a significant effect of hearing loss, $F(1, 255) = 32.84$, $p < .001$, showing a difference between children with normal hearing and those with early-identified hearing loss. The SECOND ANOVA showed significant main effects of age of ID, $F(1, 229) = 29.90$, $p < .001$, and signs, $F(1, 229) = 11.45$, $p = .001$, as well as a significant Age of ID × Signs interaction, $F(1, 229) = 17.28$, $p < .001$.

Finally, Cohen's ds were computed on these five SALT measures, using

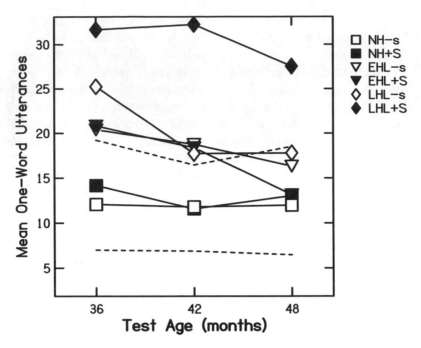

Figure 8–5. Mean numbers of one-word utterances derived from SALT for each group at each test age for six groups of children. See legend for Figure 8–1 for details.

means of children with normal hearing and those with early-identified hearing loss. These are shown in Figure 8–6. Effect size was large for each of these measures, making them well suited to gauge progress of children with hearing loss as they develop language. Although time consuming, it might well be worth the investment of effort for clinicians to use these sorts of analyses for tracking the language acquisition of their young clients. Results presented in this chapter provide a solid base of normative data.

Vocalizations

In the last chapter we found that children with hearing loss were producing nonword vocalizations longer into childhood than were children with normal hearing. Young, typically developing children produce nonword vocalizations when they babble, but those sorts of productions tend to diminish once a child starts producing real words, generally early in the 2nd year of life. We wondered if there might be something to be learned about the language development of children with hearing loss from these vocalizations, and so we explored their form in greater detail.

To do that we analyzed all communication acts scored as vocalizations in the complete 20-minute unstructured language samples from the 24- to 48-month test sessions. Laboratory staff listened to the videotaped recordings of all children with hearing loss and 40

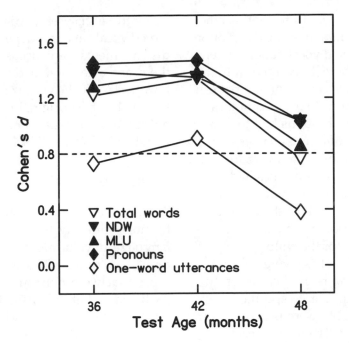

Figure 8–6. Cohen's *d* for each measure derived from SALT, computed using means for children with normal hearing and those with early-identified hearing loss. The dashed line at 0.8 separates the space into values that represent large effects (*above the line*) from those that show moderate to weak effects (*below the line*).

children with normal hearing. For the vocalization analyses done on samples from the 36- to 48-month test sessions, the children with normal hearing included in this analysis were the same ones as those on whose language samples SALT was done. For the 24- and 30-month language samples, 40 children with normal hearing were randomly selected for this analysis.

For current purposes, all communication acts that had been marked as vocalizations during the analysis described in Chapter 7 were recategorized using a more fine-grained system, partially based on the metaphonological classification system described by Oller (1986). These new categories were:

- *Crying, laughing, screaming, and squealing.*
- *Nonconstricted vocalizations:* These were vocalizations that lacked any vocal tract closure or narrowly constricted segment, and so were entirely vocalic. Sometimes these vocalizations were not fully resonant.
- *Constricted vocalizations:* These were vocalizations that contained at least one vocal tract closure or narrow constriction, that is, vocalizations that had at least one syllable margin. In descriptions of the babbled productions of young infants, these sorts of vocalizations are termed *reduplicated* or *variegated babble.*

■ *Jargon:* In terms of form, this kind of vocalization met the description of constricted vocalizations given above. Where it diverged from that category was in intonation pattern and function. To be classified as jargon, vocalizations had to be a minimum of three syllables long, although most were much longer. These vocalization types had to have stress and intonation patterns typical of English, and had to appear to be functioning as real-word utterances for the child.

■ *Protowords:* These were vocalizations that were used consistently by the child to refer to specific objects or actions, but were unique in form to the child. The form of each protoword could share no more than one consonant or vowel with the adult form of the word used to refer to that object or action. Productions that were more similar in form to adult versions than this were generally counted as real-word communication acts.

■ *Sound effects:* These were vocalizations used as substitutes for drinking, pouring, vehicle noises, animal sounds, and so on. To be included in this category, a vocalization needed to include a vocal tract constriction or closure: For example, if the sound made for a train was *choochoochoo*, it was counted as a sound effect; if it was *u-u-u* it was counted as a nonconstricted vocalization.

■ *Word replacements:* These were vocalizations that are commonly occurring substitutions for real words, even among adults, such as *uh-huh* (as an acknowledgement) or *mmmmm* (when eating).

For these analyses, two staff members scored vocalizations independently. Any disagreements were discussed between them, and a decision made jointly about how to classify the vocalization in question. If the two original scorers could not agree on a classification, a third staff member was asked to serve as referee.

Results of Vocalization Analysis

Some of the categories listed above led to more clinically useful insights into language development for these children than others. Those vocalization types that were not found to provide particularly helpful insights included cries, laughs, screams, and squeals. All children produced roughly the same numbers of these sorts of vocalizations, regardless of hearing status, sign use, and age of ID of hearing loss. Similarly, all children used sound effects to a similar extent. Less than one instance of protowords was recorded, on average, per recording session, and so that category provided no special insights, either.

The number of word replacements counted in samples from children with normal hearing and those with hearing loss differed, and so these numbers provided some interesting information regarding differences in language development between these two groups of children. In particular, a larger proportion of vocalizations for children with normal hearing consisted of word replacements: At 48 months of age children with normal hearing produced exactly 10 word replacements during the 20-minute recording, on average, which represented 34% of all their vocalizations. Children with hearing loss produced just five word replacements, on average, which accounted for 18% of all their vocalizations. This form of vocalization involves a more sophisticated level of language ability than other kinds of vocalizations examined by us: The speaker must understand the communication conventions of his native language community, and know which nonword replacements are acceptable in each of several specific contexts. Children with normal hearing apparently grasped these concepts regarding their native language earlier and more completely than did children with hearing loss.

That information regarding word replacements is interesting, but the three kinds of vocalizations that provided the most information about how language development differed for children with hearing loss from that of children with normal hearing were nonconstricted vocalizations, constricted vocalizations, and jargon. Nonconstricted vocalizations are very immature forms of vocal production. They are generally observed in the first few months of a child's life, with constricted vocalizations taking over as the predominant kind of babbled production around 7 months of age.

Figure 8–7 displays the mean number of nonconstricted vocalizations produced

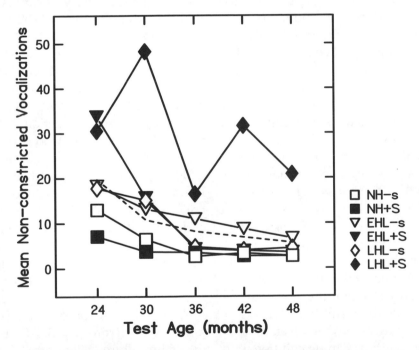

Figure 8–7. Mean numbers of nonconstricted vocalizations for each group at each test age examined for six groups of children: NH–s (normal hearing, no signs); NH+S (normal hearing, signs); EHL–s (early-identified hearing loss, no signs); EHL+S (early-identified hearing loss, signs); LHL–s (late-identified hearing loss, no signs); and LHL+S (late-identified hearing loss, signs). The dotted line shows + one standard deviation from the mean, according to data from children with normal hearing in this study. Minus one standard deviation reached the value of zero.

by each group of children from 24 to 48 months of age, and these numbers are shown in Table 8–7 at the end of the chapter. Most children, both with and without hearing loss, produced few vocalizations of this kind after 24 months of age. The exception to this pattern is that signing children with late-identified hearing loss continued to use high numbers of nonconstricted vocalizations for the duration of the project period. Nonetheless, when statistical analyses were performed on these numbers, the FIRST ANOVA did reveal a significant effect of hearing status for data from children with normal hearing and those with early-identified hearing loss, $F(1, 412) = 49.90, p < .001$. So even though none of these children produced a great number of nonconstricted vocalizations, children with early-identified hearing loss were generally producing more than children with normal hearing. No other effects or interactions were significant in that analysis.

The SECOND ANOVA resulted in significant main effects of age of ID, $F(1, 289) = 25.77, p < .001$, and signs, $F(1, 289) = 24.74, p < .001$, as well as a significant Age of ID × Signs interaction, $F(1, 289) = 42.33, p < .001$. A SEA done on these numbers for early- and late-identified children separately revealed only a significant sign effect for the late-identified children, $F(1, 273) = 26.66, p < .001$. As has been seen so often in early chapters, signing children with late-identified hearing loss performed much differently from all other groups of children. In this instance they were producing this kind of immature vocal production at higher rates later into childhood than were other children in the study.

Figure 8–8 displays mean numbers of constricted vocalizations for each group of children. These values are also provided in Table 8–8 at the end of the chapter. This figure resembles Figure 8–7, but shows that children with early-identified hearing loss, regardless of whether they used signs or not, and nonsigning children with late-identified hearing loss continued to produce constricted vocalization in higher numbers longer into this study than did children with normal hearing. Nonetheless, the statistical analyses showed the same pattern of results as those found for nonconstricted vocalizations: The FIRST ANOVA revealed a significant effect of hearing status, $F(1, 412) = 39.32, p < .001$, but nothing else.

The SECOND ANOVA showed significant main effects of age of ID, $F(1, 289) = 23.03, p < .001$, and signs, $F(1, 289) = 5.45, p = .020$, as well as a significant Age of ID × Signs interaction, $F(1, 289) = 15.87, p < .001$. A SEA done on these numbers for early- and late-identified children separately revealed only a significant sign effect for the late-identified children, $F(1, 273) = 11.05, p = .001$. So children with hearing loss produced more constricted vocalizations than children with normal hearing, with signing children whose losses were identified late producing the most of any group.

Although we do not have data on the kinds of nonword vocalizations produced by children with normal hearing when they were younger than 24 months of age, it seems safe to surmise that these children produced more nonconstricted and constricted vocalizations at those younger ages than they did after 24 months of age. They would have had to, given that those kinds of produc-

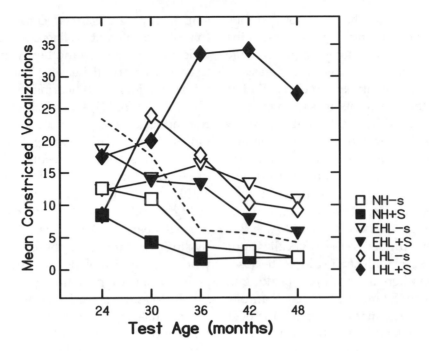

Figure 8–8. Mean numbers of constricted vocalizations for each group at each test age examined. See legend for Figure 8–7 for details.

tions are considered precursors to later language development. Consequently, in counting these two kinds of vocalizations we were not revealing evidence that children with hearing loss showed a different *kind* of vocal production from what is found for children with normal hearing; they were simply delayed in *when* they used high numbers of these production types. That sort of developmental delay for speech and language was anticipated at the outset of this study.

The third type of nonword vocalization that we examined paints a different picture of vocal development for deaf children because it is one that is not found in typical language development. The use of phonetically complex vocal-izations as substitutes for real-word, meaningful utterances is not commonly observed for typically developing young children, even though the modern media often portrays it as such. For example, a recent television commercial for greeting cards that allow senders to record a message shows a mother following her young son around trying to record him saying *Merry Christmas*. We hear him producing many examples of jargon, but no samples of the desired phrase (until the end of the commercial when tearful grandparents open the card). In reality, that kind of jargon is infrequently used by typically developing children. Instead, most children rapidly adopt the speech patterns of their linguistic community, such that just as they start having a lot that they want to communicate they possess the language abilities to do so. If language development is delayed, it is easy to imagine a scenario in which a child has more that he wants to say than he is able to say. When we look at Figure 8–9 and Table 8–9, at the end of the chapter, we see very few occurrences of jargon for children with normal hearing, and we have no reason to suspect that they produced these sorts of vocalizations at younger ages. What we do see is a greater number of these vocalizations for children with hearing loss. The absolute numbers are not high, peaking at 6 to 10 per 20-minute language sample. Nonetheless, that is more than is ever found for children with normal hearing. For this vocalization type, the only

statistically significant effect found was that of hearing status. There was a significant difference found between children with normal hearing and those with early-identified hearing loss in the FIRST ANOVA, $F(1, 412) = 26.23, p < .001$, but none of the analyses involving only children with hearing loss produced any significant results. Consequently, we are left to conclude that all children with hearing loss used jargon at higher rates than did children with normal hearing. We suggest that this finding indicates that these children, who were typically developing in all areas other than language, had as much to say as did children with normal hearing, understood the functions and conventions of communication, and had acquired some degree of

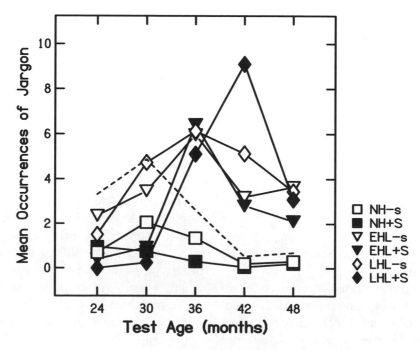

Figure 8–9. Mean occurrences of jargon for each group at each test age examined. See legend for Figure 8–7 for details.

phonetic capabilities. But they were delayed in how they could organize those phonetic abilities to produce appropriate lexical and syntactic strings. The use of jargon may arise due to the mismatch between development of cognitive/pragmatic abilities and language abilities.

Chapter Summary

In this chapter, we explored the form of children's vocal productions in detail. Regarding productions that consist of real words, we learned that children with hearing loss were seriously delayed in learning how to incorporate words into syntactically and grammatically complex productions. Using Brown's stages we found that children with hearing loss were on average between 1 and 2 years delayed in language acquisition, depending on age of ID and use of signs. Regarding nonword productions, children with hearing loss were found to continue using certain nonverbal forms of vocalization (i.e., nonconstricted and constricted) after children with normal hearing had stopped doing so. In addition, children with hearing loss used jargon, a form of nonword vocalizations that is phonetically complex and meaningful. This form of vocalizations is rarely observed in the productions of children with normal hearing. In general we learn from the data presented in this chapter that results of more conventional metrics of language development, such as those reported in earlier chapters, may be underestimating the amount of delay experienced by many children with hearing loss.

Table 8–2. Mean total words from SALT given at each test age, with standard deviations in parentheses and group numbers in italics.

Test Age (Months)	NH–s	NH+S	Early		Late	
			HL–s	HL+S	HL–s	HL+S
36	153.93 (32.28) *20*	161.90 (36.63) *20*	112.73 (41.49) *33*	111.06 (39.00) *12*	92.79 (25.20) *15*	78.31 (23.61) *9*
42	168.47 (19.83) *20*	177.85 (42.29) *20*	125.63 (38.36) *36*	127.16 (36.42) *15*	115.94 (29.92) *23*	78.92 (27.76) *10*
48	177.95 (24.60) *20*	171.05 (40.19) *20*	137.66 (39.15) *33*	162.32 (39.59) *18*	132.84 (31.84) *25*	104.95 (54.93) *12*

Table 8–3. Mean number of different words (NDW) given at each test age, with standard deviations in parentheses and group numbers in italics.

Test Age (Months)	NH–s	NH+S	Early		Late	
			HL–s	HL+S	HL–s	HL+S
36	71.47 (18.20) *20*	74.12 (11.50) *20*	52.36 (16.24) *33*	49.59 (13.01) *12*	47.24 (13.33) *15*	38.63 (15.42) *9*
42	76.49 (11.53) *20*	77.79 (9.75) *20*	56.20 (18.18) *36*	61.15 (15.38) *15*	53.39 (14.84) *23*	42.71 (12.95) *10*
48	79.41 (11.27) *20*	82.36 (11.62) *20*	61.41 (19.47) *33*	71.39 (16.02) *18*	59.41 (15.16) *25*	47.89 (21.02) *12*

Table 8–4. Means for mean length of utterance (MLU) given at each test age, with standard deviations in parentheses and group numbers in italics.

Test Age (Months)	NH–s	NH+S	Early		Late	
			HL–s	HL+S	HL–s	HL+S
36	3.43 (0.71) *20*	3.54 (0.83) *20*	2.40 (0.95) *33*	2.34 (0.88) *12*	1.99 (0.58) *15*	1.59 (0.48) *9*
42	3.70 (0.46) *20*	3.96 (0.92) *20*	2.70 (0.90) *36*	2.74 (0.84) *15*	2.48 (0.70) *23*	1.61 (0.59) *10*
48	3.99 (0.53) *20*	3.87 (0.91) *20*	3.02 (0.92) *33*	3.55 (0.91) *18*	2.90 (0.76) *25*	2.22 (1.23) *12*

Table 8–5. Mean number of pronouns given at each test age, with standard deviations in parentheses and group numbers in italics.

Test Age (Months)	NH–s	NH+S	Early		Late	
			HL–s	HL+S	HL–s	HL+S
36	34.13 (8.52) *20*	36.94 (10.59) *20*	18.76 (12.71) *33*	17.25 (16.57) *12*	12.14 (8.28) *15*	5.33 (6.72) *9*
42	41.80 (9.18) *20*	41.68 (12.19) *20*	23.10 (14.41) *36*	24.91 (12.70) *15*	19.64 (10.34) *23*	5.67 (9.76) *10*
48	40.96 (8.90) *20*	37.91 (9.71) *20*	25.26 (12.86) *33*	32.36 (12.63) *18*	25.67 (12.82) *25*	18.54 (20.58) *12*

Table 8–6. Mean one-word utterances given at each test age, with standard deviations in parentheses and group numbers in italics.

Test Age (Months)	NH–s	NH+S	Early		Late	
			HL–s	HL+S	HL–s	HL+S
36	12.07 (7.06) *20*	14.16 (4.94) *20*	20.41 (10.52) *33*	20.84 (9.25) *12*	25.27 (9.61) *15*	31.68 (12.36) *9*
42	11.80 (4.22) *20*	11.58 (5.43) *20*	18.80 (8.19) *36*	18.42 (10.75) *15*	17.77 (7.69) *23*	32.25 (14.35) *10*
48	11.98 (4.31) *20*	13.04 (7.45) *20*	16.33 (7.15) *33*	13.14 (6.42) *18*	17.81 (7.32) *25*	27.54 (15.67) *12*

Table 8–7. Mean nonconstricted vocalizations given at each test age, with standard deviations in parentheses and group numbers in italics.

Test Age (Months)	NH–s	NH+S	Early		Late	
			HL–s	HL+S	HL–s	HL+S
24	13.00 (10.69) *20*	7.15 (7.65) *20*	18.35 (11.47) *26*	33.80 (26.92) *10*	17.75 (14.66) *4*	30.50 (3.54) *2*
30	6.45 (7.31) *20*	3.70 (3.06) *20*	13.14 (13.16) *35*	15.71 (23.55) *14*	15.09 (17.75) *11*	48.25 (46.45) *4*
36	2.65 (2.76) *20*	3.50 (6.66) *20*	10.91 (14.01) *33*	4.33 (4.83) *12*	4.73 (4.23) *15*	16.44 (13.13) *9*
42	3.35 (4.38) *20*	2.62 (3.25) *21*	8.72 (9.20) *36*	3.93 (2.89) *15*	4.04 (4.96) *23*	31.60 (38.17) *10*
48	2.75 (3.37) *20*	2.75 (2.55) *20*	6.67 (6.66) *33*	3.61 (3.03) *18*	4.52 (5.21) *25*	20.83 (28.17) *12*

Table 8–8. Mean constricted vocalizations given at each test age, with standard deviations in parentheses and group numbers in italics.

Test Age (Months)	NH–s	NH+S	Early		Late	
			HL–s	HL+S	HL–s	HL+S
24	12.60 (13.66) *20*	8.45 (12.02) *20*	18.54 (13.57) *26*	12.30 (8.64) *10*	8.50 (11.68) *4*	17.50 (24.75) *2*
30	10.95 (13.21) *20*	4.30 (3.21) *20*	14.09 (15.35) *35*	13.71 (13.15) *14*	23.91 (21.58) *11*	20.00 (15.34) *4*
36	3.60 (4.31) *20*	1.65 (2.06) *20*	16.27 (18.18) *33*	13.17 (12.89) *12*	17.73 (14.83) *15*	33.56 (25.70) *9*
42	2.85 (3.91) *20*	1.76 (2.55) *21*	13.22 (17.72) *36*	7.73 (7.27) *15*	10.35 (13.62) *23*	34.20 (18.39) *10*
48	1.90 (2.02) *20*	1.85 (2.62) *20*	10.70 (13.86) *33*	5.61 (7.44) *18*	9.24 (12.31) *25*	27.33 (21.84) *12*

Table 8–9. Mean occurrences of jargon given at each test age, with standard deviations in parentheses and group numbers in italics.

Test Age (Months)	NH–s	NH+S	Early		Late	
			HL–s	HL+S	HL–s	HL+S
24	0.70 (1.08) *20*	0.95 (3.38) *20*	2.35 (5.31) *26*	0.40 (0.52) *10*	1.50 (1.91) *4*	0.00 (0.00) *2*
30	2.05 (4.30) *20*	0.75 (2.31) *20*	3.46 (7.73) *35*	0.93 (2.06) *14*	4.73 (5.04) *11*	0.25 (0.50) *4*
36	1.35 (2.25) *20*	0.30 (0.92) *20*	5.97 (8.42) *33*	6.42 (9.21) *12*	6.13 (6.95) *15*	5.11 (6.95) *9*
42	0.20 (0.52) *20*	0.05 (0.22) *21*	3.19 (4.33) *36*	2.80 (4.93) *15*	5.13 (6.49) *23*	9.10 (15.65) *10*
48	0.30 (0.47) *20*	0.20 (0.41) *20*	3.64 (5.73) *33*	2.11 (3.43) *18*	3.44 (6.06) *25*	3.08 (4.40) *12*

References

Brown, R. (1973). *A first language: The early stages.* Cambridge, MA: Harvard University Press.

Miller, J., & Chapman, R. (2006). *Systematic Analysis of Language Transcripts (SALT): Version 9.* Madison, WI: University of Wisconsin-Madison, Language Analysis Laboratory.

Oller, D. K. (1986). Metaphonology and infant vocalizations. In B. Lindblom & R. Zetterstrom (Eds.), *Precursors of early speech* (pp. 21–35). Hampshire, UK: Macmillan Press.

9

Treatment Effects

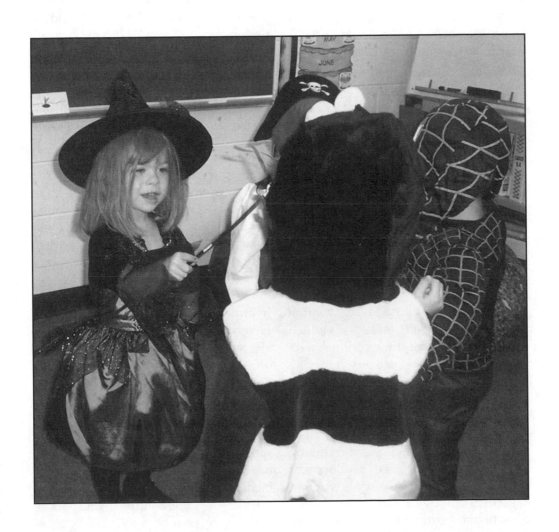

By now we have learned something about the effects of hearing loss, age of identification of that hearing loss, and the use of signs on language outcomes for children. We have discovered that children with hearing loss, on average, continue to perform more poorly on language measures than their peers with normal hearing, in spite of having had their hearing loss identified early in many cases and having received the best auditory prostheses currently available. This situation was found to exist for the children participating in this study, even though they all were being served by intervention programs that any objective standards would indicate are quite good. We must therefore conclude that, as a profession, either we have failed to identify intervention methods that ensure that children with hearing loss will overcome barriers to language acquisition imposed by that sensory deficit, or we are simply failing to provide that level of care to all affected children. This last suggestion—that we have not discovered how to deliver consistently good intervention to children and their families—is added because there were some children with hearing loss tested at every age who performed as well as children with normal hearing on at least one language measure. That means that there may have been something about the intervention these children were receiving that facilitated language development particularly well. Professionals working with deaf children certainly have ideas about what treatment factors best facilitate positive language outcomes, and in this chapter we examine those ideas.

We are generally finding that mean scores for children with hearing loss are at or slightly more than one standard deviation below the means of scores for children with normal hearing on all language measures. Variance, as indexed by standard deviations, was similar across groups for all measures. This means that some children with hearing loss, roughly those in the top 10 to 15%, were performing as well as the average child with normal hearing on any measure, at any test age. What accounted for the good performance of those few deaf children? Were they always the same children performing that well, or did some quasirandom group just happen to score well on a measure or two at each test age? In other words, are there genuine "stars" among these children, or is it more accurate to describe the performance of all children with hearing loss as being generally depressed, with a couple children spuriously doing well once in a while? Answering these questions could help us know what treatment variables to be examining in order to move our current intervention methods forward so that we might improve language outcomes for all children with hearing loss.

In this chapter, the effects of specific treatment variables are investigated. First, we examine how outcomes were affected by factors related to the type of prostheses children had. Next, we look explicitly at whether an intervention strategy focused on the use of hearing leads to better language skills than strategies more globally encouraging spoken communication. Specific factors related to the use of signs are examined, and finally we ask if there are true stars among the children who participated in this study.

Prosthesis Effects

When the application for funding for this study was written in 2002, children with moderate hearing loss used hearing aids and children with severe-to-profound hearing loss typically received a cochlear implant. There was little deviation from those two amplification options, and the type of amplification a child received was almost entirely dependent on the degree of hearing loss that child had. Consequently, we thought there would be very little in the way of interesting results related to the configuration of children's auditory prostheses coming out of these analyses. We thought we would find that children with hearing aids were faring better than children with cochlear implants, but that it would be impossible to disentangle that apparent prosthesis effect from an effect of auditory sensitivity. Little did we know how quickly options for auditory stimulation would change in the course of a few years.

Shortly after this study began, professionals began to consider alternatives to the two basic options outlined above. Consequently, children started showing up at test time with a variety of prosthesis combinations: The children with BE-PTAs between 50 and 70 dB all continued to use only hearing aids, but children with poorer BE-PTAs differed in whether they had one implant, bilateral implants, or an implant on one ear and a hearing aid on the other ear. This last configuration is generally termed *bimodal stimulation*, and that terminology is used here.

As soon as these various prosthesis options appeared on the scene we recognized the need to examine outcomes related to the types of prostheses, and combinations of those prostheses, that children used. To do that we decided to examine outcomes at 48 months for children with hearing loss because that marked the end of the developmental period examined by us. Ninety children with hearing loss were tested at that last session, but 12 of them were late-identified signers. Those children performed so differently on all language measures compared to all other children with hearing loss that we decided to exclude their results from these analyses. There was one other child who had an extremely unusual sequence of prostheses, and so we excluded that child's data from this particular analysis, as well. Thus, we were left with 77 children with hearing loss for this particular investigation.

We selected six dependent language measures to examine: auditory comprehension, as measured by the Auditory Comprehension subtest of the PLS-4; expressive vocabulary, as measured by the EOWPVT; the number of real-word utterances (RW-Us) observed in the 20-minute videotape of unstructured play; the mean length of utterance (MLU) from the SALT; the numbers of pronouns computed by SALT; and the numbers of different words (NDW) calculated with SALT. These measures were all considered sensitive to variability in outcomes because they each had Cohen's ds of greater than 0.80 for a considerable period of the study when scores for children with normal hearing and those with hearing loss were compared.

Age of Implantation

The first question asked was whether the age of implantation, for the first implant, significantly affected language abilities at 48 months of age. The first row of Table 9–1 shows Pearson product-moment correlation coefficients (r) for each of these six language measures and age of the child's first implant. The

Table 9–1. Pearson product-moment correlation coefficients (*r*) between each dependent language measure and age of first implant for all children who had implants and were tested at 48 months of age, those who had electric-only stimulation, and those who had some acoustic stimulation. Also shown are *p* values and the number of children whose data contributed to the calculation of that *r*.

		Auditory Compre-hension	EOWPVT	RW-U	MLU	Pronouns	NDW
All Children	*r*	−.142	−.167	−.057	−.320	−.077	−.294
	p	.316	.237	.691	.022	.589	.037
	N	52	52	51	51	51	51
Electric Only	*r*	−.473	−.392	−.071	−.514	−.255	−.524
	p	.013	.043	.731	.007	.208	.006
	N	27	27	26	26	26	26
Some Acoustic	*r*	.002	−.074	−.062	−.178	−.037	−.187
	p	.994	.724	.770	.395	.860	.371
	N	25	25	25	25	25	25

Note. EOWPVT = Expressive One-Word Picture Vocabulary Test; RW-U = real-word utterances obtained in the 20-minute child language sample; MLU = mean length of utterance in morphemes; NDW = number of different words from SALT analysis. Numbers are different for RW-U, MLU, Pronouns, and NDW because one child did not have a useable language sample at that test age.

second and third rows of Table 9–1 show these coefficients separately for children who no longer wore hearing aids after receiving their first implants (*electric only*) and for those who kept wearing their hearing aids on the un-implanted side after receiving their first implants (*some acoustic*). As can be seen, significant correlations were found only for those children who stopped wearing a hearing aid once they received an implant. Children who continued to use a hearing aid after getting an implant appear to have continued language learning uninterrupted by the change in prosthesis. Children who no longer used a hearing aid once they received an implant, on the other hand,

were apparently affected strongly by the change in auditory input: For them the age at which they received that implant explained significant amounts of variance on most language measures. The signal components these children were using to begin deciphering the speech signal were apparently disrupted seriously enough when they changed prostheses that they needed to restart the language learning process.

The *What* and *How Many* of Prostheses

Next, language scores at 48 months of age were examined based on what kind of stimulation configuration children had for the majority of their young lives. Of course, it would have been ideal from a methodological perspective if we had been able to design this study so that children with severe-to-profound hearing loss were randomly assigned to a stimulation configuration at 12 months of age: One third would have received one implant only; one third would have received simultaneous bilateral implants; and one third would have had bimodal stimulation. But real life does not happen that neatly. While we were busy conducting our research, parents were making decisions about what kind of stimulation to provide to their children in consultation with their otologists and audiologists. As a result, we needed to form groupings of children based on what actually happened to them. The greatest confound in sorting children into groups involved the fact that they received second implants, if they were to get them, at various ages. We considered grouping children in various ways, and finally settled upon the following groups. The first three of these are generically classified as having *electric-only* stimulation because none of them wore hearing aids once they received a first cochlear implant. The latter three groups are termed *some-acoustic* stimulation because they all had access to acoustic hearing through hearing aids for much of their young lives, either alone or in combination with an implant.

- *One CI:* These children received one implant before 24 months of age and discontinued wearing a hearing aid at that time. These children did not receive a second implant while participating in this study. There were 14 children in this group tested at 48 months.

- *CICI:* These were the children who received two implants simultaneously. There were only five children fitting this criterion who were tested at 48 months. All five were early identified and received their bilateral implants before 18 months of age. The small group size reflects the fact that simultaneous implantation was a relatively new phenomenon in 2004, when these children were implanted. Three other children in this study received two implants simultaneously, but they were all late-identified signing children.

- *CI-CICI:* These were children who received one cochlear implant early in their lives, and discontinued wearing a hearing aid. After 24 months of age these children received a second implant. There were eight children meeting these criteria at 48 months.

- *HACI:* These children received one implant at a young age and retained their hearing aid in the other ear. They continued with this configuration for the duration of time they were in this study. Sixteen children fit into this group at 48 months.

- *HACI-CICI:* These children fit the criteria for the group above, but then received a second implant during the time that this study was being conducted. Nine children fit into this group at 48 months.

- *HA-only:* These were the children who had bilateral hearing aids for the duration of the study. There were 25 children in this group at 48 months.

Table 9–2 shows means for relevant independent variables for each group. Looking across these participants, there can be found no consistent pattern of who received which kind of prosthesis combination based on BE-PTAs, other than the fact children with moderate losses were in the *HA-only* group. Among the five groups of children who had at least one implant, there was no statistically significant differ-

ence in BE-PTA. We also kept track of auditory thresholds at 250 Hz for these children. It appears that children in the *CICI* and *CI-CICI* groups may have had slightly poorer thresholds at this frequency. However, these values are based on results from fewer participants for these groups than for the other groups, and from thresholds that were obtained earlier in the children's lives. It was rare for children to have unaided

Table 9–2. Means for independent variables across six groups of prosthesis configurations, with standard deviations in parentheses and group numbers in italics.

	One CI	CICI	CI-CICI	HACI	HACI-CICI	HA Only
SES	27.71 (14.23) *14*	38.80 (16.16) *5*	33.38 (14.01) *8*	36.06 (14.46) *16*	31.67 (12.33) *9*	28.92 (10.38) *25*
BE-PTA	104 (16) *14*	101 (6) *5*	108 (13) *8*	100 (16) *16*	98 (10) *9*	65 (11) *25*
Aided PTA	38 (19) *12*	33 (8) *5*	32 (14) *8*	32 (9) *16*	33 (5) *9*	30 (6) *16*
250 Hz	87 (19) *10*	98 (8) *4*	99 (4) *4*	89 (13) *13*	89 (9) *7*	51 (11) *19*
ID-Age	5.17 (4.81) *14*	3.47 (1.45) *5*	6.33 (4.11) *8*	10.40 (6.41) *16*	7.48 (5.54) *9*	8.23 (8.88) *25*
Age First Implant	15.21 (5.78) *14*	13.20 (1.30) *5*	14.00 (5.10) *8*	20.63 (7.38) *16*	14.78 (2.95) *9*	
Age Second Implant			35.75 (4.64) *8*		31.78 (4.84) *9*	

Note. Auditory thresholds at 250 Hz were not available for all children. All age-related values are given in months; all auditory thresholds are given in dB HL.

thresholds measured once they received an implant, unless they were wearing a hearing aid on one ear. In any event, the small difference in 250-Hz thresholds shown here was not statistically significant. We were unable to identify any consistent trend in any independent variable that explained which children received which configuration of prosthesis.

Table 9–3 displays means and standard deviations of scores for each of the six language measures at 48 months of age. ANOVAs were computed on these scores with prosthesis configuration as the main effect. None was found to be statistically significant. Next, analyses of covariance (ANCOVAs) were performed on scores for children with at least one cochlear implant, excluding children in the *HA-only* group, using age of first implant as the covariate. Only scores for NDW showed a significant group effect, $F(4, 45) = 2.62$, $p = .047$. Post hoc comparisons were done, but none showed significance when a correction for multiple contrasts was applied. Consequently, we are unable to ascribe any of the variability in language outcomes for these deaf children to the kind of prosthesis they had. Even children with moderate losses who

Table 9–3. Mean raw scores at 48 months for each group, with standard deviations in parentheses and group numbers in italics.

	One CI	CICI	CI-CICI	HACI	HACI-CICI	HA Only
Auditory Comprehension	40.21 (10.48) *14*	40.4 (7.09) *5*	44.5 (8.04) *8*	43.38 (8.80) *16*	46.11 (10.03) *9*	45.16 (9.56) *25*
EOWPVT	26.86 (9.14) *14*	31.20 (15.27) *5*	34.50 (4.50) *8*	30.88 (9.06) *16*	34.44 (6.84) *9*	35.04 (9.62) *25*
RW-U	121.08 (33.75) *13*	85.00 (36.68) *5*	107.69 (19.00) *8*	109.41 (30.54) *16*	113.28 (30.82) *9*	113.85 (30.17) *24*
MLU	2.96 (1.13) *13*	2.27 (0.67) *5*	3.50 (0.51) *8*	2.88 (0.81) *16*	3.16 (0.58) *9*	3.34 (0.96) *24*
Pronouns	24.89 (15.03) *13*	12.27 (7.48) *5*	29.32 (7.89) *8*	26.14 (13.48) *16*	29.84 (12.79) *9*	29.93 (12.66) *24*
NDW	56.85 (23.30) *13*	45.65 (19.83) *5*	71.61 (9.48) *8*	60.56 (16.62) *16*	66.46 (14.93) *9*	67.54 (15.78) *24*

wore bilateral hearing aids were doing no better at 48 months of age than children with more significant hearing loss wearing other kinds of auditory prostheses. It will be recalled that earlier analyses of language measures, reported in previous chapters, generally showed prosthesis effects for children with early-identified hearing loss: Children with hearing aids developed language outcomes more rapidly than children who received an implant. However, the analyses in this chapter indicate that performance at 48 months did not differ for children based on type of prosthesis. Apparently, children with cochlear implants "caught up" by 48 months of age.

Finally, mean scores for each of the six prostheses groups were plotted for each of the six dependent measures across test ages. These results are shown in Figures 9–1 through 9–6. For these

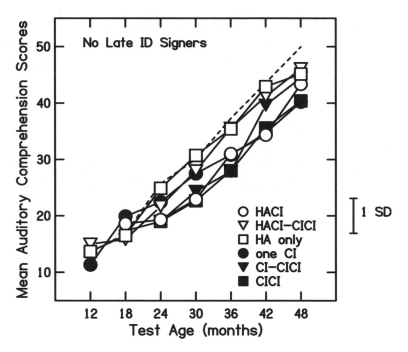

Figure 9–1. Mean scores for Auditory Comprehension for children with hearing loss. Groups are based on the kind of stimulation configuration children had for the majority of their lives: *One CI* (one CI, discontinued use of HA after implant); *CICI* (simultaneous, bilateral implants); *CI-CICI* (received one CI early in life and discontinued use of HA, then later received a second CI); *HA-CI* (one CI, one HA); *HACI-CICI* (received one CI early in life and continued using HA, then later received a second CI); *HA only* (bilateral HAs). The dotted line marks one standard deviation below the mean of scores for children with normal hearing. A bar representing one standard deviation is shown to the right of the figure. This pooled standard deviation was obtained from the original analysis of scores for children with normal hearing and those with early-identified hearing loss reported in Chapter 6.

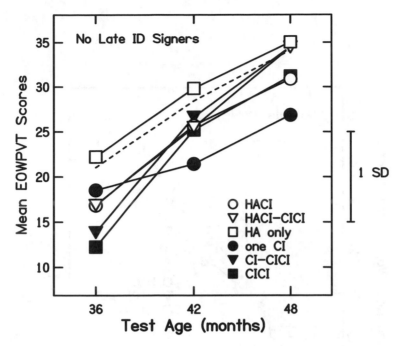

Figure 9–2. Mean scores for EOWPVT for children with hearing loss. Groups are based on the kind of stimulation configuration children had for the majority of their lives. The dotted line marks one standard deviation below the mean of scores for children with normal hearing. A bar representing one standard deviation is shown to the right of the figure. This pooled standard deviation was obtained from the original analysis of scores for children with normal hearing and those with early-identified hearing loss reported in Chapter 6.

plots, all children with hearing loss were included, regardless of whether they were tested at 48 months or not. The same criteria were used to place the children not tested at 48 months into groups as those used for the 48-month participants. Here we show only the boundary of one standard deviation below the mean of normal-hearing children with a dotted line: Means for all groups of deaf children are at or below this line, so it would not have been useful to display a wider range of possible scores. To provide a metric for gauging variance, we have marked one standard deviation to

the right of the plot. This is the pooled standard deviation obtained from the original analysis of each dependent measure, for children with normal hearing and early-identified hearing loss, as reported in earlier chapters.

These figures illustrate a couple trends that are apparent in Table 9–3: First, no evidence is found to support the practice of early simultaneous, bilateral implantation for children with hearing loss. Those who received two implants at the same time were certainly not performing any better on these language measures than were children

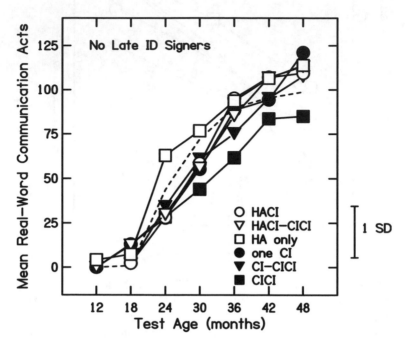

Figure 9–3. Mean scores of real-word communication acts for children with hearing loss. Groups are based on the kind of stimulation configuration children had for the majority of their lives. The dotted line marks one standard deviation below the mean of scores for children with normal hearing. A bar representing one standard deviation is shown to the right of the figure. This pooled standard deviation was obtained from the original analysis of scores for children with normal hearing and those with early-identified hearing loss reported in Chapter 7.

with other sorts of prosthesis configurations. In fact, when measures derived from the unstructured language sample (RW-U) and subsequent SALT (MLU, Pronouns, and NDW) are examined, children in the *CICI* group appear to be performing poorest, even though the statistical analyses did not show significant effects. This finding is important: Implanting a child is a much more invasive treatment than giving a child a hearing aid. Consequently, there should be evidence of its effectiveness above and beyond what is provided by less invasive procedures. No such evidence was found here.

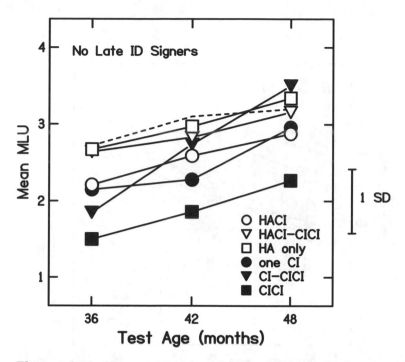

Figure 9–4. Mean scores for MLU for children with hearing loss. Groups are based on the kind of stimulation configuration children had for the majority of their lives. The dotted line marks one standard deviation below the mean of scores for children with normal hearing. A bar representing one standard deviation is shown to the right of the figure. This pooled standard deviation was obtained from the original analysis of scores for children with normal hearing and those with early-identified hearing loss reported in Chapter 8.

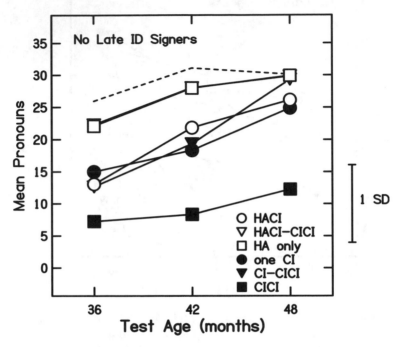

Figure 9–5. Mean scores for Pronouns for children with hearing loss. Groups are based on the kind of stimulation configuration children had for the majority of their lives. The dotted line marks one standard deviation below the mean of scores for children with normal hearing. A bar representing one standard deviation is shown to the right of the figure. This pooled standard deviation was obtained from the original analysis of scores for children with normal hearing and those with early-identified hearing loss reported in Chapter 8.

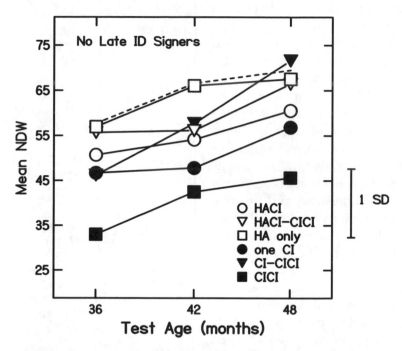

Figure 9–6. Mean scores for NDW for children with hearing loss. Groups are based on the kind of stimulation configuration children had for the majority of their lives. The dotted line marks one standard deviation below the mean of scores for children with normal hearing. A bar representing one standard deviation is shown to the right of the figure. This pooled standard deviation was obtained from the original analysis of scores for children with normal hearing and those with early-identified hearing loss reported in Chapter 8.

Auditory Oral or Auditory Verbal?

Max Goldstein imported a method of teaching deaf children that placed a strong emphasis on hearing. The belief at that time, roughly a hundred years ago, was that the auditory system is much like a muscle, and so it can be strengthened through use. That approach flourished in North America through the 20th century, and is now generally recognized with the moniker of Auditory-Verbal Therapy (AVT). A similar approach to intervention adheres just as strongly to the belief that deaf children can learn to understand and produce spoken language well enough to participate fully in mainstream society, without using signs, but does not put as great an emphasis on requiring that instruction be done through the auditory system alone. This latter approach is often labeled Auditory Oral (AO), and so it will be here. We examined whether one or the other of these two approaches to educating deaf children without the use of signs was associated with better language outcomes.

Again, we elected to examine scores for the 48-month test age. There were a total of 60 children tested at 48 months who were in one or the other sort of nonsigning program. Children were considered to be in an AVT program only if administrators of the program identified themselves as such, and if there was at least one professional with certification in AVT on staff. Accordingly, 45 children were considered to be in AO programs, and 15 children were considered to be in AVT programs. Table 9–4 shows means for each group

Table 9–4. Means at 48 months for BE-PTA, aided PTA, socioeconomic status (SES), and ID-age for each group with standard deviations in parentheses and group numbers in italics.

	AO	AVT
BE-PTA	90 (21) *45*	90 (18) *15*
Aided PTA	36 (13) *39*	32 (7) *14*
SES	32.07 (13.33) *45*	27.67 (12.23) *15*
ID-Age	9.39 (7.86) *45*	7.73 (5.92) *15*

Note. Socioeconomic status is given using the two-factor index described in the text. All age-related values are given in months; all auditory thresholds are given in dB HL.

of children of BE-PTA, aided PTA, SES, and ID-age. As can be seen, groups were well matched on each of these demographic variables.

The same dependent language measures as those used to test for effects of prosthesis configurations were used to test for possible differences between these two groups. As in the earlier analysis, scores from the 48-month test session were used. These are shown on Table 9–5. A series of *t*-tests was performed to check for possible differences between these two intervention methods, but no significant differences were found. Children performed similarly regardless of whether they were in AO

Table 9–5. Mean raw scores at 48 months for each group, with standard deviations in parentheses and group numbers in italics.

	AO	AVT
Auditory Comprehension	43.78 (8.84) *45*	41.00 (10.87) *15*
EOWPVT	32.93 (8.68) *45*	29.80 (11.87) *15*
RW-U	116.52 (32.06) *43*	107.90 (34.99) *15*
MLU	2.95 (0.79) *43*	3.00 (1.02) *15*
Pronouns	25.42 (12.23) *43*	25.51 (14.55) *15*
NDW	61.12 (17.55) *43*	58.92 (18.37) *15*

or AVT programs. To illustrate this point, scores for all six measures were plotted across test ages on Figures 9–7 through 9–12. For these figures, scores were included for all children in non-signing programs tested at each age, according to whether their intervention program was AO or AVT: Across all participants tested at all ages, 54 were in AO and 20 in AVT programs. Also plotted in these figures are scores for children in signing programs, if their hearing loss was identified early. These figures show just how similar developmental trajectories were for children with hearing loss, on average, as long as they were not part of the late-identified signing group.

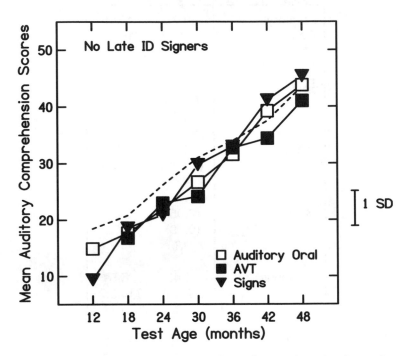

Figure 9–7. Mean scores for Auditory Comprehension for early-identified children in nonsigning programs tested at each age, according to type of intervention program (AVT = Auditory-Verbal Therapy). Also included are mean scores for early-identified children in signing programs. The dotted line marks one standard deviation below the mean of scores for children with normal hearing. A bar representing one standard deviation is shown to the right of the figure. This pooled standard deviation was obtained from the original analysis of scores for children with normal hearing and those with early-identified hearing loss reported in Chapter 6.

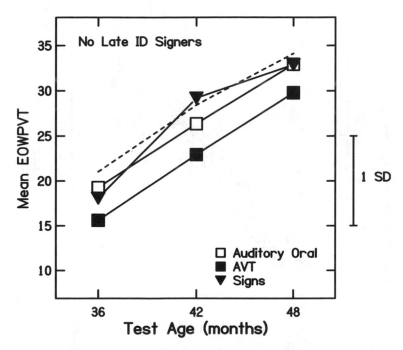

Figure 9–8. Mean scores for EOWPVT for early-identified children in nonsigning programs tested at each age, according to type of intervention program. Also included are mean scores for early-identified children in signing programs. The dotted line marks one standard deviation below the mean of scores for children with normal hearing. A bar representing one standard deviation is shown to the right of the figure. This pooled standard deviation was obtained from the original analysis of scores for children with normal hearing and those with early-identified hearing loss reported in Chapter 6.

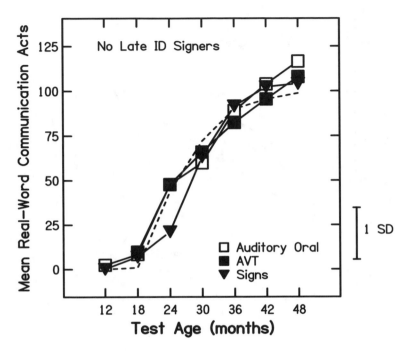

Figure 9–9. Mean scores of real-word communication acts for early-identified children in nonsigning programs tested at each age, according to type of intervention. Also included are mean scores for early-identified children in signing programs. The dotted line marks one standard deviation below the mean of scores for children with normal hearing. A bar representing one standard deviation is shown to the right of the figure. This pooled standard deviation was obtained from the original analysis of scores for children with normal hearing and those with early-identified hearing loss reported in Chapter 7.

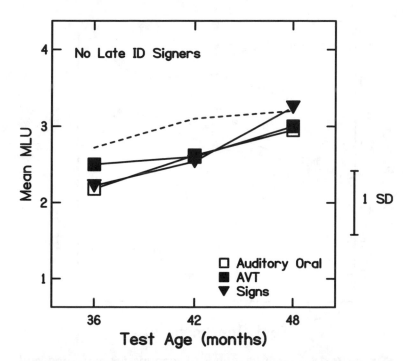

Figure 9–10. Mean scores for MLU for early-identified children in nonsigning programs tested at each age, according to type of intervention. Also included are mean scores for early-identified children in signing programs. The dotted line marks one standard deviation below the mean of scores for children with normal hearing. A bar representing one standard deviation is shown to the right of the figure. This pooled standard deviation was obtained from the original analysis of scores for children with normal hearing and those with early-identified hearing loss reported in Chapter 8.

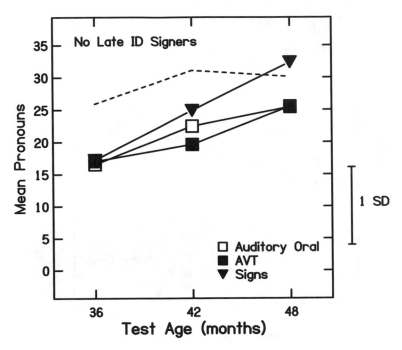

Figure 9–11. Mean scores for Pronouns for early-identified children in nonsigning programs tested at each age, according to type of intervention. Also included are mean scores for early-identified children in signing programs. The dotted line marks one standard deviation below the mean of scores for children with normal hearing. A bar representing one standard deviation is shown to the right of the figure. This pooled standard deviation was obtained from the original analysis of scores for children with normal hearing and those with early-identified hearing loss reported in Chapter 8.

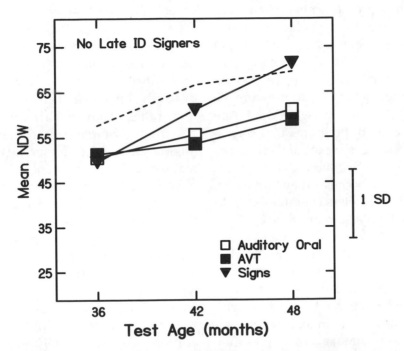

Figure 9–12. Mean scores for NDW for early-identified children in nonsigning programs tested at each age, according to type of intervention. Also included are mean scores for early-identified children in signing programs. The dotted line marks one standard deviation below the mean of scores for children with normal hearing. A bar representing one standard deviation is shown to the right of the figure. This pooled standard deviation was obtained from the original analysis of scores for children with normal hearing and those with early-identified hearing loss reported in Chapter 8.

Signing Effects

Is More Better?

Figure 4–2 illustrated that the proportion of time that parents and children accompanied their spoken language with signs decreased as children got older. By 48 months of age, neither parent nor child was signing very much during their communications with one another. Of course, these children were all in preschool programs that consistently used signs as part of their curricula. We know that these children were able to sign because they did so in school. Nonetheless, Figure 4–2 indicates that both parents and children decreased the proportion of communication time with each other during which they used signs. On average, we have already found that these children performed similarly to children who were not using signs in conjunction with their spoken language, as long as they were not identified late. But there was variability in language outcomes for these children, as well as variability in the proportion of time that they and their parents used signs to accompany their spoken communication. We wanted to know whether variability across those two measures was related.

This question was somewhat tricky to investigate precisely because the amount of time that parents and children signed to each other generally decreased as children got older. That meant that age (and so spoken language abilities in general) and time spent signing were strongly and inversely correlated. As a result we needed to examine this relation at discrete test ages: To combine test ages would have confounded the effects of decreases in signing as children got older with variability in the amount of time different parent-child dyads used signs at any one test age. This meant that our sample sizes were quite small, especially because only 67% of signing parents provided estimates of the time they spent signing at any one test age. And signing children with late-identified hearing loss could not be included in these analyses because they were so distinctly different in their performance from other children. That further decreased our sample sizes. Nonetheless, this question seemed important enough that we wished to examine it.

We used the same set of six dependent language measures that were used in the two earlier analyses reported in this chapter. Individual scores were plotted as a function of the proportion of time that mothers reported they used signs with their children, and are shown on Figures 9–13, through 9–18. Four of the six measures (EOWPVT, MLU, numbers of pronouns, and NDW) were plotted for all three test sessions at which they were analyzed: 36 to 48 months. For the two measures obtained from all seven test sessions (auditory comprehension and RW-U), we elected to use scores from three test times: 24, 36, and 48 months. Scores for each test age are represented with different symbols. If we look closely we find that there was no relation between children's language outcomes and the proportion of time that their parents signed with them. A series of correlational analyses supported this conclusion: Pearson product-moment correlation coefficients computed at each test age between each language measure and proportion of time parents signed to their children were all close to zero.

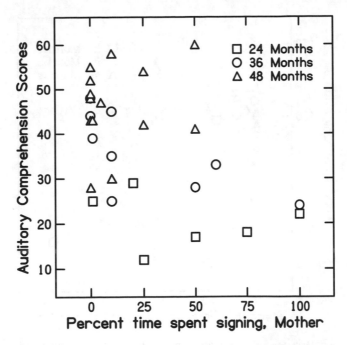

Figure 9–13. Scores for Auditory Comprehension and percent time mother signed to child, at 24, 36, and 48 months.

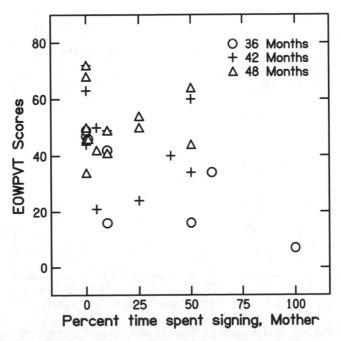

Figure 9–14. Scores for EOWPVT and percent time mother signed to child, at 36, 42, and 48 months.

245

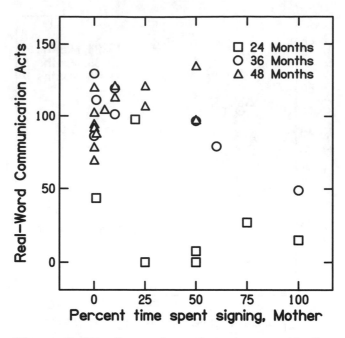

Figure 9–15. Scores for real-word communication acts and percent time mother signed to child, at 24, 36, and 48 months.

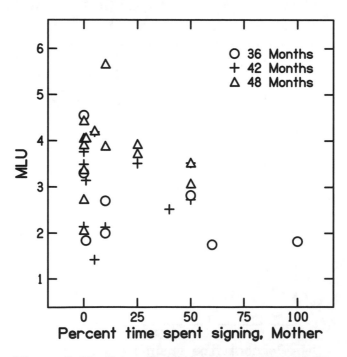

Figure 9–16. Scores for MLU and percent time mother signed to child, at 36, 42, and 48 months.

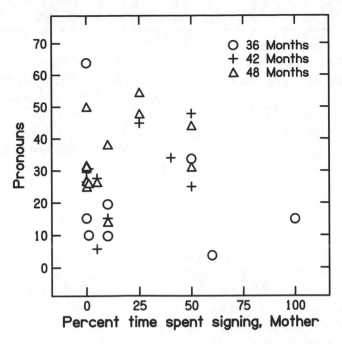

Figure 9–17. Scores for Pronouns and percent time mother signed to child, at 36, 42, and 48 months.

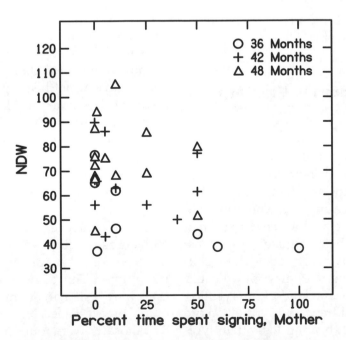

Figure 9–18. Scores for NDW and percent time mother signed to child, at 36, 42, and 48 months.

Type of Signs: English versus American Sign Language

A total of 44 children with hearing loss used signs. Of those children, 30 were exposed to American Sign Language (ASL): 18 who were identified early, and 12 who were identified late. Fourteen children in this study were exposed to manually coded English: 11 who were identified early and three who were identified late. We were curious to know if one method of signs led to better spoken language outcomes than the other. To examine that question we performed *t*-tests for each of the six language measures discussed earlier in this chapter for children with early-identified hearing loss, based on whether they were exposed to ASL or manually coded English. None of these tests produced significant results. Consequently, we conclude that there were no differences in outcomes for the type of signs children were exposed to.

Stardom is Fleeting

Educators, clinicians, and scientists interested in childhood hearing loss have long been interested in children considered to be "stars"—those children with hearing loss who appear to be functioning as children with normal hearing in their language use. If we could identify what makes these children stars, the reasoning is, we could provide the same kind of intervention to other children, and so help more children with hearing loss attain typical language abilities. Accordingly, we sought to identify the stars within this study.

In most discussions of stars, there is no objective metric used for defining who they are: A star is labeled as such based on subjective impressions that the child is communicating as well as children with normal hearing. We wanted to be more objective in our approach. We began to think about how to define potential stars while analyzing data from the 36-month test age, and so we developed some criteria at that time and continued using them. We chose to define stars using four measures from SALT because these measures provide the most sensitive indices of native language ability. Children with hearing loss had to score *better than* half a standard deviation below the mean of children with normal hearing on three SALT measures: MLU, total number of words, and number of different words. For one measure, the number of one-word utterances, high numbers indicated more immature language patterns. On this measure, children with hearing loss were required to score *below* half a standard deviation *above* the mean of children with normal hearing in order to be categorized as a star. Although these criteria did not include the measure of auditory comprehension, which has turned out to be consistently sensitive to differences between children with normal hearing and those with hearing loss, it served us well.

Over the three test ages of 36, 42, and 48 months, 15 children were found to meet all four requirements at one or more times. Thirteen of these 15 children were tested at a minimum of two of the three test ages. Nonetheless, only 5 of those 13 were found to be stars at both times. Ten children were tested at all three ages, and only one of those 10 children was found to be a star all three times. So, out of all participants with hearing loss, very few were consistently performing as well as children with normal hearing on this set of language measures.

Table 9–6 displays characteristics of the 15 children designated as stars. On one hand it is not surprising to see that seven of these 15 children had moderate hearing loss; on the other hand, 25 children in this study met that description, and were tested at least once between the ages of 36 and 48 months. Eighteen of those children failed to qualify as stars even once. Therefore, we cannot conclude that having only a moderate hearing loss is protection against the language problems that can arise due to hearing loss.

One trend that seems clear from Table 9–6 is that almost all of these children were identified, fit with hearing aids, and started in intervention early in life. So although we have observed that children with late-identified hearing loss are doing as well as children with early-identified hearing loss, on average, there certainly does seem to be an advantage to being identified as soon as possible. If we hope to some day eliminate entirely the negative consequences of hearing loss, we will need to ensure that children are identified as young as possible. The challenge we face is to develop intervention strategies that can move children through the language learning process as rapidly as children with normal hearing move through that process.

After completing data collection for all test ages, we decided that it was worth exploring how the set of children identified as stars would have been different if we had used another set of criteria. In particular, we wanted to see

what would happen if we used the set of six language measures that we have generally used in this chapter to examine differences based on treatment: that is, auditory comprehension, EOWPVT, number of real-word utterances, MLU, NDW, and number of pronouns. We went back through our data at each of the test ages of 36, 42, and 48 months of age, and identified the children with hearing loss who scored at or better than ½ standard deviation below the mean of children with normal hearing on all six of those measures. This analysis resulted in fewer stars. There were only three stars at each of 36 and 42 months of age, with no overlap among these children. At 48 months of age there were four stars, and only one of these children had been classified as a star at a younger age (36 months) using these criteria; this was the same child who was a star at all three test ages using the earlier method. Only 30% of the children classified as stars according to the first method were reclassified using the new criteria.

The point to be made with these analyses is that there were very few children with hearing loss who were acquiring language at a similar rate to that of the average child with normal hearing. The typical situation for these children was that they were delayed in their language development, but could perform well on some of the measures some of the time. However, we do learn one important lesson from these analyses, and that is that getting an early start in intervention is important if we ever hope to eliminate the language delay currently being experienced by children with hearing loss: As with the analysis described above, the only factor that the children identified as stars in this new

Table 9–6. Characteristics of children designated as "stars" at one or more test times between 36 and 48 months of age.

Star #	Times Tested	Times Star	Age When Star (Months)	SES	BE-PTA (dB HL)	ID-Age (Months)	Prosthesis	Age 1st Implant (Months)	Age 2nd Implant (Months)	Intervention Type
1	3	3	All	36	58	2.67	HA only			Signs (English)
2	3	2	36, 48	36	95	3	HACI	12		AVT
3	3	2	36, 42	30	87	4	HACI-CICI	13	30	AVT
4	3	2	42, 48	42	50	13	HA only			AO
5	3	1	42	30	62	2.33	HA only			AO
6	3	1	36	35	107	2	HACI	13		AO
7	3	1	48	36	105	4	One CI	10		Signs (English)
8	3	1	48	16	92	9.33	CI-CICI	12	38	AO
9	3	1	48	30	108	2.33	One CI	9		Signs (ASL)
10	3	1	42	42	65	7.33	HA only			AVT
11	2	2	42, 48	56	120	1.33	CI-CICI	12	42	Signs (ASL)
12	2	1	42	42	57	4	HA only			AO
13	2	1	48	42	70	2.33	HA only			AO
14	1	1	48	49	120	2.67	HACI	17		Signs (English)
15	1	1	48	64	57	24	HA only			Signs (ASL)

formulation had in common with one another, and with the children identified as stars using the earlier criteria, was that they were all identified before 1 year of age, with one exception, and that child had only a moderate hearing loss.

Are There Differences in Geography?

Even after all of these analyses, we were left wondering if there might be something about specific intervention methods that could explain particularly positive outcomes. We thought that if we could identify one or two test sites where children with hearing loss were performing consistently well, we could look at the intervention methods used in those areas for ideas about how to design intervention for the future. To do this we plotted mean scores at 48 months of age on each of the six language measures used in this chapter for all children with hearing loss, for each test site where two or more children were tested at that age. These scores are shown in Figures 9–19 through 9–24. Scores at every test site for children with hearing loss were within plus/minus one standard deviation of the overall mean for all children with hearing loss, with one exception: Children at one site slipped below that cutoff on the real-word

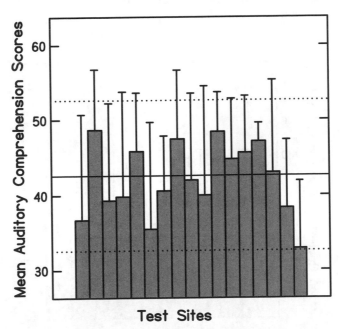

Figure 9–19. Mean scores for Auditory Comprehension at 48 months of age for all children with hearing loss, for each test site where two or more children were tested at that age. Solid line shows mean for all children with hearing loss, and dotted lines show +/– one standard deviations. Error bars show within-group standard deviations for all children at that site.

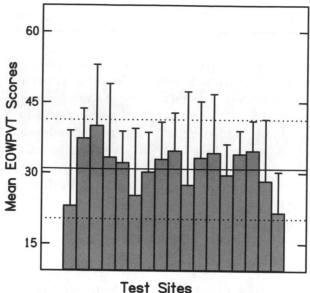

Figure 9–20. Mean scores for EOWPVT at 48 months of age for all children with hearing loss, for each test site where two or more children were tested at that age. Solid line shows mean for all children with hearing loss, and dotted lines show +/– one standard deviations. Error bars show within-group standard deviations for all children at that site.

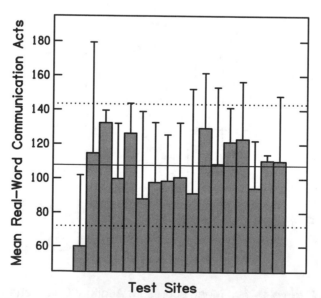

Figure 9–21. Mean scores for real-word communication acts at 48 months of age for all children with hearing loss, for each test site where two or more children were tested at that age. Solid line shows mean for all children with hearing loss, and dotted lines show +/– one standard deviations. Error bars show within-group standard deviations for all children at that site.

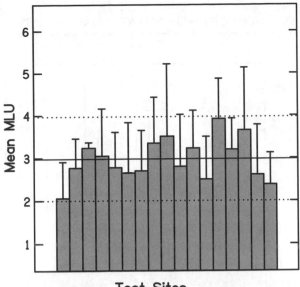

Figure 9-22. Mean scores for MLU at 48 months of age for all children with hearing loss, for each test site where two or more children were tested at that age. Solid line shows mean for all children with hearing loss, and dotted lines show +/– one standard deviations. Error bars show within-group standard deviations for all children at that site.

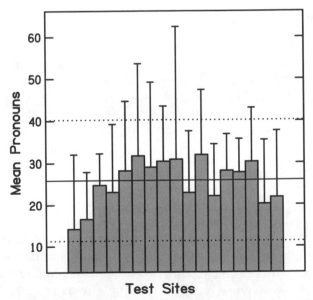

Figure 9-23. Mean scores for Pronouns at 48 months of age for all children with hearing loss, for each test site where two or more children were tested at that age. Solid line shows mean for all children with hearing loss, and dotted lines show +/– one standard deviations. Error bars show within-group standard deviations for all children at that site.

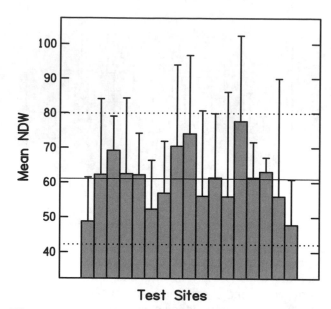

Figure 9–24. Mean scores for NDW at 48 months of age for all children with hearing loss, for each test site where two or more children were tested at that age. Solid line shows mean for all children with hearing loss, and dotted lines show +/− one standard deviations. Error bars show within-group standard deviations for all children at that site.

communication acts. In general, however, we were unable to identify any site where children were consistently outperforming children at other sites.

Chapter Summary

This chapter explored specific aspects of treatment regimens that might account for variability in language outcomes for children with hearing loss. In previous chapters we have seen that children with hearing loss, on average, are not performing as well as children with normal hearing. But that is *on average*. It was our hope that by examining specific aspects of the treatment these children were receiving we might

be able to identify components of those treatments that seem to promote better outcomes. Clearly, that was not what happened.

In this chapter we learned that the configuration of children's prostheses accounted for little variance in language outcomes. Of primary concern, no advantage was observed for the practice of early, simultaneous implantation. Cochlear implantation involves surgery, and is costly. Finding that there is no advantage to language development of receiving two implants simultaneously could have significant effects both on the treatment we provide to children with hearing loss and on how we design and fit prostheses in the future. Perhaps of graver concern, it was found that children with moderate losses were faring no better than children with severe-to-profound losses. Quite obviously, factors other than auditory sensitivity explain language outcomes.

It was also found that nonsigning intervention strategies that place a particular emphasis on developing auditory skills provided no special benefits.

The amount of time that parents signed with their children also did not influence outcomes, nor did the kind of signs parents were using.

Finally, we observed that although there were children with hearing loss at each test age who performed similarly to the average child with normal hearing on one or a few measures, these appear to be fleeting moments of stardom: Only one child performed at that level consistently across test sessions. Nonetheless, the children who enjoyed even one session as a star were most clearly marked by the young age at which their hearing losses were identified. No particular kind of auditory prosthesis or type of intervention marks this group of children as different from the wider sample.

At the start of this chapter the suggestions were made that either we have not identified treatment regimens that help children overcome the barriers to language acquisition imposed by hearing loss, or we are simply not delivering those services to all children. Results of this chapter support the first of these suggestions. We, as a profession, need to be addressing the very real need for improved services for children with hearing loss.

In sum, we have not yet identified the factors that may allow us to eliminate the deleterious consequences of hearing loss on language learning. In the next chapter, we will turn our attention to what parents are doing that may explain variance in language outcomes.

10

All about Parents

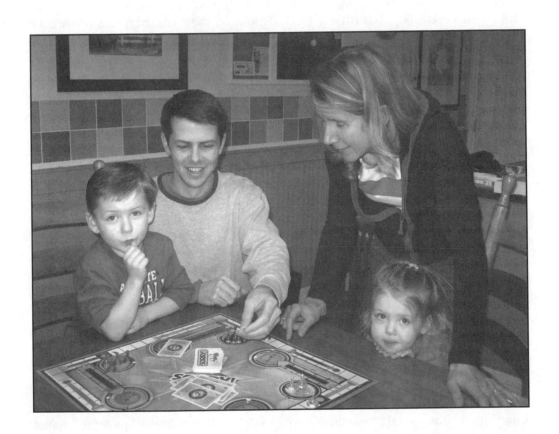

Parents are the most important influence in their young child's life. Any intervention that we may develop will only be as effective as parents' abilities to implement it. Parents are also the people who will most intensely feel the consequences of the success or failure of their intervention choices. Long after the professional providing early intervention to a child has moved on to other things (new students, a new job, or even a new career), the parents of that child will be dealing with the effects that the intervention had on their child's development. For these reasons it is critical that we consider the role of parents in their children's intervention. For the purposes of this study we wanted to know how parents were coping with having a young child with hearing loss, and how they were interacting with their children.

All parents in this study had normal hearing. Except possibly for the two children who had deaf relatives in their extended families, all parents were caught by surprise when told of their children's hearing loss: None of them would have chosen to have a deaf child. But just as they were grieving over the news that their children have a serious sensory deficit, these parents were faced with having to make important decisions regarding amplification and intervention for their children. The combination of emotional, financial, and informational factors might be expected to result in extra stress for parents of children with hearing loss, above that which all new parents experience just by having a baby. In the first half of this chapter, the possibility that parents may have experienced increased stress is examined.

In the second half of this chapter, we report on our examination of the form and function of parents' language when they were talking to their children. The way parents interact with their children has significant effects on language development, even for children with normal hearing. The best evidence of that comes from studies of children growing up in abject poverty. For example, Hart and Risley (1995) found that parents in extremely low socioeconomic conditions spoke to their children less often than other parents, and used different communication styles. Clearly, conditions of poverty affect how parents communicate with their children. We wondered whether the condition of having a child with hearing loss might have similar effects, and so we examined the nature of parental language input to these children.

Parenting Stress

We used the Parenting Stress Index, Third Edition (PSI; Abidin, 1995) to evaluate how much stress parents were experiencing. The PSI is a measure of stress in the parent-child relationship. It was standardized for use with parents of children from 1 month to 12 years of age. The PSI is administered as a checklist of 101 written items that parents respond to using a rating scale. Sample items are *My child makes more demands on me than most children* and *I enjoy being a parent.* Parents must indicate on the response form how strongly the statement applies to them, using a five-point rating scale. Answers to these questions receive weights between 1 and 5, and weighted scores are summed separately for each of 14 subtests. Higher scores indicate greater stress. Six of those subtests are related to stress arising from the child's behavior (distractibility/hyperactivity, adaptability, how well the child reinforces parents, how demanding the child is, mood, and acceptability of child to parents). The sum of scores across these six subtests is known as the Child Domain. The PSI also generates weighted scores on eight subscales related to the parent's feelings about her own situation (competence, isolation, attachment, health, role restriction, depression, spousal support, and life stress). The composite score from these subscales indexes the proportion of stress related to the parent's situation and is known as the Parent Domain. Scores for these two subscales can be summed to obtain a Total Stress Score, which serves as the primary indicator of whether the parent-child relationship is in danger of dysfunctional parenting or child behavior problems.

A subset of items on the PSI is used to evaluate whether parents are responding defensively or not. A defensive response pattern is one in which a parent is unable to recognize or unwilling to admit that there are problems in the parent-child relationship. Summing across these select items generates a score that indicates whether parents were likely to be defensive in their responses. A defensive approach to responding can lead to underestimates of the amount of stress parents are actually experiencing, and so render the instrument invalid. For this study, scores were examined first for defensive responding, and any test indicating that the parent completing the form may have responded defensively was eliminated from further scoring. Table 10–1 displays the numbers of tests that met that criterion, for each group at each test age. Across all groups and test ages, 19% of the responses to this instrument met the criterion of possibly being defensive.

Table 10–1. Count of defensive responders for each group at each test age.

Test Age (Months)	NH–s	NH+S	Early HL–s	Early HL+S	Late HL–s	Late HL+S	Total
12	6			3			9
18	11	3	5	4			23
24	4	3	4	2	1	1	15
30	4	3	5	3	2	2	19
36	6	5	6	2	4	4	27
42	8	3	5	2	7	4	29
48	5	2	5	4	9	3	28
Total	44	19	30	20	23	14	150

Specific percentages for groups were, across test ages: 21% for *NH–s*, 11% for *NH+S*, 14% for *EHL–s*, 23% for *EHL+S*, 28% for *LHL–s*, and 38% for *LHL+S*.

The PSI also requires that respondents indicate at the time of testing which of several stress-evoking situations they recently experienced. The list includes items such as *death of a parent*, *divorce*, and *loss of job*. Disproportionately high scores for these items can indicate that the parent is experiencing stress for reasons unrelated to the parent-child relationship, and so render results invalid. Mean scores for life stress were similar across all groups and close to the published mean for the test. No parent had a life stress score that was considered clinically significant.

The PSI has been used in earlier studies to examine parenting stress in hearing parents of deaf children. In Quittner et al. (1990), mothers of children between 2 and 5 years of age (mean = 48 months) completed the PSI: Some mothers had children with normal hearing, and others had children with hearing loss. Results showed that mothers of children with hearing loss rated their children as being more hyperactive, demanding, moody, and less adaptable than did mothers of children with normal hearing. When scores for individual subscales were summed across the Child Domain, the mean for mothers of children with HL were at the 85th percentile, a level considered to be clinically significant— although just barely.

In the current study, parents completed the PSI as part of the protocol at each test session. Because parents complete this form on their own, no special training of testers was required for them to administer this instrument. All scoring was done at the central facility by two independent scorers, and reliability checked. Statistical tests were then performed on scores of stress resulting from the Child Domain and stress resulting from the Parent Domain.

Parenting Stress Outcomes: Child Domain

Table 10–2, at the end of the chapter, shows mean scores on the Child Domain obtained for all groups in this study, and Figure 10–1 displays these means for these six groups of participants. The dotted line on this figure represents the raw score corresponding to the 85th percentile for this metric according to the test authors. This is the boundary for clinical significance. Clearly, no mean score for any group was even close to this boundary. Nonetheless, the FIRST ANOVA showed a significant main effect of hearing status, $F(1, 542) = 9.24$, $p = .002$, indicating that parents of children with early-identified hearing loss were experiencing more stress associated with their children than were parents of children with normal hearing. There were no changes in the amount of stress parents reported across test ages, and no differences based on whether parents used signs with their children or not. The SECOND ANOVA revealed no significant effects. In particular, there were no differences found for parents of children with hearing loss depending on whether the loss was identified early or late. Looking at scores from 48 months only, parents of children with normal hearing had a mean score on the Child Domain of 92 (33rd percentile), and parents of children with hearing loss had

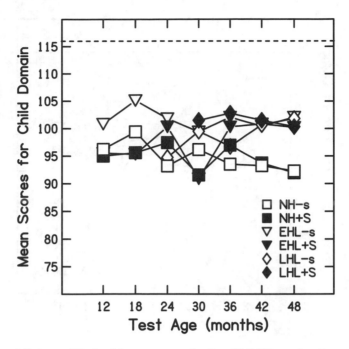

Figure 10–1. Mean scores for the Child Domain portion of the Parenting Stress Index for each group at each test age. NH–s (normal hearing, no signs); NH+S (normal hearing, signs); EHL–s (early-identified hearing loss, no signs); EHL+S (early-identified hearing loss, signs); LHL–s (late-identified hearing loss, no signs); and LHL⁺S (late-identified hearing loss, signs). The dotted line marks the boundary of clinical significance.

a mean score of 101 (55th percentile). So, although parents of children with hearing loss showed evidence of slightly more stress in the Child Domain than did parents of children with normal hearing, they were well within normal boundaries.

Parenting Stress Outcomes: Parent Domain

Table 10–3, at the end of the chapter, shows mean scores on the Parent Domain obtained for all groups in this study, and Figure 10–2 displays these means for these six groups of participants. The dotted line on this figure represents the raw score that corresponds to the 85th percentile, the boundary of clinical significance. No mean score for any group was close to this level. The FIRST ANOVA showed only a significant main effect of hearing status, $F(1, 542) = 12.23$, $p = .001$, and the SECOND ANOVA showed no significant effects. There were no changes in the amount of stress parents reported in the Parent Domain across test ages. There were no differences found between signing and

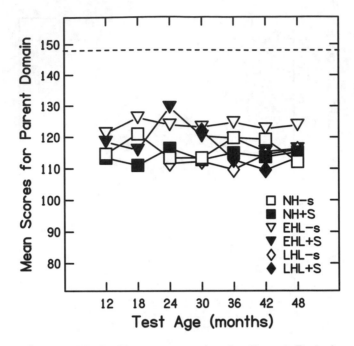

Figure 10–2. Mean scores for the Parent Domain portion of the Parenting Stress Index for each group at each test age. NH–s (normal hearing, no signs); NH+S (normal hearing, signs); EHL–s (early-identified hearing loss, no signs); EHL+S (early-identified hearing loss, signs); LHL–s (late-identified hearing loss, no signs); and LHL+S (late-identified hearing loss, signs). The dotted line marks the boundary of clinical significance.

nonsigning parents, and there were no differences for parents of children with hearing loss depending on whether the loss was identified early or late. Across all test ages, parents of children with normal hearing had a mean score on the Parent Domain of 114 (39th percentile), and parents of children with hearing loss had a mean score of 119 (48th percentile). So, although parents of children with early-identified hearing loss showed evidence of slightly more stress related to feelings about their own situations than did parents of children with normal hearing, they were well within normal boundaries.

How These Results Compare to Earlier Findings

These results indicate that the parents in this study who had children with hearing loss were not experiencing clinically relevant levels of stress. We wanted to explore how our results compared to those of others who have examined parenting stress in parents of deaf children, especially Quittner et al. (1990), who used the same instrument. Specifically, we compared scores for parents in this study to those of parents in the Quittner et al. study for the subscales on which Quittner et al. observed that parents of children with hearing loss were experiencing levels of stress significantly higher than those found for a control group of parents of children with normal hearing. Scores from the 48-month test session were used because that was the mean age of children in the Quittner et al. study, although the range of children's ages was greater in that study than in our study: Quittner et al. included parents of children as old as 5 years of age, which likely means they may have been close to 6 years old. That would make those children 2 years older than the children in this study. Table 10–4 shows comparisons of scores across the two studies: The first five subscales are from the Child Domain, and the last three are from the Parent Domain. In most cases, parents

Table 10–4. Mean scores on the Parenting Stress Index (PSI) from Quittner et al. (1990) and from the present study for subscales found to have significant differences between parents of 48-month-old children with normal hearing or with hearing loss by Quittner et al.

Subscale	Normal Hearing		Hearing Loss	
	This Study	Quittner et al.	This Study	Quittner et al.
Adaptability	24.00 (4.70)	24.54 (4.57)	25.99 (5.66)	29.87 (5.57)
Acceptability	11.41 (2.82)	12.73 (2.95)	12.43 (3.70)	14.73 (3.76)
Demanding	16.98 (3.32)	18.81 (4.12)	20.01 (5.48)	25.31 (5.69)
Child Mood	9.82 (2.30)	10.12 (2.97)	10.32 (2.77)	11.30 (3.27)
Distractibility-Hyperactivity	21.23 (4.67)	22.48 (4.92)	24.13 (5.32)	27.57 (5.54)
Attachment	10.73 (2.63)	12.26 (2.97)	11.36 (2.74)	13.75 (3.49)
Role Restriction	18.23 (4.55)	18.05 (5.00)	19.14 (4.38)	21.61 (5.49)
Competence	24.68 (4.48)	28.48 (5.98)	25.84 (5.64)	31.68 (5.80)

Note. Mean scores from this study were from the 48-month test session; all children with hearing loss were included. The first five subscales are from the Child Domain; the last three are from the Parent Domain. Some data from Chronic Parenting Stress: Moderating versus Mediating Effects of Social Support, by A. L. Quittner, R. L. Glueckauf, & D. N. Jackson, 1990, *Journal of Personality and Social Psychology, 59*, pp. 1266–1278.

of children with normal hearing in the two studies showed similar mean scores. Parents of children with hearing loss in the Quittner et al. study had higher scores than did the parents of children with hearing loss in this study on all subscales, and there are a couple that really stand out: the adaptability score and the score indexing how demanding the children were. For both these subscales, the scores from parents of children with hearing loss in the Quittner et al. study are clinically significant. Clearly those parents felt that their deaf children did not adapt easily to change, and that they were highly demanding. That was not so for the parents of children with hearing loss in this study: Only two subscales of the PSI showed significant differences in scores for parents of children with normal hearing and those with hearing loss in our study: Demandingness, $t(111) = 3.30$, $p = .001$, and Distractibility-Hyperactivity, $t(111) = 2.96$, $p = .004$. For both subscales, parents of children with hearing loss rated their children higher. However, in neither case did mean scores for children with hearing loss reach levels considered to be clinically significant. The difference in findings between the two studies could be due to Quittner et al. including parents of slightly older children. It could be due to the fact that some children in their study were apparently not identified as having hearing loss until later than 30 months of age. Finally, Quittner et al. did not describe what kind of intervention the families in their study were receiving, or how frequently they received it. All families in the current study were receiving intervention at least once per week for the duration of the study. Perhaps meeting with an intervention provider who understood the problems of having a child with hearing loss had an ameliorating effect on stress levels.

Correlations with Independent Variables

We computed correlation coefficients between the same set of independent variables used in earlier chapters and scores for the Child and Parent Domains of the PSI: For children with normal hearing, that meant only SES was examined; for children with hearing loss, that meant that SES, BE-PTA, ID-Age, and frequency of intervention, both before and after 36 months were examined. None of these correlation coefficients indicated that significant amounts of variance in parenting stress were explained by the independent variables. The failure to find a significant correlation with frequency of intervention suggests that even if the fact that parents in this study were receiving intervention at least once per week accounted for differences between outcomes in this and the Quittner et al. study, once a week was sufficiently frequent to reap the benefits of that intervention.

Parenting Stress Summary

In summary, parents of children with hearing loss in the current study did not demonstrate deleterious levels of stress. There was no evidence that learning of their children's hearing loss close to birth evoked particularly high levels of stress, although these data were not collected close to the time of identification for those children. Stress levels of parents may have been higher around the time their children were first identified. Clearly, however, if that were the case, stress dissipated within a short time after intervention was started. Similarly, there was no evidence that parents experienced more stress if they did not learn of their children's hearing loss until after age 12 months but before 30 months.

Parental Language

Past research studies conducted in this laboratory examined parental language style by asking each parent to build a Tinkertoy model with her child (e.g., Nittrouer, 2002; Nittrouer & Burton, 2005). Those interactions were videotaped and subsequently scored for parental language acts, such as inquiries and directives. However, that procedure is appropriate for children only after they have reached the age of roughly 3 years, when they can pay attention to that kind of constructive activity for a minimum of 10 minutes. Therefore, the procedure of having parent and child build a Tinkertoy model together was used only in test sessions when children were 36 to 48 months of age. This procedure is illustrated in Figure 10–3. A different model was provided at each test age. When children were younger than 36 months of age, we had the parent and child play together on the floor with a set of toys different from those used for scoring children's language. Each parent-child dyad was given a Fisher Price toy farm and two books in the *Carl* series by Alexandra Day: *Carl's Birthday* (1995) and *Carl's Afternoon in the Park* (1991). These books have no words, so

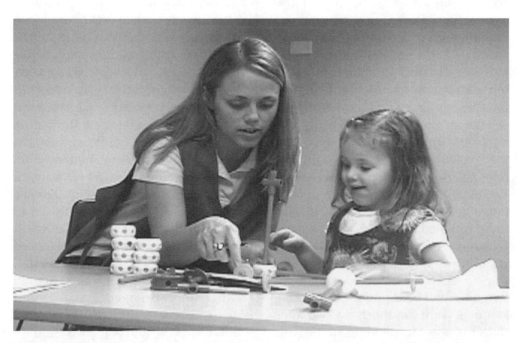

Figure 10–3. Parent and child working on a Tinkertoy model for the parental language task.

the parent and/or child had to create their own language for the pictures. The toy farm typically has batteries in it that allow some of its parts to make sound. Batteries, however, were not installed for this project. In this way, any stimulation from the farm was strictly visual, and so children with NH were no more affected in their play by sound than were children with HL.

At all ages, the parent-child dyads were videotaped for 11 minutes. During this time the parent wore the FM transmitter. Once the videotapes arrived back at the central site, 10 minutes of the interaction (starting after the first minute) were transferred to a DVD, and a time code laid down as had been done for the children's language samples. Two scorers independently watched each sample of the parent and child interacting, judged parental language input during the observation intervals, and recorded their responses on paper forms. The categories used for scoring parental language input have been used previously in our laboratory and are shown in Appendix D. Two individuals entered the recorded data for each scorer into the database independently, as was done for the scoring of children's language, and reliability was calculated as it was for measures of children's language (Chapter 7). These values were 99.1% for reliability of judging that a communication act occurred, and 79.0% for judging which of the 16 acts it was.

Twenty samples of parental language style were unusable, for largely the same reasons that samples of children's language had been unusable: Recorded samples were too short, the FM transmitter was not functioning, or the video signal was poor.

How Much Input

The first question we were interested in was whether the total amount of parental language input differed across groups. Table 10–5, at the end of the chapter, shows mean numbers of parental language acts for each group of participants. Figure 10–4 displays these results for parents from all six groups. The FIRST ANOVA showed a significant main effect of hearing status, $F(1, 634) = 4.70$, $p = .031$, as well as a significant main effect of signs, $F(1, 634) = 4.70$, $p = .031$. The Hearing Status × Signs interaction was also significant, $F(1, 634) = 4.08$, $p = .044$, which prompted a SEA looking at the effect of signs for children with normal hearing and those with hearing loss separately. A significant effect of signs was found for children with normal hearing only, $F(1, 634) = 14.98$, $p < .001$. Signing parents of normal-hearing children produced fewer communication acts overall than did nonsigning parents. That was true through the entire study, except for the very last test age. The SECOND ANOVA showed no significant main effects or interactions for children with hearing loss, and so we may conclude that all parents of children with hearing loss communicated with their children about the same amount.

In sum, we find that although the effect of hearing status was found to be significant in the FIRST ANOVA, there were no great differences observed across children with hearing loss and those with normal hearing. When all children are considered, across all test times, the mean numbers of total communication acts from parents were 100.8 ($SD = 17.8$) for parents of children with

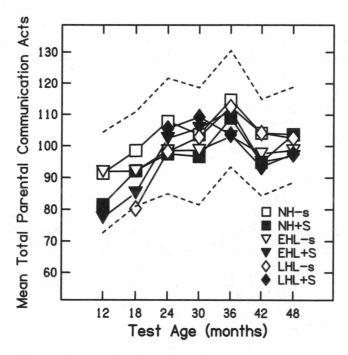

Figure 10–4. Mean numbers of total parental communication acts observed during the 10–minute language sample. NH–s (normal hearing, no signs); NH+S (normal hearing, signs); EHL–s (early-identified hearing loss, no signs); EHL+S (early-identified hearing loss, signs); LHL–s (late-identified hearing loss, no signs); and LHL+S (late-identified hearing loss, signs). The dotted lines show +/– one standard deviation from the mean, according to data from children with normal hearing in this study.

normal hearing and 99.4 for parents of children with hearing loss ($SD = 17.9$).

It's a Matter of Style

Roughly speaking, a hundred communication acts were observed for these 10-minute samples for most test ages: Although some variation was found based on hearing status and signs (for parents of children with normal hearing), it was small. When we investigated which specific acts comprised those

totals, we found that inquiries and explanation/descriptions each accounted for about 30% of those totals (26 inquiries and 31 explanation/descriptions per language sample, on average), and those percentages were consistent across all participant groups: No statistically significant effects were found. Directives accounted for roughly another 20% (18 per sample, on average), and again that was consistent across all groups.

Only the numbers of verbal responses that parents provided in response to their children's communicative attempts differed across groups. Table 10–6, at the end of the chapter, shows means for each group at each test age, and Figure 10–5 displays these means for all six groups. In the FIRST ANOVA, we found only a significant main effect of hearing status, $F(1, 634) = 41.94$, $p < .001$, indicating that parents of children with early-identified hearing loss produced fewer verbal responses than did parents of children with normal hearing. The SECOND ANOVA revealed a significant main effect of signs for children with hearing loss, $F(1, 289) = 11.13$, $p =$ .001, as well as a significant Age of ID × Signs interaction, $F(1, 289) = 14.30$, $p < .001$. The SEA that was performed to evaluate the main effects of signs, prosthesis, and test age for children with early-identified and late-identified hearing loss separately showed only a significant main effect of signs for children with late-identified hearing loss, $F(1, 273) = 11.33$, $p < .001$. There were no significant main effects or interactions for the numbers of verbal responses obtained from parents of children with early-identified hearing loss, and no

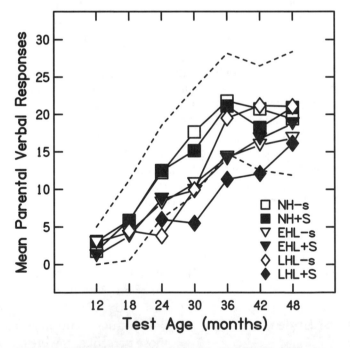

Figure 10–5. Mean numbers of verbal responses observed during the 10–minute parental language sample. NH–s (normal hearing, no signs); NH+S (normal hearing, signs); EHL–s (early-identified hearing loss, no signs); EHL+S (early-identified hearing loss, signs); LHL–s (late-identified hearing loss, no signs); and LHL+S (late-identified hearing loss, signs). The dotted lines show +/– one standard deviation from the mean, according to data from children with normal hearing in this study.

other significant effects for those parents of children with late-identified hearing loss. So for parents whose children's hearing losses were identified late, parents who did not sign with their children produced more verbal responses than parents who signed. Unlike other measures for which we find a difference between late-identified signing and nonsigning children, however, here the trend is that those nonsigning parents of late-identified children demonstrated a particularly high number of these behaviors. That outcome is quite apparent in Figure 10–5. Of all parents whose children had hearing loss, these were the only ones who responded verbally to their children's communicative attempts as frequently as did parents of children with normal hearing. In evaluating this result, it is important to recall that all children initiated communication with their parents with roughly the same frequency, a result reported in Chapter 7 (Figure 7–4). This difference in absolute numbers of verbal responses, therefore, cannot be explained by any particular group of parents having more or less communicative attempts from their children to respond to. Apparently, parents of children whose losses were identified late, and who did not sign with their children, were particularly responsive. That may have had a facilitative effect in helping these children develop language.

Correlations with Independent Variables

Only one measure of parental language style showed a significant difference among these groups of parents: how verbally responsive parents were to their children's communicative attempts. This

measure has been shown repeatedly to influence children's language acquisition (e.g., Baumwell, Tamis-LeMonda, & Bornstein, 1997; Clarke-Stewart, 1973; Hart & Risley, 1995; Nittrouer, 1996), and so we wanted to know what accounted for variability in parental verbal responsiveness among these particular parents. However, when the correlational analyses were performed, we could find no significant proportion of variance in responsiveness explained by the set of independent variables we examined: not SES for parents of either normal-hearing or deaf children, and not BE-PTA, ID-Age, or numbers of intervention visits for children with hearing loss.

Correlations with Dependent Measures of Language Abilities

Even though none of the independent variables was found to correlate with this measure of parental verbal responsiveness, earlier studies have demonstrated that this variability may affect how well children develop language. For that reason, we decided to examine whether the number of times that parents responded verbally to their children's communicative attempts explained any of the variance in children's language measures. To do so, we computed correlation coefficients between the number of verbal responses within a parental language sample and outcomes of the six language measures examined in Chapter 9, obtained from that parent's child at that test session: (a) Auditory Comprehension scores; (b) expressive vocabulary scores (EOWPVT); (c) numbers of real-word utterances from the children's language samples (RW-Us); (d) mean length of utterance (MLU);

(e) numbers of pronouns; and (f) numbers of different words (NDW). These correlation coefficients were computed for children with normal hearing and for those with hearing loss separately, and are shown in Table 10–7. A significant and large proportion of variance in auditory comprehension scores and in numbers of real-word utterances was explained for both children with normal hearing and for those with hearing loss by the frequency with which their parents responded verbally. For children with hearing loss, a significant and large proportion of variance in all dependent language measures was explained by how frequently parents responded to their children's communicative attempts. This means that language development was particularly sensitive to this parental behavior among children with hearing loss, which makes it especially unfortunate that parents of these children seem to engage in the behavior less, on average, than do parents of children with normal hearing. It also means that the enhancement in verbal responsiveness demonstrated by those nonsigning parents of children with late-identified hearing loss would have been especially facilitative.

Parents of the Stars

We were curious to know if the parents of the "stars" discussed in Chapter 9 were particularly responsive to their children's communicative attempts, and so we computed the mean number of verbal responses for all parents whose

Table 10–7. Correlation coefficients for scores on dependent language measures and numbers of parental verbal responses.

	Auditory Comprehension	EOWPVT	RW-U	MLU	Pronouns	NDW
Normal Hearing						
r	.685	.060	.741	-.061	-.046	.001
p	<.001	.455	<.001	.574	.674	.992
N	376	159	374	87	87	87
Hearing Loss						
r	.642	.389	.761	.390	.448	.447
p	<.001	<.001	<.001	<.001	<.001	<.001
N	403	236	399	237	237	237

Note. EOWPVT = Expressive One-Word Picture Vocabulary Test; RW-U = real-word utterances obtained in the 20-minute child language sample; MLU = mean length of utterance in morphemes; NDW = number of different words from SALT analysis. Correlations were computed on test scores from 12 to 48 months for RW-U and Auditory Comprehension scores; they were performed on scores from 36 to 48 months for EOWPVT, MLU, Pronouns, and NDW.

children were categorized as stars at each of the three test ages. Results were impressive: the mean at 36 months = 19.5; the mean at 42 months = 22; and the mean at 48 months = 21. If these values are compared to those on Table 10–6, it is apparent that they are greater than means for parents of most children with hearing loss at each age. The only exception is the group of nonsigning children with late-identified hearing loss: Parents of those children responded verbally to their children's communicative attempts about as frequently as did the parents of the stars, most of whom were identified early. Clearly, one thing intervention providers can be doing to help facilitate positive language outcomes for children with hearing loss is to be encouraging parents to respond as frequently as possible to their children's communicative attempts.

Parental Language Summary

Perhaps the most informative correlation obtained in this analysis was that between the number of parental verbal responses and the number of utterances that a child produced with real words, at that test session: More than half of the variance in the number of real-word utterances produced by a child was explained by how verbally responsive the parent was. This was true both for children with normal hearing and for those with hearing loss. In research on human behavior, that is a very large chunk of variance to be able to explain. Why was this relation between parental and child behavior so strong? Perhaps the answer rests with the fact that communication is a social activity. Most of us enjoy social interactions, especially with people whom we care about. These

children responded to their parents' offerings of verbal responses to their communicative attempts by generating more real-word language productions. Again, the overall numbers of communicative attempts on the part of children were similar across all groups. What differed as a function of parental verbal responsiveness was how many of those attempts consisted of at least one real word. That is a critical piece of information to help us understand how these children acquired language because a child must start generating some language before we can begin to mold it. We need something to work with. Apparently, we can positively influence the number of attempts a child makes at communicating using real words by increasing the number of times we respond verbally to any attempt at communication.

Good and Poor Language Users: What Differentiates Them?

We were bolstered in our search for factors that might explain language development in children with hearing loss by the finding that simply the number of times that a parent responds verbally to a child's communicative attempt explains a large share of variance in the numbers of communication acts with real words. As a result of that finding, we decided to explore the relation between the behaviors of these communication partners more closely. We wanted to know if the behavior of the parent really accounted for the child's language development so strongly, and if so, what sorts of behaviors we might be instructing parents to use.

For this analysis, we looked at small, well-matched groups. We selected one test age (36 months), and identified just 15 parent-child pairs to examine in more detail. Two groups of these children had hearing loss. We selected five children with early-identified hearing loss who wore cochlear implants, and who scored *better than* ½ standard deviation below the mean of children with normal hearing on the number of real-word utterances they produced during the 20-minute child language sample (the Good-HL group). These were among the best performers in that group. We then matched these children with five children with hearing loss who wore cochlear implants and showed the fewest number of real-word utterances (the Poor-HL group—a term used here to describe language abilities only). Children in these two groups were matched as closely as possible on gender, sign use, SES, and BE-PTA. All had received their cochlear implants before the age of 18 months (mean = 12.7 months; standard deviation = 3.1 months). Some children had a single implant (Good-HL = 3, Poor-HL = 2), some had bilateral implants (one in each group), and others had a cochlear implant/hearing aid combination (Good-HL = 1, Poor-HL = 2). Finally, we identified children with normal hearing who scored within ½ standard deviation of their group's mean for real-word utterances at 36 months. We then identified all children in that subset who were matched to children in the two groups of children with hearing loss on gender, sign use, and SES. Five of those children were randomly selected for closer examination in this analysis.

The first step in these analyses was to examine how well numbers of real-word utterances differentiated these three groups on other language measures, and so we gathered scores for these children at 36 months of age on three other measures: (a) MLU, (b) numbers of pronouns, and (c) NDW. Means for the five children in each group are shown in Figure 10–6. Children in the Good-HL group had scores similar to those of children with normal hearing on these language measures. Children in the Poor-HL group scored much more poorly.

Next we examined the ways in which the parents of these 15 children interacted with their children using a more fine-grained analysis than we had previously used. We were interested in how well parental interaction style can predict future language behavior of children, and so we looked at parental behavior 1 year earlier than when these measures of children's language were collected (i.e., at 24 months). These measures were made on the 20-minute videotape samples that had been used to score children's behavior, not the 10-minute samples used to score parents' behavior, described earlier in this chapter. Ten minutes of those samples were analyzed, starting at the 6-minute mark. Form and function of the parents' language were examined. Two graduate students transcribed the entire 10-minute sample of parental language. Both students had experience with scoring and transcription as part of the broader study. These transcripts were submitted to SALT, as described in Chapter 8. From those analyses of parental language, we examined four measures similar to those obtained from samples of children's language: (a) total numbers of words, (b) MLU, (c) pronouns, and (d) NDW. Means for these four language forms are shown in Figure 10–7.

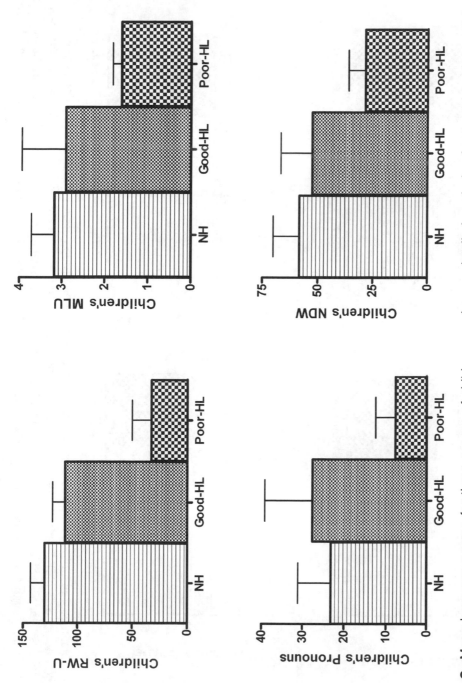

Figure 10–6. Mean language scores for three groups of children on whom a detailed analysis of parental language style was done. Groups are identified by children's hearing status and language ability: NH (normal hearing); Good-HL (good language, hearing loss); and Poor-HL (poor language, hearing loss). RW-U = real-word utterances; MLU = mean length of utterance, in morphemes; Pronouns = number of pronouns; and NDW = number of different words.

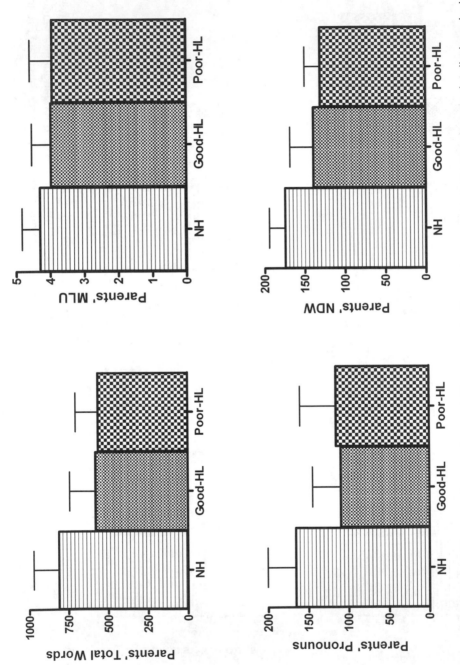

Figure 10–7. Mean scores for language forms of parents' language, for three groups of parents on whom a detailed analysis of parental language style was done. Groups are identified by children's hearing status and language ability: NH (normal hearing); Good-HL (good language, hearing loss); and Poor-HL (poor language, hearing loss). Total Words = total number of words produced in the 10-minute scoring interval; MLU = mean length of utterance, in morphemes; Pronouns = number of pronouns; and NDW = number of different words.

There are differences in the numbers of these behaviors between the parents of children with normal hearing and those with hearing loss, but none between the two hearing-loss groups. Parents were providing similar language models to their children with hearing loss, regardless of group. So what accounted for differences between these two groups of children in terms of how mature their language forms were?

In addition to these transcripts, the two scorers also evaluated the pragmatic function of each parental language act, explicitly counting four kinds of acts: (a) the number of times parents verbally responded to their children, (b) the number of times they praised their children, and (c) the number of times they recast something their children said. Table 10–8 provides specific definitions for these categories. Finally, (d) the number of *Wh-* question words used by these parents was obtained from SALT, and counted as indicating open-ended questions, a kind of pragmatic function. Figure 10–8 shows mean numbers of these pragmatic language functions for these three groups of parents. What we find is that the way in which parents interacted with their children differed greatly. The children with hearing loss who were showing mature language forms in their communication acts had parents who asked them lots of open-ended questions that required the child to generate a response. They had parents who responded verbally to their communicative attempts, and who praised them for those attempts. Finally, they had parents who reformulated their language attempts in different and/or expanded forms. In general, what we observe is that a parental communication style that encourages the child to produce language, responds sensitively to those attempts, and provides alternative or expanded models of the language the child is explicitly trying to produce facilitates better language outcomes in children with hearing loss. Regarding this last finding, it is emphasized that no differences were observed in terms of the language forms being modeled by the parents. In fact, we also counted the number of times that a

Table 10–8. Description of category labels for pragmatic function of parental language acts used in a detailed analysis of parental interaction style.

Function	Definition
Verbal response	Parent verbally responds to a question, statement, or action by the child directed to the parent. Does not include praise or recasts.
Praise	Parent verbally encourages child to continue with the course of action, and/or expresses approval aloud to the child. Statement is clearly about the child's behavior, not the object.
Recast	Parent restates or expands a child's immature production, integrating part or all of the child's production. Does not include correction of articulation errors.

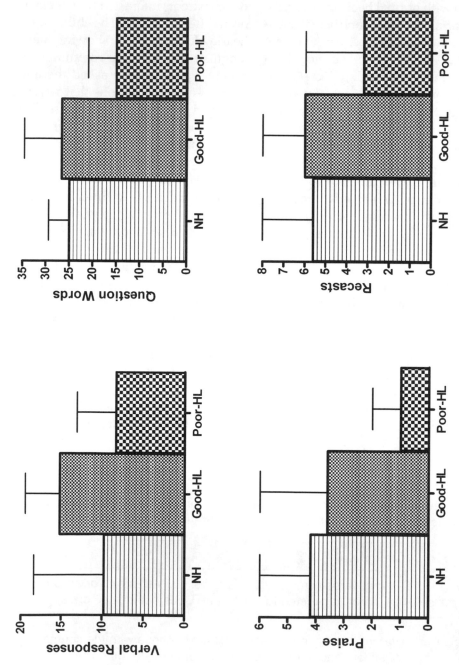

Figure 10–8. Mean numbers of parental language acts in each of four pragmatic function categories. NH (normal hearing); Good-HL (good language, hearing loss); and Poor-HL (poor language, hearing loss).

276

parent provided language to a child, without a prior attempt by the child. We called those behaviors language *models*, and we did not find differences in those numbers. So, a critical component of recasts is that they must contain at least part of the language the child produced. Although these differences in outcomes were observed for a small number of parent-child dyads, the conclusions mirror those of numerous other investigators for broader populations of children (e.g., Baker & Nelson, 1984; Hart & Risley, 1995; McNeill & Fowler, 1999; Newport, Gleitman, & Gleitman, 1977).

Chapter Summary

In this chapter, we reported on outcomes for the parents of children with hearing loss. We asked how well these parents were coping with the knowledge that their children have hearing loss, and how well they were able to handle accommodations required by their children's condition. We also asked if there were specific styles of parental interaction that facilitated children's language development better than others, and if parental language style was affected by having a child with hearing loss.

The first thing we learned was that parents do not feel undue levels of stress by learning of their infant's hearing loss. Stress levels were not affected by the age at which a child's hearing loss was identified, or by whether parents used signs or not with their children.

When it comes to parental language styles, we found that these parents provided language input that was generally consistent with what we know about the kind of language typically provided in middle-class families. Examined from a global perspective, all parents, regardless of their children's hearing status, asked roughly the same numbers of questions, and issued similar numbers of directives. A significant difference was observed, however, in how frequently these parents responded verbally to their children's communicative attempts. Parents of children with hearing loss generally responded less to their children's communicative attempts than did parents of children with normal hearing. That difference is especially deleterious because we also learned that language acquisition is more sensitive to parents' responsiveness for children with hearing loss than it is for those with normal hearing. Finally, it was observed that the critical factor influencing children's language development is how generally responsive parents are to their children's communicative attempts, rather than the specific kinds of language models that they present. An interaction style on the part of parents that encourages children to generate language, responds sensitively, and expands upon the language the child is explicitly trying to produce best serves language development for children with hearing loss.

Table 10–2. Mean scores from the Parenting Stress Index (PSI) associated with the Child Domain for each group at each test age. Standard deviations are in parentheses, and group numbers are in italics.

Test Age (Months)	NH–s	NH+S	Early		Late	
			HL–s	HL+S	HL–s	HL+S
12	96.22 (14.80) *23*	95.00 (15.15) *12*	100.82 (12.70) *11*	95.50 (17.68) *2*	*0*	*0*
18	99.41 (13.17) *32*	95.60 (14.19) *25*	105.11 (14.87) *19*	95.33 (22.05) *9*	117.00 (22.63) *2*	*0*
24	93.21 (13.55) *28*	97.45 (15.21) *22*	101.81 (12.56) *26*	100.33 (18.93) *9*	94.75 (15.20) *4*	105.00 (0.00) *1*
30	96.19 (12.40) *21*	91.58 (16.15) *24*	99.41 (16.65) *32*	90.91 (16.60) *11*	99.50 (10.08) *10*	101.50 (4.95) *2*
36	93.52 (15.19) *25*	96.96 (15.61) *25*	102.07 (18.24) *29*	100.30 (17.58) *10*	96.73 (16.54) *11*	102.80 (14.92) *5*
42	93.26 (13.68) *19*	93.74 (12.92) *23*	100.42 (17.73) *33*	100.85 (23.78) *13*	100.69 (22.22) *16*	101.50 (15.73) *6*
48	92.29 (15.91) *21*	91.96 (16.77) *23*	102.07 (19.84) *29*	100.21 (17.36) *14*	101.82 (21.79) *17*	100.33 (19.62) *9*

Table 10–3. Mean scores from the Parenting Stress Index (PSI) associated with the Parent Domain for each group at each test age. Standard deviations are in parentheses, and group numbers are in italics.

Test Age (Months)	NH–s	NH+S	Early HL–s	Early HL+S	Late HL–s	Late HL+S
12	114.70 (16.84) *23*	113.42 (11.97) *12*	121.27 (17.46) *11*	118.50 (6.36) *2*	*0*	*0*
18	121.09 (14.29) *32*	111.16 (13.14) *25*	126.21 (18.03) *19*	116.00 (16.06) *9*	138.00 (5.66) *2*	*0*
24	113.50 (15.49) *28*	116.55 (17.31) *22*	123.96 (19.18) *26*	129.56 (17.79) *9*	111.75 (16.01) *4*	105.00 (0.00) *1*
30	113.48 (14.31) *21*	112.88 (14.04) *24*	123.22 (20.80) *32*	120.36 (13.97) *11*	112.30 (15.00) *10*	122.00 (26.87) *2*
36	119.80 (19.82) *25*	115.00 (20.07) *25*	124.66 (22.95) *29*	119.70 (15.31) *10*	109.64 (11.09) *11*	112.80 (11.52) *5*
42	119.32 (15.73) *19*	113.70 (15.80) *23*	122.67 (22.62) *33*	115.38 (17.36) *13*	114.44 (15.92) *16*	109.50 (11.79) *6*
48	112.14 (18.05) *21*	115.22 (16.74) *23*	123.83 (24.87) *29*	116.29 (16.71) *14*	116.06 (13.75) *17*	113.44 (14.69) *9*

Table 10–5. Mean numbers of parental communication acts for each group at each test age. Standard deviations are in parentheses, and group numbers are in italics.

Test Age (Months)	NH–s	NH+S	Early		Late	
			HL–s	HL+S	HL–s	HL+S
12	91.38 (13.79) *29*	81.46 (18.80) *12*	91.95 (15.33) *11*	77.40 (33.29) *5*	*0*	*0*
18	98.54 (12.87) *40*	92.18 (16.98) *28*	92.09 (16.57) *22*	85.23 (20.51) *13*	80.25 (5.30) *2*	*0*
24	107.75 (14.30) *32*	97.50 (21.38) *25*	98.50 (18.00) *29*	102.40 (10.24) *10*	98.20 (10.50) *5*	105.50 (21.92) *2*
30	103.58 (16.37) *24*	96.69 (20.04) *26*	98.65 (18.95) *36*	105.61 (13.82) *14*	102.82 (20.29) *11*	109.13 (7.16) *4*
36	114.63 (17.36) *31*	108.91 (19.57) *28*	103.10 (16.94) *34*	111.27 (13.06) *11*	112.43 (17.27) *15*	103.67 (16.46) *9*
42	104.17 (13.93) *26*	94.92 (15.53) *25*	97.64 (17.60) *36*	95.00 (9.73) *15*	104.22 (18.89) *23*	93.44 (14.94) *9*
48	103.79 (15.13) *26*	103.65 (15.54) *24*	98.70 (20.20) *33*	96.88 (10.63) *17*	102.58 (20.60) *26*	97.54 (12.76) *12*

Table 10–6. Mean numbers of parental verbal responses for each group at each test age. Standard deviations are in parentheses, and group numbers are in italics.

Test Age (Months)	NH–s	NH+S	Early		Late	
			HL–s	HL+S	HL–s	HL+S
12	1.78 (2.15) *29*	3.08 (4.05) *12*	2.95 (2.68) *11*	1.20 (1.44) *5*	*0*	*0*
18	5.89 (5.27) *40*	5.86 (5.50) *28*	4.27 (4.44) *22*	3.77 (3.15) *13*	4.50 (2.83) *2*	*0*
24	12.22 (5.97) *32*	12.50 (6.53) *25*	8.19 (5.90) *29*	8.70 (3.44) *10*	3.80 (2.71) *5*	6.00 (4.24) *2*
30	17.65 (6.74) *24*	15.15 (7.35) *26*	10.76 (7.26) *36*	9.86 (4.60) *14*	9.95 (4.53) *11*	5.50 (4.60) *4*
36	21.79 (7.42) *31*	21.11 (5.91) *28*	14.29 (7.02) *34*	14.05 (5.47) *11*	19.50 (7.10) *15*	11.33 (6.29) *9*
42	20.73 (6.84) *26*	18.24 (7.03) *25*	15.88 (6.74) *36*	16.73 (6.54) *15*	21.17 (7.57) *23*	12.11 (6.44) *9*
48	19.40 (8.29) *26*	20.92 (8.33) *24*	16.80 (7.70) *33*	18.76 (4.59) *17*	21.06 (7.13) *26*	16.13 (8.87) *12*

References

Abidin, R. R. (1995). *Parenting Stress Index* (3rd ed.). Lutz, FL: Psychological Assessment Resources.

Baker, N. D., & Nelson, K. E. (1984). Recasting and related conversational techniques for triggering syntactic advances by young children. *First Language, 5,* 3–22.

Baumwell, L., Tamis-LeMonda, C. S., & Bornstein, M. H. (1997). Maternal verbal sensitivity and child language comprehension. *Infant Behavior and Development, 20,* 247–258.

Clarke-Stewart, K. A. (1973). Interactions between mothers and their young children: Characteristics and consequences. *Monographs of the Society for Research in Child Development, 38,* 1–109.

Day, A. (1991). *Carl's afternoon in the park.* Farrar, Canada: Douglas & McIntyre.

Day, A. (1995). *Carl's birthday.* Farrar, Canada: Harper Collins Canada.

Hart, B., & Risley, T. R. (1995). *Meaningful differences in the everyday experience of young American children.* Baltimore: Paul H. Brookes.

McNeill, J., & Fowler, S. (1999). Let's talk: Encouraging mother-child conversations during story reading. *Journal of Early Intervention, 22,* 51–69.

Newport, E. L., Gleitman, H., & Gleitman, L. (1977). Mother, I'd rather do it myself: Some effects and non-effects of maternal speech style. In C. E. Snow & C. A. Ferguson (Eds.), *Talking to children: Language input and acquisition* (pp. 109–149). Cambridge, UK: Cambridge University Press.

Nittrouer, S. (1996). The relation between speech perception and phonemic awareness: Evidence from low-SES children and children with chronic OM. *Journal of Speech and Hearing Research, 39,* 1059–1070.

Nittrouer, S. (2002). From ear to cortex: A perspective on what clinicians need to understand about speech perception and language processing. *Language, Speech and Hearing Services in Schools, 33,* 237–251.

Nittrouer, S., & Burton, L. T. (2005). The role of early language experience in the development of speech perception and phonological processing abilities: Evidence from 5-year-olds with histories of otitis media with effusion and low socioeconomic status. *Journal of Communication Disorders, 38,* 29–63.

Quittner, A. L., Glueckauf, R. L., & Jackson, D. N. (1990). Chronic parenting stress: Moderating versus mediating effects of social support. *Journal of Personality and Social Psychology, 59,* 1266–1278.

11

Putting It All Together: A Latent Measure of Language Acquisition

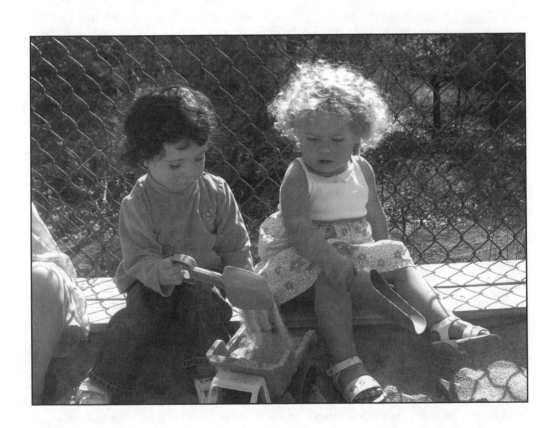

In earlier chapters, we learned something about a great number of separate measures of language development for the children in this study. These measures all tell a similar story about the effects of hearing loss and treatment variables on language development. But language is more than any one of these measures can evaluate on its own. Each measure might tell us about some aspect of language processing, but none of those measures on its own tells us about the underlying construct. When discrete measures are used to gauge the language development of a specific group of children, or to assess progress for an individual child, the question really being asked is how well that particular group, or individual child, performs compared to the canonical typically developing child. Typically developing children exhibit a restricted range of scores on any one measure—say, a measure of expressive vocabulary—but that range of scores is not the whole of language development. The range of scores associated with the canonical typically developing child is simply that: the scores that typical children tend to get on that one measure. Just because any one child obtains a score within that range on that one measure does not mean that he is typical in his language development overall. The goal of the analysis reported in this chapter was to try to create a composite variable of language development that is comprehensive in nature. We did this by creating a latent language measure meant to capture the underlying phenomenon from all these separate measures.

An advantage offered by the procedure reported in this chapter is that it allowed us to evaluate more accurately the contributions of separate sources of variance to the underlying phenomenon. As discussed in Chapter 4, there are many sources of variance in any measure that is made. Some of these sources of variance are the very effects that we want to assess, things like hearing loss, sign use, age of identification of hearing loss, auditory sensitivity, and so on. However, there are always sources of variance that influence scores at any one time that we are not interested in: Is the child cranky because she missed a nap? Is he getting a new tooth? Does the accompanying parent have a cold? These sources of variance introduce error into any one measure, at any discrete test, for any particular child. A goal of research methods is to estimate the amount of error due to these factors so that valid estimates of the effects of interest can be obtained. The analysis method reported in this chapter achieved that goal.

Overview of Model Building

Until now we have presented and analyzed changes across time in aggregates of scores for groups of participants. These procedures have represented standard statistical procedures that have been used for decades to examine sources of variance. A simple model for representing these effects is shown in Equation 1.

In this formula, S is the score obtained for a specific dependent measure for an individual participant (i) at a discrete test time (t). Each x is a source of variance from a factor such as gender, SES, age of ID, and so forth, and

---

Equation 1

$$S_{it} = \beta_0 + \beta_1 x_{1i} + \beta_2 x_{2i} + \beta_3 x_{3i} \ldots\ldots + \varepsilon_{it}$$

---

the β parameters represent the size of the impact of each of these factors. These are usually factors that we know about, and that have similar effects across participants who share values of that factor. The ε in this instance represents error variance and is unique to each participant at each test time. This might include factors such as whether the child is teething or missed a nap, as well as testing factors such as whether the test time was late in the afternoon that day or early in the morning. These are sources of variance that are difficult to account for.

Many approaches to modeling developmental changes over time involve looking at trends across test ages for groups of children. Very much as we have done in earlier chapters, group means are examined as they change over test ages. This approach is valuable, and has been used successfully to extend our understanding of how factors such as hearing loss and cochlear implantation affect language development. However, there are other statistical approaches that provide different perspectives regarding the impact of these types of factors on the abstract construct of language. In this chapter, we used one of these other approaches: latent growth modeling.

Latent growth models have important differences from the types of models used in previous chapters. With latent growth models we are not concerned specifically with aggregate results at discrete test ages or across test ages. Rather, we are interested in characterizing developmental trajectories of individual children. In a standard latent growth model, a latent dependent measure is modeled for each participant with a subject-specific intercept and slope. Subsequently, this intercept and slope are modeled as functions of predictor variables. As a result, the ways in which those variables generally affect the intercept and slope for the latent dependent variable can be estimated. In this way we obtain estimates of the effects of those predictor variables on the growth trajectory of that dependent measure.

From this perspective, the equation for any dependent measure for an individual participant at a discrete test age is shown in Equation 2.

In this formulation, the score for this individual at this test time is modeled as being based on an intercept (β_{0i}) and a slope (β_{1i}) over time, with some error variance. Both the intercept and the slope are linked to individual values of the predictor variables through Equations 3 and 4.

Equation 2

$$S_{it} = \beta_{0i} + \beta_{1i} t + \varepsilon_{it}$$

Equation 3

$$\beta_{0i} = \alpha_{00} + \alpha_{01}(SES_i) + \alpha_{02}(G_i) + \alpha_{03}(Hear_i)... + \zeta_{0i}$$

Equation 4

$$\beta_{1i} = \alpha_{10} + \alpha_{11}(SES_i) + \alpha_{12}(G_i) + \alpha_{13}(Hear_i)... + \zeta_{1i}$$

Each α represents an effect of a predictor variable on either the intercept (β_{0i}) or on the slope (β_{1i}), and ζ is the error term. In these equations only the effects of SES, gender (G), and hearing status (Hear) are explicitly shown, but many others can be included. We see that both the intercept and the slope are affected by our predictor variables. It is these effects that we are most interested in quantifying in the modeling reported in this chapter.

Once this technique is understood, it is easy to see that our decision not to insist that this study be strictly longitudinal in design presented no problems for the approach. Variability was inherent in developmental trajectories of all participants, for many reasons. Missing a test session was just one more source of that variability.

This Specific Model

A schematic representation of the overall model used is shown in Figure 11–1, and is explained in the sections below. The variables that we chose to examine as predictor variables in this model were ones that have been shown in earlier chapters to affect the growth of language acquisition. Six of these factors are constant across time, and three vary across test ages.

The First Linkage: Constant Sources of Variance

Some of the factors that contribute to variance in language outcomes remain constant over time. The constant factors contributing to variance in language outcomes, shown to the left on Figure 11–1, are these:

Hearing status: This variable simply indicated whether a child had normal hearing or had a hearing loss. For modeling purposes it is denoted *HL*. For this variable, children with normal hearing are coded as 0 and children with hearing loss as 1.

Age of ID: This variable was set using a binary code separating children whose hearing loss was identified before 6 months of age from those whose hearing loss was identified after 1 year of age. For modeling purposes it is denoted *LID*, for late identification. For this variable, children with early-identified hearing loss or with normal hearing are coded as 0 and late-identified children are coded as 1.

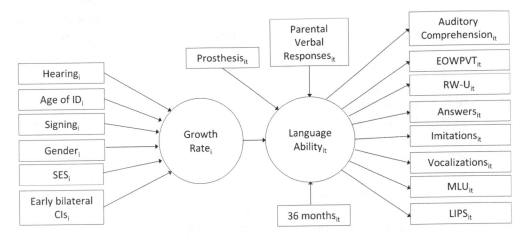

Figure 11–1. Diagram of latent growth model used in this chapter.

Signing status: This variable indicated whether a child's parents used signs or not. For modeling purposes it is denoted S. For this variable, nonsigners are coded as 0 and signers as 1.

Gender: This variable indicated whether a child was a boy or a girl. For modeling purposes it is denoted G. For this variable, boys are coded as 0 and girls as 1.

SES: Socioeconomic status was found in earlier analyses to influence language acquisition only for children with normal hearing. Nonetheless, it was examined in this model because it is considered by most clinicians and investigators to have an influence on outcomes for children with hearing loss. We sought to increase the sensitivity of this factor by modeling it as a binary variable, rather than as the continuous variable it has been considered to be in earlier chapters. Here a child was categorized as low SES if this score was equal to or below 15 and to be mid/high SES if this score was greater than 15. Although somewhat arbitrary, this cutoff has generally been found in earlier work to mark a

natural boundary. Having an SES of greater than 15 means that the primary income earner in the household had at least a high-school diploma and a job that involved skilled labor. Scores at or below 15 indicate a home in which the primary income earner generally did not graduate from high school and worked as an unskilled laborer or was unemployed. These are conditions that severely constrain a child's opportunities for language experiences. Incorporating SES in this way meant that we were evaluating the effects of having low SES only; we could not examine the effect, if any, of having an especially high SES. For modeling purposes this variable is denoted *SES*. For this variable, low-SES children are coded as 0 and mid-/high-SES children as 1.

Early, bilateral CIs: This variable was set using a binary code separating the children who received two implants before 18 months of age. For modeling purposes it is denoted C. For this variable, children with early bilateral implants are coded as 1 and all others are coded as 0.

Most latent growth models explore changes in both the intercept and in the slope of the regression lines, but we set the intercept to zero for all participants. This simply means that we assumed children had no language abilities at birth. Therefore, only the effects of predictor variables on the slope of language development were explored. Examining these constant effects was termed the *first linkage*, and the equation for this is shown in Equation 5.

Here, β is the slope of the line representing latent language ability for an individual participant. We set it to 1 for a "canonical" participant, whom we arbitrarily coded as a nonsigning male with normal hearing and low SES. This means that this canonical participant shows growth on this latent language measure of 1 for each test time, or each 6 months of age. Consequently, we quantify deviations from that slope of 1 (α) that arise due to these predictor variables. Table 11–1 defines each parameter that we quantified in the first linkage.

Figure 11–2 illustrates the role these parameters play in the model by showing examples of the expected growth rate that would be observed for three different children. In this figure the center diagonal line shows how we set average growth rate for our canonical group of children, which consisted of nonsigning males with normal hearing and low SES. The lower diagonal line shows the growth rate for a similar

child with hearing loss rather than normal hearing. In this case, α_1 quantifies the change in the slope of the line. A significantly negative α_1 indicates that, all other things being equal, a child with hearing loss acquires language more slowly than a child with normal hearing. The upper diagonal line shows the growth rate for a girl who is otherwise identical to the canonical group. In this case, α_6 quantifies the change in the slope of the line. A significantly positive value for α_6 indicates that, all other things being equal, girls with normal hearing acquire language faster than boys.

The Second Linkage: Time-Varying Sources of Variance

In the second part of the model, the growth rate is linked to actual language ability using a linear form. At this stage of the model, three factors that change across time or at discrete times and are believed to impact language ability are introduced: parental verbal responsiveness, prosthesis, and change in intervention at 36 months. Introduction of the parental verbal response measure is straightforward; it is brought into the model as a simple linear effect that has a different value depending on the child's hearing status. The number of instances of parental verbal responses is used here.

Equation 5

$$\beta_i = 1 + \alpha_1(HL_i) + \alpha_2(LID_i) + \alpha_3(S_i) + \alpha_4(HL_i)(S_i) + \alpha_5(LID_i)(S_i)$$
$$+ \alpha_6(G_i) + \alpha_7(HL_i)(G_i) + \alpha_8(SES_i) + \alpha_8(HL_i)(SES_i) + \alpha_{10}(C_i) + \zeta_i$$

Table 11–1. Description of each parameter quantified in the first linkage of the model. These are parameters that remained constant across test ages.

Parameter	Interpretation
α_1	*Hearing status:* Difference in average growth rate between nonsigning children with normal hearing and nonsigning children with early-identified hearing loss
α_2	*Age of ID:* Difference in average growth rate between nonsigning children with early-identified hearing loss and nonsigning children with late-identified hearing loss
α_3	*Signing, NH:* Effect of signing on growth rate for children with normal hearing
α_4	(Added to α_3) *Signing, early-identified HL:* Effect of signing on growth rate for children with early-identified hearing loss
α_5	(Added to α_3 and α_4) *Signing, late-identified HL:* Effect of signing on growth rate for children with late-identified hearing loss
α_6	*Gender, NH:* Difference in average growth rate between females and males with normal hearing
α_7	(Added to α_6) *Gender, HL:* Difference in average growth rate between females and males with HL
α_8	*SES, NH:* Effect of SES greater than 15 on growth rate for children with normal hearing
α_9	(Added to α_8) *SES, HL:* Effect of SES greater than 15 on growth rate for children with hearing loss
α_{10}	*Early, bilateral implants:* Additional effect on growth rate of getting two CIs before 18 months of age

In contrast, the inclusion of a prosthesis effect is complex. Before presenting the mathematic form for this linkage, we explain some of the theoretical reasons for our choice of model for the prosthesis effect.

The governing principle behind the modeling of the prosthesis effect is that an individual's language growth curve can change in slope, by either accelerating or decelerating, when the configuration of the individual's prostheses is modified. So, for example, a child with a hearing aid (or dual hearing aids) up to the age of 24 months might receive his first cochlear implant at that time. Consequently, at 24 months the child's language growth rate might change. Such changes in growth rate are allowed to occur at the time of first cochlear implantation, with different modifications for those who keep a hearing aid on the other ear and for those who do not. Similar modifications are incorporated for

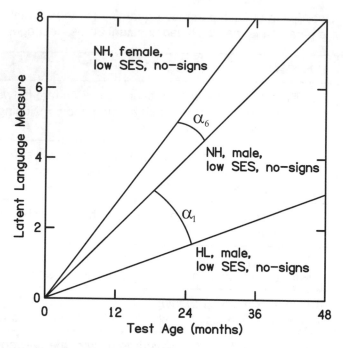

Figure 11–2. Illustration of expected growth rates based on parameters in the first linkage for three fictitious children. The trajectory in the middle is for a non-signing boy with normal hearing and low SES. The top trajectory is for a child who meets the same criteria, except is a girl. The bottom trajectory is for a child who meets the same criteria as the boy represented in the middle, but has a hearing loss.

the time of the second cochlear implantation. No consideration is required for early, simultaneous implantation because all children with early, simultaneous implantation were accounted for in the first linkage of the model.

It is easy to see how this modeling offers greater precision in estimating the effects of cochlear implantation than traditional statistical approaches. When individual scores across children are considered, as in previous chapters, it is impossible to examine effects temporally tied to the implantation because age at which the implantation occurred varied for these children. Using these

modeling techniques, we can estimate the effect on the trajectory of language growth associated with implantation for each child individually, and then use those individual values to estimate the effect across children.

Also, an effect is placed in the model to determine whether children with hearing loss exhibit a change in their rate of language growth at 36 months, the time at which they typically begin attending school. Statistical methods used in early chapters did not allow us to investigate this change in intervention.

The resulting model incorporating these time-varying effects is shown in

Equation 6, where t is the number of 6-month periods since birth; L_{it} is the latent language ability of child i at time t; f_{1i} and f_{2i} denote the time of first and second cochlear implantation, respectively; I is the indicator function that takes a value of 1 if its argument is true and a value of 0 otherwise; X_i is an indicator that is true if child i was allowed to keep his hearing aid upon receiving his first cochlear implant; and P_{it} is the (centered) parental verbal response score for the parent of child i at time t. P_{it} is centered so that the other parameters can be interpreted as corresponding to their effect at the average level of parental verbal response.

To illustrate the role these parameters play in the model, Figure 11–3 shows an example of a growth pattern

---

Equation 6

$$L_{it} = \beta_i t + \gamma_1 \left((t - f_{1i}) I_{\{t \geq f_{1i}\}} \right) + \gamma_2 \left((t - f_{1i}) I_{\{t \geq f_{1i} \& X_i\}} \right) + \gamma_3 \left((t - f_{2i}) I_{\{t \geq f_{2i}\}} \right)$$
$$+ \gamma_4 \left((t - f_{2i}) I_{\{t \geq f_{2i} \& X_i\}} \right) + \gamma_5 \left((t - 6) I_{\{t \geq 6\}} \right) (HL_i) + \gamma_6 (P_{it}) + \gamma_7 (P_{it})(HL_i)$$

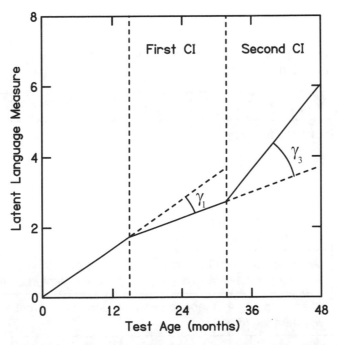

Figure 11–3. Illustration of expected growth rates based on parameters in the second linkage for one fictitious child who received a first implant at age 14 months and a second implant at age 31 months. Although not shown, the effect of changing intervention at 36 months of age was modeled in the same way.

that might be taken by a child who sequentially receives bilateral implants. The solid line represents the final growth curve for this child. Suppose this child received his first implant at the age of 14 months and his second implant at the age of 31 months. Also, suppose that he did not keep his hearing aid after the first implant. At the time of the first implant, the language acquisition rate changes, resulting in a change in the slope of the line. This change in slope is quantified by γ_1. In this case, the change was negative, and the child's language acquisition slowed upon receiving the first implant. At the time of the second implant, there is another change in the rate of language acquisition, quantified by γ_3. In the illus-

tration, the change is positive, indicating that the child's language acquisition sped up upon receiving the second implant.

For children who did not receive a first or second cochlear implant during the study period, the corresponding values of f_{1i} and/or f_{2i} are set to an arbitrarily large value. As a result, these children do not receive any contribution from the corresponding terms in γ_1 through γ_4.

For children with normal hearing, the latent language ability at time t is only impacted by the first term ($\beta_i t$) and the first parental verbal response term. The parameters in this level of the model can be interpreted as described in Table 11–2.

Table 11–2. Description of each parameter quantified in the second linkage. These are time-varying parameters.

Parameter	Interpretation
γ_1	Change in slope of language acquisition with first CI when not keeping HA
γ_2	(Added to γ_1) Change in slope of language acquisition with first CI when keeping HA
γ_3	Additional change in slope of language acquisition with second CI when not keeping HA at time of first implant
γ_4	(Added to γ_3) Additional change in slope of language acquisition with second CI when keeping HA at time of first implant
γ_5	Change in slope of language acquisition at 36 months for children with hearing loss
γ_6	Impact of parental verbal response score on language level for children with normal hearing
γ_7	(Added to γ_6) Impact of parental verbal response score on language level for children with hearing loss

Dependent Measures Used in the Latent Language Measure

An important chore in developing the model was to decide which language measures should be used to construct the latent language variable. Several considerations came into play. It is necessary to use enough measures and to use measures that are sufficiently representative of the underlying construct (language) to derive an accurate picture of that underlying construct. Using a lot of separate measures is a good idea if the only goal is to derive an accurate picture of that underlying construct because any redundancy in contributions of those measures does not negatively impact the variance estimates obtained for predictor variables. However, the more dependent measures that are used to construct the latent variable, the longer the actual processing time that is required to fit the model. So there is an advantage to keeping the set of dependent measures used to construct the latent measure as lean as possible.

After careful thought and some pilot work, we arrived at a set of eight measures to be used in the construction of the latent measure. Each of these measures is listed below along with a description of the reason we chose it. Following each is the equation used to model the relationship between the overall latent language variable and the individual measure. We emphasize that we did sufficient pilot work to assure ourselves that the inclusion of additional dependent measures did not perturb the variance estimates that we got for predictor variables.

Auditory Comprehension

This was the most sensitive measure of how well children understand language. It has a linear developmental function, and was measured at all seven test ages. The formula used to model this measure is shown in Equation 7, where R_{it} is the auditory comprehension raw score for child i at measurement time t. N denotes the normal distribution with mean (θ) and variance (σ^2) arguments, and the θ and σ^2 parameters are unknown. In other words, as language ability increases over time, a child's auditory comprehension score increases as a linear function of that language ability, and the actual observation is normally distributed around that linearly predicted value.

EOWPVT Scores

We wanted a measure of expressive vocabulary. This measure has a linear developmental function, although it was only measured at three test ages. We tried including LDS scores, as well, but found that they added no new information, so we removed those scores from the final model. The formula for this effect is seen in Equation 8, where E_{it} is the expressive vocabulary score for child i at measurement time t. All other terms are similarly explained as they were for auditory comprehension.

Equation 7

$$R_{it} \sim N(\theta_{R0} + \theta_{R1} L_{it}, \sigma_R^2)$$

Equation 8

$$E_{it} \sim N(\theta_{E0} + \theta_{E1}L_{it}, \sigma_E^2)$$

Real-Word Utterances

The number of utterances consisting of real words produced in the 20-minute language sample provided a metric of how well children actually used language in their communication with others. It is a robust measure that was obtained at all test ages, and was sensitive to differences among groups. It has an S-shaped function, and so the formula chosen for this effect is shown in Equation 9, where W_{it} is the number of real-word utterances for child i at measurement time t and $\text{logit}^{-1}(x) = \exp(x)/(1 + \exp(x))$ where exp is the exponential function. In this equation, θ_{W0} corresponds to the number of real-word utterances at which the average child plateaus, θ_{W1} controls the shift of the curve to the left or right, and θ_{W2} controls the steepness of the curve.

Answers

The number of answers children produced in the 20-minute language sample was used to provide a metric of how responsive children were in a meaningful way. This variable showed an S-shaped developmental trajectory. We chose the formula shown in Equation 10 for answers, where A_{it} is the number of answers for child i at measurement time t. In this equation, θ_{A0} corresponds to the number of answers at which the average child plateaus, θ_{A1} controls the shift of the curve to the left or right, and θ_{A2} controls the steepness of the curve.

Imitations

We included this category because we wanted to have a couple variables on which the children developing language more slowly had higher scores than those children developing language more quickly. This variable showed a curvilinear developmental trajectory, and the nonsigning children with late-identified hearing loss had a higher

---

Equation 9

$$W_{it} \sim N(\theta_{W0}\text{logit}^{-1}(\theta_{W1} + \theta_{W2}L_{it}), \sigma_W^2)$$

Equation 10

$$A_{it} \sim N(\theta_{A0}\text{logit}^{-1}(\theta_{A1} + \theta_{A2}L_{it}), \sigma_A^2)$$

Equation 11

$$K_{it} \sim N(\theta_{K0} + \theta_{K3}(HL_i)(LID_i)(1 - S_i) + \theta_{K1}L_{it} + \theta_{K2}L_{it}^2, \sigma_K^2)$$

Equation 12

$$V_{it} \sim N(\theta_{V0} + \theta_{V3}(HL_i)(LID_i)(S_i) + \theta_{V1}L_{it} + \theta_{V2}L_{it}^2, \sigma_V^2)$$

peak than other groups. The formula chosen is shown in Equation 11, where K_{it} is the number of imitations for child i at measurement time t. In other words, as language ability increases over time, the number of a child's imitations will follow a curvilinear pattern, and children with late-identified hearing loss who are not exposed to signs will show a similar curvature, albeit with a higher peak.

Number of Vocalizations

The total number of vocalizations produced during the 20-minute language sample was included to provide another metric on which children developing language more slowly had higher scores than those children developing language more quickly. We tried including more specific measures of vocalizations, such as the number of constricted vocalizations, but they added no unique information to the latent language measure, and so we removed them. This measure had a curvilinear developmental trajectory, and signing children with

late-identified hearing loss had a higher peak than other children. For these reasons we used the formula shown in Equation 12, where V_{it} is the number of vocalizations for child i at measurement time t.

MLU

Mean length of utterance was one of the SALT measures that showed significant differences among groups. Growth is linear for this measure, and so we used the formula shown in Equation 13, where M_{it} is the MLU for child i at measurement time t.

LIPS Classification Score

We wanted to include a cognitive facet to our latent language measure, and

Equation 13

$$M_{it} \sim N(\theta_{M0} + \theta_{M1}L_{it}, \sigma_M^2)$$

> ## Equation 14
>
> $$F_{it} \sim N(\theta_{F0} + \theta_{F1} L_{it}, \sigma_F^2)$$

this score was found to differ across our groups. It was only measured at one test time. As a result, it was reasonable to model it using a linear function shown in Equation 14, where F_{it} is the Leiter classification score for child i at measurement time t.

Choice of Methodology

The previous sections give all the information needed to link the data together using the latent growth framework. However, specification of the model is not complete until we provide information on our prior knowledge about parameters. Such specification of prior knowledge is required because we have chosen to perform the analysis using Bayesian methodology (Gelman, Carlin, Stern, & Rubin, 1995). Bayesian methodology offers a number of advantages over Classical (sometimes called Frequentist) approaches to modeling of data. An introduction to a comprehensive list of advantages would require an entire chapter, but it is worth mentioning some of the most important ones. First, the Bayesian methodology allows for very intuitive interpretation of parameters and uncertainty. In contrast to Classical statistical methods that rely on confidence intervals to describe uncertainty, Bayesian methods rely on credible sets. A credible set is an interval in which we can state that the true parameter value falls with some known

probability. For example, we might find that the parameter α_1 has a 95% credible set of (−.2, −.1). The interpretation would be that there is a 95% probability that the true effect of hearing loss on the rate of language acquisition is between −.2 and −.1. In contrast, a finding of the same interval using a Classical approach would yield a more complex interpretation: If the study were repeated an infinite number of times with newly and randomly selected children from the population of interest, and intervals were constructed using the same methodology used here, 95% of the constructed intervals would contain the true parameter.

A second advantage to using Bayesian methodology is that estimation of parameters and their uncertainties can be performed using an algorithmic technique known as Markov chain Monte Carlo (MCMC), which draws samples from the distribution of the parameters conditional on the data without relying on asymptotic approximations like most Classical approaches. MCMC can be used in some Classical models, but some theoretical complications can arise in trying to do so (Robert & Casella, 1999). Finally, Bayesian methods provide a consistent approach to probability and modeling in that conclusions are not based on unobserved data or experimenter intention, two things that can influence Classical approaches (Berger & Berry, 1988; Berger & Wolpert, 1984).

With all that said, however, for our model we chose not to assign informative prior distributions to the parameters. Before observing the data we specified that we had no knowledge whatsoever about the estimated values the parameters would take once we fit the model to the observed data. For the regression-type parameters (α, γ, and θ parameters), we used normal distributions centered at zero with a variance of 1000. For the variance parameters (the σ^2 parameters), we used gamma distributions with a mean of 1 and a variance of 1000. In spite of our decision not to specify prior distributions, the use of a Bayesian approach provided advantages to this modeling.

Execution of the Model

The model was fit using an MCMC algorithm executed in the R programming language (R Development Core Team, 2007). The BRugs package, which relies on the WinBUGS software, provided the functionality for running the algorithm. The MCMC algorithm was run for 600,000 iterations, the first 200,000 of which were discarded for burn-in. The result was a remaining 400,000 samples from the joint posterior distribution of the parameters (i.e., the distribution of the parameters conditional on the observed data). These samples were thinned by a factor of 200 in order to conserve storage space, resulting in a final random sample size of 2,000 from the posterior distribution.

Results

The parameters in the model are summarized separately for each of the two linkages. For each linkage, a table is presented containing the unknown parameters in the model, as well as some functions of multiple parameters. Examining effects for multiple param-

eters is required to provide an understanding of some of the interactions we have observed in this study, such as that involving late-identified hearing loss and signing. For each parameter, a summary is created including the posterior mean (a point estimate of the true value) in Column 2, a 95% credible set in Column 3, and a brief interpretation of the parameter's value in Column 4. Interpretation is based both on the posterior mean and the extent to which the credible set crosses zero, if it does at all. Two effects may have the same posterior mean. If the credible set of one does not cross zero, or does so only slightly, the conclusion may be that the effect is likely not equal to zero for the larger population. If the credible set of the other effect sits squarely over zero, then it more likely does not influence language growth in the larger population.

The First Linkage

Parameter values for the first linkage are presented in Table 11–3. Below we describe the important effects reported in this table.

Hearing loss: In Row 1 of Table 11–3 we see that nonsigning children with early-identified hearing loss had language growth rates .27 lower, on average, than their nonsigning counterparts with normal hearing. For nonsigning boys with low SES, this translates into a 27% difference in the average rate of language growth between children with normal hearing and those with hearing loss. So a child with early-identified hearing loss has a rate of growth on our latent language variable of .73, compared to a similar child with normal hearing whose rate of growth is 1.00.

Table 11-3. Parameter values and their interpretation for the constant variables examined in the first linkage.

Parameter	Posterior Mean	Posterior 95% Credible Set	Interpretation
α_1	−.27	(−.44, −.07)*	Among nonsigning children, HL children had language growth rates .27 lower than their NH counterparts.
α_2	−.05	(−.16, .05)	Among nonsigning HL children, there was no difference between those identified early and those identified late.
α_3	.11	(.01, .22)*	Among NH children, signing led to a .11 increase in the rate of language growth.
α_4	−.09	(−.24, .05)	Among early-identified HL children, the effect of signing was .09 less than the effect of signing for NH children.
$\alpha_3 + \alpha_4$	.02	(−.08, .12)	Among early-identified HL children, signing did not affect their rate of language growth.
α_5	−.22	(−.4, −.05)*	Signing led to a −.22 decrease for late-identified HL children, compared to early-identified HL children.
$\alpha_4 + \alpha_5$	−.27	(−.42, −.13)*	Among signing HL children, those who were identified late had a growth rate .27 lower.
$\alpha_3 + \alpha_4 + \alpha_5$	−.20	(−.36, −.06)*	Among late-identified HL children, signers had a growth rate .20 lower than nonsigners.
α_6	.09	(0, .2)	Among NH children, females had growth rates .09 greater than males.
α_7	−.04	(−.18, .08)	For HL children, the difference between females and males was .04 less than for NH children.
$\alpha_6 + \alpha_7$	.05	(−.03, .13)	Among HL children, females had growth rates .05 greater than males.
α_8	.12	(−.04, .35)	Among NH children, mid/high SES was associated with a .12 greater rate of language growth.

Table 11–3. *continued*

Parameter	Posterior Mean	Posterior 95% Credible Set	Interpretation
α_9	.05	(–.17, .22)	For HL children, the difference in growth rates between mid-/high- and low-SES children was .05 more than the difference for NH children.
$\alpha_8 + \alpha_9$	.17	(.06, .28)*	Among HL children, mid/high SES was associated with a .17 greater rate of language growth.
α_{10}	–.17	(–.42, .06)	Children who had early simultaneous implantation of two CIs had a language growth rate .17 less than HL children without early implantation of two CIs.
σ_β^2	.04	(.03, .07)*	Within a single group of children (e.g., within male, low SES, HL/EID–s), the variance in growth rates was .04.

Note. Effects for which the 95% interval does not cross zero are indicated with * in Column 3.

Age of ID: In Row 2 we see that age of ID had only a minimal effect (–.05) on growth rates, at least for nonsigning children. If we look at Row 7, we see that being identified late caused a .27 decrease on the rate of language growth for signing children with hearing loss.

Signing, normal hearing: In Row 3 we find that for children with normal hearing, signing was associated with a .11 increase in the rate of language growth. For nonsigning males with low SES, this corresponds to an 11% increase in the rate of language growth as a result of signing. We had thought that this outcome might be obtained because of our decision to include in the latent language variable two measures of behaviors on which the children learn-

ing language poorly showed higher scores than other children: Signing children with normal hearing scored lower on these measures than did nonsigning children with normal hearing. However, when we investigated the effect further we were unable to completely account for it with those two measures. Of course, it will be recalled that the only measure on which signing children with normal hearing performed better than nonsigning children with normal hearing (i.e., had significantly higher scores) was auditory comprehension. The fact that we included that measure in the latent language measure surely helps account for the finding reported here: For children with normal hearing, those whose parents used signs with them did indeed have slightly greater developmental trajectories. This finding highlights the strength of this model. We see that an effect was uncovered that would have gone largely unreported otherwise.

Signing, early-identified hearing loss: In Row 5 we see that signing had no effect on language growth for children with early-identified hearing loss. Thus, we learn that we can make no inferences regarding potential benefits of using signs with deaf children from results obtained with hearing children. We suspect that the reasons parents choose to use signs with their children differ depending on whether their children have normal hearing or hearing loss. It may be that parents who choose to sign with their children with normal hearing are distinct from other parents, perhaps being hypervigilant in their parenting style. In that case, these parents might be providing other forms of support that account for the difference in the rate of language acquisition for children with normal hearing. In the case of children with hearing loss, many parents who choose to use signs would not do so if their children did not have those hearing losses. Therefore, any differences between signing and nonsigning parents of hearing children would not exist for these parents. In any event, the effects of signing were not consistent across these two groups of children.

Signing, late-identified hearing loss: The next several rows show that among all children with hearing loss, those who were late-identified and used signs had slower rates of growth than did nonsigning children with late-identified hearing loss or children with early-identified hearing loss, both signing and nonsign-

ing. For example, when compared to signing children with early-identified hearing loss, signing children with late-identified hearing loss had a decrease of .27 in their language growth rate (Row 7). When compared to nonsigning children with late-identified hearing loss, signing children with late-identified hearing loss have a decrease of .20 in their growth rate (Row 8).

This finding further complicates our ability to interpret the use of signs with children as an independent effect. Clearly, it interacts with how much risk a child is at for delays in language acquisition, such that the greater the risk, the more interfering is the effect of signing. This idea is potentially important because signs are used so commonly with children, even those with normal hearing, who are at risk for delays in language acquisition. Perhaps we, collectively, need to reconsider that practice. It may be better to focus our intervention efforts on promoting the development of spoken language with these children, if indeed our goal for them is to develop spoken language.

Gender: Gender was found to have a moderate impact on the language growth rates of children both with normal hearing and with hearing loss. Among children with normal hearing, girls had a growth rate .09 greater than boys (Row 9), and among children with hearing loss, girls had a growth rate .05 greater than boys (Row 11).

SES: In this analysis, SES was found to have a moderate impact on the language growth rates of children with normal hearing and a strong impact on the growth rates of children with hearing loss. Among children with normal hearing, those with SES scores greater than 15 had growth rates .12 greater than children with SES scores lower than or equal to 15 (Row 12). Among children with hearing loss, those with SES scores greater than 15 had growth rates .17 greater than children with SES poorer than or equal to 15 (Row 14).

Early, bilateral implants: Children who had early simultaneous implantation of two cochlear implants had an average language growth rate .17 less than corresponding children with hearing loss who did not undergo early, simultaneous bilateral implantation (Row 15).

The Second Linkage

The summary of parameter values for the second linkage is presented in Table 11–4. Below we describe the important effects reported in this table.

First CI: The first three rows have to do with the effects of getting a first implant. Neither children who kept their hearing aid upon receiving their first implant nor children who did not keep

their hearing aid upon receiving their first implant showed an increase in language acquisition rate at the time of receiving the first implant. Of course, we need to recall that most children in this study received a cochlear implant early in life. Those children who kept two hearing aids generally performed similarly to children who received implants. Thus, the effect of receiving a first implant would be hard to separate from the general effect of being a child with a hearing loss in this model.

Second CI: The fourth through the sixth rows have to do with the effect of getting a second implant. Receiving a second implant produced a .17 increase in the rate of language growth for children who did not keep their HA at the time of first implant implantation. For children who kept their HA at the time of the first implant, receiving a second implant produced a .40 increase in the rate of language acquisition. This effect is only found for children who did not have early bilateral implantation.

Table 11–4. Parameter values and their interpretation for the constant variables examined in the second linkage.

Parameter	Posterior Mean	Posterior 95% Credible Set	Interpretation
γ_1	.01	(−.12, .15)	When they got their first CI, children who did not keep their HA showed no change in the rate of language acquisition.
γ_2	−.04	(−.21, .13)	When they got their first CI, children who kept their HA showed no difference in the change of rate of language acquisition from those who did not keep their HA.

continues

Table 11–4. *continued*

Parameter	Posterior Mean	Posterior 95% Credible Set	Interpretation
$\gamma_1 + \gamma_2$	−.03	(−.18, .13)	When they got their first CI, children who kept their HA showed no change in the rate of language acquisition.
γ_3	.17	(−.07, .42)	When they got their second CI, children who did not keep their HA when they got their first CI showed an increase of .17 in the rate of language acquisition.
γ_4	.23	(−.11, .59)	When they got their second CI, children who kept their HA when they got their first CI showed an increase .23 larger than those who did not keep their HA.
$\gamma_3 + \gamma_4$	.40	(.16, .69)*	When they got their second CI, children who kept their HA when they obtained their first CI showed an increase of .40 in the rate of language acquisition.
γ_5	.16	(.03, .29)*	Among children with hearing loss, an average increase of .16 in the rate of language growth occurs at 36 months.
γ_6	.04	(.02, .05)*	Among children with normal hearing, an increase of 1 parental verbal response in a 10-minute period is associated with a .04 increase in language ability.
γ_7	.01	(−.01, .02)	Among children with hearing loss, an increase of 1 parental verbal response in a 10-minute period is not associated with any greater increase in language ability than for children with normal hearing.
$\gamma_6 + \gamma_7$	.04	(.03, .06)*	Among children with hearing loss, an increase of 1 parental verbal response in a 10-minute period is associated with a .04 increase in language ability.

Note. Effects for which the 95% interval does not cross zero are indicated with * in Column 3.

36-month effect: Row 7 indicates that children with hearing loss showed an increase of .16 in the rate of language growth at 36 months when they entered preschool programs. This effect was not possible to observe using the methods reported in earlier chapters.

Parental verbal responses: For children both with normal hearing and with hearing loss, the influence of parental verbal responses was significantly, positively related to the rate of language growth. An increase of just one parental verbal response in the 10-minute language sample was associated with an increase of .04 in language ability. It is easy to imagine that if this trend is extrapolated to parental interactions over the course of an entire day, this factor would greatly influence children's language development.

Chapter Summary

This chapter brought together some ideas and information that have been suggested by the data presented in earlier chapters. Here we built a latent language variable that was meant to represent the complex entity underlying most of our separate measures that is language. Rather than examining scores obtained at discrete test ages, we explicitly tried to quantify the sources of variance accounting for the rate of acquisition of that complex variable, language. What we learned was complementary to bits and pieces of information gathered in earlier chapters, but made the points more elegantly.

First, we learned that just by virtue of having a hearing loss, children's rate of language acquisition was significantly impacted.

The use of signs to supplement language input to these children was found to have only minimal effects, in specific instances. Children with normal hearing appeared to benefit from the addition of signs to their language experiences. However, the use of signs did not have consistent effects across all participants, which makes it difficult to attribute this outcome explicitly to the use of signs. This effect might be accounted for by some unknown variable unrelated to signing. There may be something that defines parents who decide to use signs with their children in the absence of hearing loss that could explain this outcome. For children with late-identified hearing loss, the use of signs was deleterious to language acquisition. That suggests that there might be something akin to a critical period in language acquisition: As children get older, they are less capable of learning language when two languages are being presented. For children with early-identified hearing loss, there simply was no effect, either positive or negative, observed for the use of signs.

We continued to find evidence that implanting children with bilateral implants very early in life does not seem like a particularly good idea. However, giving children a second implant a little later in childhood may have significant benefits, and those benefits appear to be greatest for children who continued to wear a hearing aid on the unimplanted ear between the times of the first and second implants. Possible reasons for these findings will be explored in the next chapter.

With this latent growth model we were able to observe effects not found using methods reported in earlier chapters. For example, we found an advantage for children from mid-/high-SES homes. That outcome suggests ways that we might adjust intervention for children with hearing loss: Specifically, we might ask what is different in the homes of low- and mid-/high-SES children, and try to make adjustments to the former.

We also observed an increase in the rate of language acquisition when children with hearing loss began attending preschool programs. This result again suggests where we might start looking in order to enhance language outcomes for children with hearing loss. If we could find a way to make intervention as facilitative in the years before 36 months as in those preschool years, we might be able to increase the rate of language acquisition for children with hearing loss during the first three years of life.

One of the potentially most important findings coming out of this study continues to be the enormous effect that certain styles of parental interaction appear to have on language development in children. Parents who respond verbally to any and all attempts on the part of their children to communicate seem to be contributing very strongly and positively to their children's language learning. Again, the reasons and ramifications of this effect will be explored in greater detail in the next and final chapter.

References

Berger, J. O., & Berry, D. A. (1988). Statistical analysis and the illusion of objectivity. *American Scientist*, 76, 159–165.

Berger, J. O., & Wolpert, R. (1984). *The likelihood principle.* Hayward, CA: Institute of Mathematical Statistics.

Gelman, A. B., Carlin, J. S., Stern, H. S., & Rubin, D. B. (1995). *Bayesian data analysis.* Boca Raton, FL: Chapman & Hall/CRC.

R Development Core Team. (2007). *R: A language and environment for statistical computing.* Vienna, Austria: R Foundation for Statistical Computing.

Robert, C. P., & Casella, G. (1999). *Monte Carlo statistical methods.* New York: Springer-Verlag.

12

Considering the Past,
Planning for the Future

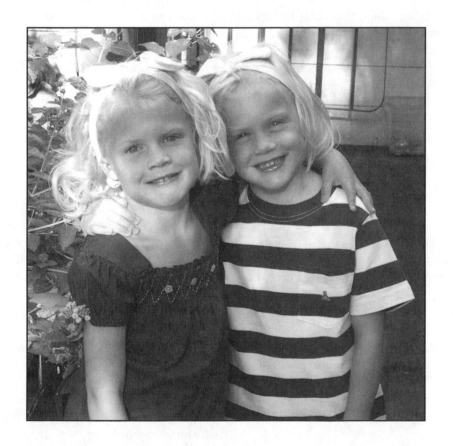

Some years ago, a young bride prepared to make her first holiday meal. It would be a large family event, with her parents and her husband's parents present. She wanted everything to be perfect, and most of all, wanted to make sure there was sufficient food for all who attended. Therefore, she bought a very large roast. When she went to cook it, however, she discovered that it was too large for the new roasting pan she had received as a wedding present. Improvising, she cut several inches off each end of the roast, and cooked them in a smaller pan.

The years passed. The woman's family grew, but not her roasting pan. Each year, she encountered the same problem: There was more meat than pan. So each year she arrived upon the same solution of cooking the ends in a smaller pan, always vowing to invest in a larger pan before the holiday rolled around again. As with many good intentions, though, she never quite got around to doing so.

Eventually, the woman's daughter married, and responsibility for preparing the holiday meal was passed to her. The wedding had been big, and the daughter had received many wonderful gifts, including a large roasting pan. Nonetheless, when she set about cooking her first holiday meal, she sliced several inches off each end of the roast, and placed them in a smaller pan.

The mother, witnessing this event, exclaimed, "What are you doing to that beautiful roast? Why didn't you put it all in the big pan?"

Astonished, the daughter replied, "But Mom, this is how a roast is cooked! It's how you always did it!"

Considering the Past

The story above illustrates why it is important to understand the historical context of what we do. In Chapter 1 we learned about the underpinnings of current strategies for intervention with deaf children. Practices in intervening with children with hearing loss and scientific investigation into speech transmission and perception were intertwined during the early years of deaf education in America. Approaches to helping deaf children learn spoken language emerged largely from the widespread perspective that the physical speech signal consists of strings of phonetic segments, with each segment defined by a specific setting on a specific acoustic cue. The setting for any one cue might exhibit some variability depending on talker characteristics and phonetic environment, but it was thought to be more or less stable. Accordingly, treatment efforts focused largely on ensuring that auditory sensitivity was adequate for each of these cues and that children responded to and produced each phonetic segment correctly. If listeners could discriminate small changes in relevant acoustic cues or features, the assumption was, they could recover phonetic structure. In other words, they could perceive speech.

These "linear" approaches to intervention received support from paradigms in the scientific community regarding speech production and perception. Scientists have traditionally framed questions concerning human speech perception to ask how the manipulation of discrete cues affects decisions about the identity of individual phonetic segments. Scientists working in the area of speech technology have been concerned with how well information about discrete phonetic segments is transmitted. Our methods of gauging success for technological innovations have involved counting the numbers of phonemes that listeners can recognize given certain transmission characteristics, such as filter settings. These assessments are done by presenting sets of speech stimuli, usually words, and asking listeners to repeat what they hear. This approach has been used since the earliest days of the telephone, and has continued through our efforts to design ever more effective cochlear implants.

Because most of us shared this view of what it means to communicate—transmitting bits of information serially—we were unprepared to interpret and use findings from experiments such as those of Remez and colleagues (1981) and Shannon and colleagues (1995) regarding speech processed to preserve only the spectral skeletons or only the temporal envelopes of speech. Those experiments demonstrated that listeners can understand spoken sentences when speech signals are processed to eliminate the properties we refer to as acoustic cues. For similar reasons, many of us did not predict the great success we have witnessed for cochlear implants. These devices have allowed many individuals with severe-to-profound hearing loss to learn to understand spoken language, even though implants fail to deliver the signal details we know as acoustic cues. The very fact that cochlear implants support speech perception as well as they do dictates that we modify our view of speech communication. Generally speaking, however, we have not done so. Cochlear implants are viewed as substitutes for natural hearing, even if the signal quality is recognized as being inferior. To evaluate performance, we continue to use standard metrics such as how many phonetic segments or features can be recognized correctly by the listener with an implant. But it is time to realize that our linear perspective of speech communication is unable to explain the perceptual phenomena we have discovered in recent years. To appreciate spoken communication and fashion a new approach to intervention for deaf children, we need to modify our view of what it means to communicate with spoken language. We need to see the child's task in learning about the speech signal as something other than developing the ability to pluck bits of the signal from the ongoing speech stream—a nasal murmur here, a fricative noise there.

Discovering Structure in the Signal

When the child comes into the world, the speech she hears from those around her is meaningless, a complex acoustic signal lacking linguistic form. Although the child is genetically predisposed to develop linguistic competency, learning is nonetheless involved. The child must learn how to take these sensory inputs and derive meaningful structure from them. This process involves something other than just learning to harvest bits of the signal; it involves discovering the linguistically meaningful form comprised of the whole signal. If it were the case that listeners harvest bits of the signal to derive phonetic structure, we would have expected the severity of the hearing loss experienced by the children in this study to correlate with their language abilities. But for no measure was a significant correlation observed between auditory sensitivity and performance. Instead, what we found was that factors other than simple auditory sensitivity explained language outcomes for these children with significant hearing loss.

In keeping with earlier linear views of speech perception, the idea was widely accepted 20 to 40 years ago that infants begin life able to discriminate all of the phonemes of all of the languages of the world. During the first year of life, the belief was, infants tune their attention to only the phonetic distinctions of the native language they are acquiring (e.g., Eimas, Siqueland, Jusczyk, & Vigorito, 1971; Jusczyk, 1995; Kuhl, 1980; Werker, 1991, 1994). Recently, this perspective has changed (Nittrouer, 2001). We no longer view the task of speech perception as one of discriminating between phonetic segments—after all, in the everyday world of communications we are never given two syllables to discriminate. Rather, the task involved in speech perception involves one of recovering meaningful linguistic structure (including but not limited to phonetic structure) from the ongoing signal. This difference may sound like a trivial shift in perspective, but it implies major changes in how we approach intervention. Even though infants with normal hearing can discriminate some of the acoustic distinctions commonly thought to underlie specific phonetic distinctions, it does not mean that they have an awareness of phonetic structure. Sensitivity to pho-

netic structure in the native language is something that continues to be refined over the first decade or so of life, not over the first year (e.g., Beckman & Edwards, 2000; Hazan & Barrett, 2000; Nittrouer, 2006; Werker & Yeung, 2005). For children with hearing loss, this means that our approaches to intervention should not focus on training them to recognize and reproduce individual phonemes, but rather should focus on helping them discover linguistic form.

Upon first consideration, it is hard to explain why the various elements that are spread widely across both the spectral and temporal domains of the speech signal are integrated into unitary percepts when we listen to speech—other than the fact that they are. Formant frequencies across the spectrum generally lack any natural relationship, and voiced signal portions are different in kind from adjacent noises, such as those associated with fricatives and stops. Yet listeners integrate these disparate acoustic ingredients so strongly when they listen to speech that they are unable to hear individual spectral components (e.g., Best, Morrongiello, & Robson, 1981; Mann & Liberman, 1983). Each child must be able to integrate the acoustic components of the signal into linguistically relevant structure if she is ever to develop native competencies in a language.

To begin to appreciate the task facing the child, we can consider traditional Gestalt principles of perception, as illustrated by Figure 12–1. From this figure, we can recover either the image of a young woman, looking away from us, or the profile of an old woman. The same information is available to our visual systems in both cases, but how we organize that information perceptually determines what we see. (Readers

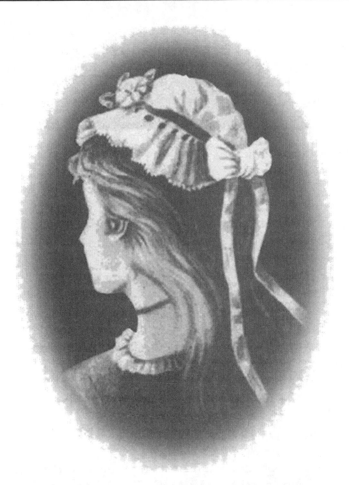

Figure 12–1. Picture illustrating how the same sensory input can be perceived differently. Here one sees either a young woman looking away or an old woman with her chin touching her chest. From "A New Ambiguous Figure," by E. G. Boring, 1930, *American Journal of Psychology, 42,* pp. 444–445. Adapted by L. L. Lohr, 2003, *Creating Graphics for Learning and Performance: Lessons in Visual Literacy.* Upper Saddle River, NJ: Pearson. Copyright 1930, University of Illinois. Reproduced with permission.

who are having difficulty recovering one or the other of the images can turn to Appendix E, which highlights the forms by using a slightly brighter shade for the skin tone than that on Figure 12–1.) By analogy, we can understand the task facing the child with impaired hearing as having to learn how to organize the sensory inputs available to her about spoken language in order to derive a meaningful form. Generally, children begin to discover how to do this very early in life, and initially use signal properties that can be labeled as "global" to derive relevant structure; these are properties that are broader spectrally and temporally than traditional acoustic cues. For children with normal hearing, this process is straightforward because they have access to the complete speech signal. Children with hearing loss, especially those wearing cochlear implants, only have access to highly impoverished signals. Therefore, we must help them discover structure in the signal by providing adequate forms of perceptual support.

Evidence that typically developing children recover global structure from the speech signal early in life came from a laboratory in France as far back as 1986. Then, Bénédicte de Boysson-Bardies and her colleagues computed long-term average spectra of speech samples from adult and infant speakers of several languages. Results for speakers of just two languages, French and Algerian, are shown in Figure 12–2. We see that the long-term spectra of adult speakers of French, both male and female, are peaked and concentrated in the low frequencies. These spectra are shown on the left of Figure 12–2. Long-term spectra of adult speakers of Algerian are flatter, covering a wider range of frequencies. These spectra are on the right of Figure 12–2. When we look at the spectra of babbled productions from 10-month-old infants, we see that their vocal output is already beginning to bear the marks of their language communities. These infants are replicating in their own productions the kinds of articulatory posturing needed to shape the signal as adults in their linguistic communities do. Again, however, the kind of structure represented in these long-term spectra is global in nature,

rather than the spectro-temporal details commonly called acoustic cues.

Linguists and psychologists studying child language theorize that young children use the kinds of global *acoustic* structure represented by long-term spectra to begin recovering *linguistic* structure in their native language. For example, children may use prosody, a property arising from the glottal source, to begin parsing the speech signal into its constituent phrases (Gleitman & Wanner, 1982; Jusczyk, 1997; Morgan & Demuth, 1996; Soderstrom, Seidl, Kemler Nelson, & Jusczyk, 2003). They may attend to the relatively slow modulations of the lower formants to start parsing those phrases into separate words (Nittrouer, Lowenstein, & Packer, 2009): Dynamic signal stretches that are frequently repeated in heard speech start to be recovered from the ongoing speech stream as distinct units, specifically words. From this perspective, it becomes apparent that even though low-frequency elements in the signal on their own may not support accurate speech recognition, these signal components serve important functions in language acquisition. This notion probably explains some of the results emerging from this study.

Low-Frequency Signal Components Guide the Way

Several findings related to the types of auditory prostheses that children were using, reported in Chapters 9 and 11, may have been surprising to readers. In particular, we found that children who received two implants shortly after their first birthdays were faring

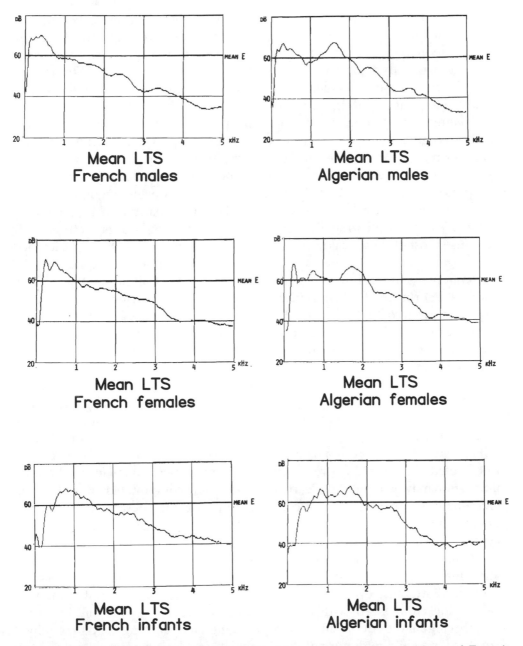

Figure 12–2. Long-term average spectra for adult and infant speakers of French and Algerian reported by de Boysson-Bardies and colleagues, 1986. From "Acoustic Investigations of Cross-Linguistic Variability in Babbling," by B. de Boysson-Bardies, L. Sagart, P. Halle, & C. Durand, 1986. In B. Lindblom & R. Zetterstrom (Eds.), *Wenner-Gren International Symposium Series: Vol. 44. Precursors of Early Speech* (pp. 113–126), New York: Stockton Press. Copyright 1986, B. de Boysson-Bardies. Reproduced with permission.

especially poorly. Children who received just one implant were even developing language more rapidly than these children, and some advantage was found for children with one implant who continued to wear a hearing aid on the unimplanted ear. Although we did not measure recognition for words presented in an open-set manner, we strongly suspect that all of these children would have performed significantly better on such a task with only their implants than with only their hearing aids. This is because most of these children were able to hear just the low-frequency signal components through their hearing aids. That information by itself is insufficient for word recognition. Put another way, if we thought these children could understand speech with hearing aids alone, they never would have received cochlear implants. Why then was the combination of one cochlear implant and one hearing aid so conducive to language learning?

The answer to that question is likely multifaceted. First, that low-frequency information may help the child learn to perceptually organize the signal components she is receiving through her implant. Again, the signal provided by an implant is highly impoverished, which makes the task of discovering meaningful structure even more difficult for the child faced with having to learn language through this device than it is for a child with normal hearing. Yet just as the normal-hearing child must discover the structure of her native language in the acoustic signal she receives, so must the child using an implant. Low-frequency hearing seems to help all listeners with hearing loss perform this kind of auditory grouping task (e.g., Zeng, 2008), and so it should

be especially important to young children just discovering how the entire spectrum of the speech signal coheres to form a unitary percept. Strong support for the idea that low-frequency signal components help the child discover the perceptual form in the implant signal comes from the finding that children who received a second implant showed a tremendous increase in the slope of their developmental trajectory for language learning if they retained their hearing aids after getting their first implants. In Chapter 11 we learned that there was a .40 increase in the slope of those trajectories for children who kept their hearing aids, compared to only a .17 increase in that slope for children who did not continue wearing a hearing aid after the first implant. That is a tremendous advantage that goes a long way towards compensating for the .27 decrease in language learning imposed on children simply because they have a hearing loss. And in addition to aiding the child's discovery of relevant perceptual form, the low-frequency components of the signal surely help the child learn about syntactic phrase structure in her native language. In general, there is every reason to strive to preserve as much of a child's acoustic hearing as possible, and to expect even a small amount of acoustic hearing to offer big dividends in language learning when combined with a cochlear implant.

Visual Information Helps Children Discover Structure, Too

The analogy of how perceivers use Gestalt principles to recover meaningful optical structure from ambiguous visual signals only goes so far in helping us understand how children discover linguistic structure in the acoustic speech signal. In 1994, Robert Remez and his colleagues published the results of a carefully conducted study in which they tried to use Gestalt principles to explain how listeners form cohesive auditory groupings from the diverse spectro-temporal components of the speech signal. Their investigation demonstrated that Gestalt principles—those based on general auditory perception—cannot explain why the signal components cohere in speech. Instead, they showed that the various parts of the spectrum cohere perceptually because listeners recognize them as arising from a single human speaker. Armed with this information, we can appreciate how any mechanism that helps us recognize the various signal components as emanating from a single vocal tract will help the child discover meaningful structure in the speech signal. Surely, the visual image of the moving vocal tract as it produces speech is one such mechanism. From this perspective it becomes clear that we should ensure that the child with hearing loss has full access to our faces when we speak—at least when it is natural to do so.

When we stop viewing the speech signal as a linear sequence of discrete phonetic segments and instead see it as a coherent structure from which relevant linguistic form must be derived, the potential role of visual input in spoken language perception becomes apparent. In Chapter 1 we learned that traditional views of lipreading held that some phonetic features may be derived from audition, even in the face of hearing loss, and other features may be

derived from vision. These two classes of features are summed to derive specific phonetic segments, or so it was thought. From this perspective, vision is not considered to provide precisely the same information as audition. That idea, however, has failed to stand the tests of time and experimentation.

One way in which we can examine how spoken language is coded by the brain is to study the immediate recall of word strings. When a series of words, such as digits, is presented in spoken form, research subjects generally recall the words in initial and final positions with more accuracy than they recall medially occurring words. These phenomena are known as the primacy and recency effects. When nonverbal images are presented in graphic form, such as numerals printed on cards, no recency effects are observed: Subjects do as poorly with the items near the ends of the series as they do with the medially presented items. In 1980, two investigators decided to examine whether words presented through lipreading alone are coded as visual signals or as auditory speech signals. To do that, they presented lists of digits in three conditions: audition only, lipreading only, and as printed numerals shown one at a time. Similar recency effects were observed for the auditory and lip-read stimuli, but no such effect was found for the printed stimuli (Campbell & Dodd, 1980). From that finding, the authors concluded that lip-read signals are processed precisely as are auditory-speech signals, and not as more general visual signals.

Another way in which we can examine the role of lip-read signals during speech perception is by using a paradigm known as phonemic restoration.

In these procedures, a portion of a spoken word is replaced with white noise, and subjects are asked to report whether they noticed the interruption or not. Generally, phonemic restoration is studied through audition alone, and experiments using the paradigm have demonstrated that listeners employ linguistic context to recover complete phonetic forms (Samuel, 1996). Recently, two investigators looked at this phenomenon by comparing recognition when lip-read signals were congruently and incongruently presented along with the auditory speech signals. Those auditory speech signals were words with varying lengths deleted from the middle and noise substituted for the missing parts. Results showed that subjects were able to restore longer stretches of missing speech when the lip-read signal continued congruently through the missing signal portion (Shahin & Miller, 2009). The conclusion of the study's authors was that lip-read signals allow the brain to fill in the missing signal portion, but the kind of "filling in" suggested by Shahin and Miller in this case does not refer to a repairing of a missing part after the fact, so to speak. Rather, these investigators have reason to assert that the brain does not register the missing part to begin with. Instead, the region of the brain that recovers the visual signal communicates with the auditory cortex where the acoustic speech signal is processed. When context, including lip-read information, is available that information is provided to the auditory cortex, which continues processing the signal just as if there was no interruption at all (Shahin, Bishop, & Miller, 2009).

This kind of finding is critical to updating our views of auditory perception and the influence that those views should have on early intervention. When Max Goldstein and other proponents of the antecedents to auditory-verbal therapy were developing their methods, they were basing their decisions about what to do on the belief that the auditory system is an encapsulated neural tract. That idea fit with views of neural organization that existed for much of the 20th century when processing of sensory information was believed to occur in a strictly bottom-up manner, passing through vertically organized structures. Higher level structures had input from lower level structures, but could not communicate to those lower structures. If signals were degraded at low levels, higher level systems could fill in the missing pieces, but could never influence processing at those lower levels. That hierarchical view of how the brain works surely spurred the assortment of models about auditory perception upon which many current intervention strategies are based: detection, then discrimination, then sensation, then recognition—or some variation on that theme. Children with hearing loss, the thinking went, should be trained to process speech in this vertical manner through the auditory system, rather than learning to depend on higher level inputs to compensate for missing signal components. To do that required that they be deprived of any information, such as lipreading, that could provide higher level compensation. We now understand that the brain functions as a well-integrated entity, with communication among the various parts occurring on a continuous basis. Visual input in the form of lipreading can only help the auditory system code the speech signal.

In this study, we found no differences in outcomes for children whose intervention was best described as auditory oral and those whose intervention was auditory verbal. We restricted participation in this study to children whose programs met certain criteria: Children and/or their parents had to be visiting with an intervention specialist at least once per week before the child was 3 years of age. The program had to have a professional trained explicitly to work with children with hearing loss at the helm, and that individual had to have at least a master's degree. By instituting these criteria, we sought to ensure that the quality of intervention was similar across children; we did not want merely to be comparing the results of good versus bad intervention in this study. Auditory-oral and auditory-verbal therapies share many of the same principles when it comes to intervention, including an emphasis on developing a child's ability to understand spoken language through hearing. However, one point where the two approaches diverge regards the extent to which access to visual information about speech should be made available to children: Traditionally, auditory-verbal therapy restricts a child's ability to see the speaker's face as much as possible, even encouraging parents and therapists to cover their mouths. The fact that no advantage was found for children receiving therapy with this emphasis indicates that it serves no special function. Here we use current knowledge about the role of visual information in speech perception to suggest that children with hearing loss should be permitted to see the speaker's face.

Experiments with the McGurk effect (McGurk & MacDonald, 1976) demonstrate that perceivers recover the same information regarding the speech signal from both vision and hearing, as

do experiments by other investigators such as Campbell and Dodd (1980) and Shahin and Miller (2009): It is not the case that some features of speech are conveyed by one modality, other features by the other modality, and then the retrieved features summed. Our goal in intervention should be to provide as complete a signal as possible to children with hearing loss. Once we recognize that listeners must perceptually organize the sensory information they receive, much as we do for the image in Figure 12–1, and one chore facing children is to learn how to organize the components of the speech signal, we can view the visual speech signal as a sensory aid. While it does not support speech recognition very well on its own, visual input helps children discover the structure of the acoustic speech signal by allowing the child to place all components within the context of the moving vocal tract.

Not All Auditory Inputs Are Equal

Having just spent considerable space explaining that various structures of the brain can communicate horizontally and even from the top down, it must now be emphasized that there do exist neural specializations, and those specializations are important in considering how to help children with hearing loss. When the auditory system was thought to be strictly vertically and hierarchically organized, the idea evolved that there are natural steps that should be followed in learning to process speech signals. For example, children should first learn to detect sound, and then they can be taught to discriminate different sounds, then learn to determine what was making the sound, and so on. There has also existed the idea that children should be taught to respond to simple, nonspeech signals before they are trained to interpret speech and other complex signals. This is a principle built into the design of many commercially available auditory training programs. The validity of that approach is challenged, however, by evidence showing that simple signals are processed in different regions of the auditory cortex than are complex signals, such as those used for communication. For example, single cell recordings from the cortices of nonhuman primates have revealed that regions at the core of the auditory cortex respond to pure tones. Communication sounds, such as the monkey calls described in Chapter 2, are processed by cells in the more lateral regions of the auditory cortex (Rauschecker, 1998; Rauschecker, Tian, & Hauser, 1995). Imaging studies have similarly demonstrated that human speech is processed at the lateral edges of the auditory cortex (Belin, Zatorre, Lafaille, Ahad, & Pike, 2000; Binder et al., 2000; Scott, Blank, Rosen, & Wise, 2000). Consequently, there is no reason to expect that training with nonspeech signals would ever help children learn to organize and comprehend spoken language.

The finding that areas of the brain outside of the auditory cortex can influence processing within the auditory cortex itself also should inform us about the kind of language we should be using with deaf children. Some therapy approaches would have us teach children phonemes one at a time. Only after they demonstrate skill at producing a circumscribed set of these items can we begin to expect them to produce phonemes correctly in words; to *generalize* is the term that is commonly used. These approaches spend a great deal of time working on isolated phonemes. However, the empirical results reviewed here concerning signal structure and neural mechanisms indicate that it is time for a change to that approach. First, it is not the case that children learn phonemes, and then learn to put them together. Rather, the child discovers phonetic structure in the speech signal, just as the child discovers other kinds of linguistically meaningful structure. That suggests that we should be presenting more complete language models than we may currently be providing in some approaches to intervention. Second, results from studies such as that of Shahin et al. (2009) showing that linguistic context can affect how the acoustic speech signal is processed in the auditory cortex means that we should be helping children learn about all levels of linguistic structure simultaneously —phonetic, syntactic, grammatical.

Learning by Doing

In the 1980s, a group of scientists working in Parma, Italy, were interested in how the brain controls motor movements in primates. To study this phenomenon, they recorded responses from single neurons in the premotor cortices of monkeys while the monkeys were performing specific hand and mouth actions. To their astonishment, they began to notice that there were responses from these same neurons when the monkeys were not being tested, but were instead watching other animals perform these tasks. There are, it turns out, certain neurons that both respond to actions by others and control actions themselves. These neurons have come to be called mirror neurons (Rizzolatti & Craighero, 2004).

The discovery of mirror neurons drew renewed attention to the connections between motor actions and the perception of those actions. There is still a great deal of work to be done before we fully understand the role of mirror neurons in perception and motor control, but regardless of how we finally come to understand that role, their discovery has helped to fuel renewed interest in the idea that there is a sensorimotor foundation to speech perception. That original position, known as the Motor Theory (e.g., Liberman, Cooper, Shankweiler, & Studdert-Kennedy, 1967), had fallen into disrepute in favor of purely auditory accounts of speech perception during much of the latter part of the 20th century. Now, at the start of the 21st century, scientists are again affirming the connection between being able to produce an action and perceive the action (e.g., Todd, Lee, & O'Boyle, 2006).

The importance of practice in producing language—and particularly in generating it—is emphasized by the findings reported in Chapter 10 concerning the contributions of parental verbal responses to child language outcomes. Parents who responded more frequently to their children's communicative attempts had children with better language skills than did parents who did not respond verbally. And this effect could not be traced to how often parents modeled language for their children: All parents tended to provide general language models to a similar extent. Instead, the effect of parental language resided precisely in how often they engaged in behavior that encouraged children to produce language on their own, or provided examples explicitly of the language that the child seemed to need at the moment to communicate a specific intent.

In results described in earlier chapters, it was repeatedly observed that language measures were not correlated with auditory sensitivity among children with hearing loss. If a child's hearing loss was poorer than 50 dB HL, it did not matter to what extent that loss exceeded that level; other factors accounted for how well the child learned language. That finding makes the results illustrated in Table 12–1 all the more

Table 12–1. Pearson product-moment correlation coefficients between each dependent language measure and CSIM scores for all children who were tested from 36 to 48 months of age.

	Auditory Comprehension	EOWPVT	RW-U	MLU	Pronouns	NDW
r	.745	.707	.531	.721	.697	.715
p	<.001	<.001	<.001	<.001	<.001	<.001
N	350	348	344	306	306	306

Note. EOWPVT = Expressive One-Word Picture Vocabulary Test; RW-U = real-word utterances obtained in the 20-minute child language sample; MLU = mean length of utterance in morphemes; NDW = number of different words from SALT analysis.

significant. There, we show correlation coefficients between scores on the Children's Speech Intelligibility Measure (CSIM), reported in Chapter 6, and scores on each of the six language measures used in Chapter 9 to gauge treatment effects. We see that in all but one instance (real-word utterances), children's intelligibility explained roughly half of the variance in their language abilities. That is a great deal of variance to be able to explain. And it will be recalled that the CSIM uses single words as stimuli, rather than sentences, precisely so that the adult judges cannot use linguistic context to comprehend what the child produced. Consequently, the intelligibility of a child's speech production reflects how well the child can produce and organize the constituent vocal-tract gestures of a word. The strength of the correlations shown on Table 12–1 between motor control for speech and language abilities suggests that the motor gestures involved in speech production do not simply provide the medium for expressing language. Instead, these gestures *are* the medium for generating language. The language in our heads is the movements of our mouths. Auditory sensitivity cannot explain variability in language ability, but motor control for speech can. Language is not an acoustic phenomenon, but rather a sensorimotor phenomenon. And finally, it is worth recalling that no deficits in general fine motor control were observed for children with hearing loss. What we find in comparing results from the SIB-R for general motor ability and from the CSIM for speech motor control is that children with hearing loss were delayed in their abilities to coordinate vocal-tract movements for speech production such

that their speech was not as intelligible as that of children with normal hearing.

The Language of the Hands Does Not Promote Development in the Language of the Mouth

Once it is recognized that language is inherently a motor activity, it becomes easy to appreciate why sign language was not found to facilitate the development of spoken language for the children in this study. There is no reason to suspect that the movements of the hands would facilitate a child's ability to perceive or produce movements of the vocal tract. Turning to the notion of mirror neurons, we can appreciate that different neurons would be involved in motor control and action perception for these two movement generators. When children have no risk factors that can disrupt their learning of spoken language, the use of manual language introduces no interference. Children can learn to produce and comprehend language through movements of both the hands and the mouth at the same time in their lives. However, as a child's risk of failing to learn spoken language increases, so apparently does the interference encountered by the presentation of signs.

When it comes to using signs, no evidence was found in these data to support their use as a means either of promoting spoken language development or of preventing emotional/behavioral problems, both rationales offered for the use of signs with young children. At the same time, no evidence was found that learning signs interferes with learning spoken language, for most children. Although we did not assess how well the signing children with hearing loss in this study could sign, by the time they were 36 months old they were all in preschool programs that consistently use signs as part of the curriculum. That means that they were generally signing 6 hours per day from Monday to Friday. We assume they must have had some level of proficiency in sign language. Consequently, if it is the wish of the parents that their children learn to use sign language so that they can participate in Deaf culture, no findings from this study suggest that there is a reason to discourage that, unless a child's hearing loss was identified after 1 year of age.

Is Earlier Better When It Comes to Identification?

A primary motivation for conducting this study was to examine whether language outcomes for children with hearing loss have improved with the advent of newborn hearing screening. The hope has been that initiating intervention soon after birth would dramatically improve outcomes over those being found when the average age of identification was 2 ½ years. None of the children in this study were identified with hearing loss quite that late in development. Generally speaking, however, little evidence was found for having one's hearing loss identified very near birth, rather than at 1 or 2 years of age.

But the emphasis here is on the phrase "generally speaking." There were results obtained in this study that suggest that once we determine the best ways to intervene with families of newborns identified with hearing loss —as we will hopefully do—identifying children very young will be one component of a broader set of procedures that will lead to optimal outcomes. In this study, the children who were doing particularly well in their language development (the "stars") all had been identified with hearing loss before the age of 1 year. That finding indicates that if we want children with hearing loss to perform similarly to children with normal hearing, we will need to be identifying hearing loss near birth. In addition, children who were not identified with hearing loss until after the age of 1 year were hobbled in their abilities to develop spoken language if their parents chose to also use signs with them. That finding suggests that there is some additional load placed on learning language if the process is not started before the first year of life such that it becomes difficult to acquire two separate languages at the same time. Finally, children identified after 1 year of age were found to be more delayed in syntactic development, using Brown's (1973) stages, than were children identified at birth. So these three results all indicate that the optimal time to begin learning language is as close to birth as possible.

Planning for the Future: What Should We Do Now?

Before reviewing what we might be doing to move the developmental trajectories of children with hearing loss closer to those of children with normal hearing, much of which is suggested by the discussion above, it is worth mentioning some of the things that we should not be doing. It is so easy to allow ourselves to become focused on activities other than the ones that really matter, if those latter activities are hard to do. For example, when faced with a report that we need to write we may find ourselves wandering down the hall to talk to a colleague, or making a phone call, or trying to decide which font the report would look nicest in, rather than actually writing. Doing what it takes to help a deaf child learn spoken language is hard. It is easy for educators and clinicians to get detoured in efforts to teach language by activities focused on other developmental domains. And of course, reinforcement is more plentiful for both student and teacher while working on nonlanguage goals because children with hearing loss typically do not have as great barriers imposed on their learning of other skills as they do on learning language. But an important message arising from the data reported here is that the problems faced by children with hearing loss all stem from an underlying deficit in language learning. These children were not found to have behavioral problems. They did not have psychosocial problems. They did not have motor problems, other than apparent difficulty involved in organizing vocal-tract gestures to produce speech. The one cognitive task on which children with hearing loss performed more poorly than children with normal hearing was one that can reasonably be asserted to rely on language processing: Classification. We learned from the correlations of various language measures with CSIM scores (see Table 12–1) that motor speech gestures are not only the medium of language expression but

the material of language. The results for the Classification test tell us that language is not just the medium for expressing our thoughts; it is the material used in thinking, as well.

We also learned that parents are stronger than they are sometimes given credit for being. At least by the time their children are 12 months of age, they are not experiencing unusual levels of stress as a consequence of having a child with hearing loss. And we learned how tremendously important their interactions with their children are to language acquisition by those children. The time we spend working with parents should focus on helping them learn how to make every interaction supportive of their child's language development.

In sum, we learned that the focus of our intervention with children with hearing loss and their parents should rest squarely on ways to promote language acquisition. The combined results of this study emphasize the great need for that kind of intervention. It is not enough to put hearing aids on a child or give her an implant and expect language development to proceed in anything close to a typical time frame. The children with hearing loss in this study were all receiving intervention, and a fair amount of it. Nonetheless, their language development was pervasively delayed. In Chapter 11 we learned that the rate of language growth increased when these children began attending preschool programs: Ramping up the intensity of intervention resulted in increases in the rate of language learning. From this finding we may conclude that we should be considering ways to increase the amount of intervention provided before the age of

3 years. If we could find a way to make intervention during those first years as intensive as it is after 3 years of age, we may be able to speed up language learning starting at a younger age.

Although data were not collected for children beyond the age of 4 years, it is also likely that the children participating in this study will need further language support as they enter the school years. As discussed in Chapter 1, results for children from low-SES backgrounds who attended Head Start programs showed that they fell behind once they left those programs. The environment needs to continue being supportive for those children in order for them to maintain the gains realized in early intervention. Given that the rate of language acquisition was tied to the amount of intervention these children with hearing loss were receiving, and the quality of language input, it is perfectly reasonable to suggest that they are going to need that level of support through at least the early school years.

Much has been made here about the fact that young children do not acquire speech by accumulating phonemes, one at a time. That said, children must eventually discover phonetic structure in the acoustic speech signal. Children with normal hearing typically become skilled at recognizing phonetic structure during the early school years, roughly kindergarten through second grade (Liberman, Shankweiler, Fischer, & Carter, 1974). That time span corresponds to the period during which children are developing early reading skills, as well. While it is difficult to determine the direction of cause and effect for those two skills, we do know that some children receive reading instruction and yet fail to acquire sensitivity to phonetic

structure (e.g., Pennington, Van Orden, Smith, Green, & Haith, 1990; Wagner, 1986; Wagner & Torgesen, 1987). That means that there must be more to acquiring sensitivity to phonetic structure than just reading instruction. On these pages we have discussed the notion that at some time during infancy and preschool, typically developing children acquire sensitivity to other kinds of structure in the signal. Because we found that children with hearing loss are generally delayed in acquiring sensitivity to those aspects of structure, it is likely that they are delayed in honing their abilities to recover phonetic structure, as well. Thus, again we find reason to suspect that these children will continue to need support through at least the early school years.

Evidence is found in these data for one other thing we should not do: We should not look to technology to solve the language-learning problems faced by children with hearing loss. Cochlear implants have moved the playing field for children with severe-to-profound hearing loss. These children can now achieve language abilities commensurate to those of children with moderate hearing loss. Unfortunately, children with moderate hearing loss demonstrated significant deficits compared to the language performance of children with normal hearing. It is extremely unlikely that the technology associated with cochlear implants will be modified any time soon so that it provides more favorable signals to severely-to-profoundly impaired listeners than what current hearing aids provide to moderately impaired listeners. It has taken the mammalian auditory system millennia to evolve into the exquisite sensory processor it is. We should not expect technology to perfectly replicate it any time soon.

On the other hand, we found that the way caregivers interacted with their children explained an enormous amount of variance in language outcomes for children with hearing loss. These two ideas—that technology is not close to completely compensating for the problems of hearing loss, but parents have a profound effect on outcomes—suggest that efforts to modify our intervention procedures should be at least as intensive as efforts trying to change technology. To improve language learning for deaf children, we need to be looking at our intervention methods. This should have implications for funding priorities in both research and clinical practice.

Preserving Acoustic Hearing

Perhaps it is precisely because cochlear implants have provided such a boost in recent years to children with severe-to-profound hearing loss that we have diminished our attention to acoustic hearing. Or perhaps this shift reflects a pervasive cultural trend towards seeking high-tech solutions to all our problems. But whatever the reason, the value of preserving and using acoustic hearing needs to be emphasized. We learned in Chapter 11 that the children who spent a period of time with combined electric (implant) and acoustic (hearing aid) stimulation enjoyed tremendous benefits when they received their second implant. The specific suggestion was made that acoustic stimulation helps the child find the perceptual object in the electric signal. The broader message we should take away from

those results is that we should provide children with a period of combined electric-acoustic hearing. It will be recalled that no children were found to have such poor auditory sensitivity that they could not benefit from having a hearing aid in combination with an implant.

One particular source of acoustic hearing that might be used more often is that provided by FM systems. Very few children in this study had FM systems available for home use, and those who did used them only sporadically. Precisely because it was found that acoustic hearing can be helpful in children's perceptual development as it regards language, these devices deserve stronger consideration.

Getting the Big Picture

A great deal of space has been devoted to the notion that children do not acquire language from the bottom up, acquiring separate phonetic segments and then figuring out how they fit together. Rather, children learn from the top down and learn everything at once. They start with global structure, and gradually come to recognize the internal structure within those larger units. Imitating parental language was found to occur for a very brief time window, and then quickly give way to more generative language. The parental style of interaction that was associated with the best outcomes was one in which parents recognized what their children were trying to communicate, encouraged them, and gave examples of language that could be used to communicate that particular intent. Parents led children into a communicative exchange, and then allowed the child to take the lead. Of course, the most effective parents remained engaged in the exchange, checking the child's language, expanding, and continuing to encourage.

Children need to learn about syntax, grammar, semantics, and phonetics. Learning in each of these areas promotes discovery in the other areas. It is only by learning how separate words fit together that children can discover word classes, and determine into which of those classes each newly discovered word fits. Psycholinguistic studies with typical children have revealed that children learn how to inflect classes of words, not how to inflect separate words one at a time (e.g., Mintz, 2003). Children discover the whole of the language system. Of course, part of that process involves learning about phonetic structure and individual words in the native language, as well. All of this knowledge helps with the very processing of the acoustic speech signal in the auditory cortex.

Identifying Hearing Loss Early

Our efforts to identify hearing loss as soon after birth as possible need to continue. The ultimate solution for how to treat childhood hearing loss—the one that will allow children with hearing loss to proceed through language learning on the same time table as children with normal hearing—will undoubtedly involve identifying children at the time they are born. However, it is clear that we need to modify the treatment we are providing to these children and their families once they are identified. The growth rate for language learning was

slow until the time these children entered preschool programs. Collectively, we need to find ways of objectively assessing and discussing our current intervention practices, even though emotions generally run high when it comes to intervention choices.

Using Signs for Signs' Sake

Unless parents want their children with hearing loss to grow up proficient in sign language, there is no reason to promote the use of signs. On the other hand, if parents wish for their children to participate in Deaf culture, then there is no reason for parents not to encourage their children's acquisition of sign language, providing the child has no additional handicaps that would put her at risk of learning language in a delayed manner. Because we observed a decline in the frequency of sign use between hearing parents and their deaf children over the first few years of the child's life, however, it seems likely that learning sign language is best facilitated by someone outside of the family.

Assessment

A great deal of information was gathered in this study about how we should be conducting assessments. It was found that the strongest effects of various independent variables were observed not for standard test measures, but for those that examined language use in a natural setting. We found that measures varied in their sensitivity to group differences across ages. We even found that sometimes more frequent rates of occurrence for behaviors that seem related to vocal production actually signaled slower rates of language acquisition. For some measures, development was not a linear function and so cannot be treated the same way at different ages. These findings highlight the need to obtain measures of language as it is used naturally by children, and to analyze those samples with objective techniques. Investigators and clinicians need to know the shape of the underlying developmental path in order to interpret results.

Chapter Summary

This chapter has focused on how results from this study should be used to shape treatment practices for children with hearing loss as we go forward into the 21st century. The pioneers of deaf education in America were well informed and dedicated to helping children with hearing loss. The methods they developed for treatment helped many generations of children. But we have learned a great deal in the past 100 years. Technology has changed. Even the very children we are trying to help have changed, if only because a higher percentage of these children are deaf since birth. We need to evaluate the treatments we are providing from unbiased perspectives, armed with knowledge about how the auditory system functions and how language is learned and processed. In this way, we may one day be able to help all children with hearing loss develop language that is commensurate to that of their normal-hearing peers. And it is only by mastering language that any child can ever achieve her fullest potential.

References

Beckman, M. E., & Edwards, J. (2000). The ontogeny of phonological categories and the primacy of lexical learning in linguistic development. *Child Development*, *71*, 240–249.

Belin, P., Zatorre, R. J., Lafaille, P., Ahad, P., & Pike, B. (2000). Voice-selective areas in human auditory cortex. *Nature*, *403*, 309–312.

Best, C. T., Morrongiello, B., & Robson, R. (1981). Perceptual equivalence of acoustic cues in speech and nonspeech perception. *Perception & Psychophysics*, *29*, 191–211.

Binder, J. R., Frost, J. A., Hammeke, T. A., Bellgowan, P. S., Springer, J. A., Kaufman, J. N., et al. (2000). Human temporal lobe activation by speech and nonspeech sounds. *Cerebral Cortex*, *10*, 512–528.

Boring, E. G. (1930). A new ambiguous figure. *American Journal of Psychology*, *42*, 444–445. [Adapted by L. L. Lohr, 2003, in *Creating graphics for learning and performance: Lessons in visual literacy*. Upper Saddle River, NJ: Pearson.]

Brown, R. (1973). *A first language: The early stages*. Cambridge, MA: Harvard University Press.

Campbell, R., & Dodd, B. (1980). Hearing by eye. *The Quarterly Journal of Experimental Psychology*, *32*, 85–99.

de Boysson-Bardies, B., Sagart, L., Halle, P., & Durand, C. (1986). Acoustic investigations of cross-linguistic variability in babbling. In B. Lindblom & R. Zetterstrom (Eds.), *Wenner-Gren International Symposium Series: Vol. 44. Precursors of early speech* (pp. 113–126). New York: Stockton Press.

Eimas, P. D., Siqueland, E. R., Jusczyk, P., & Vigorito, J. (1971). Speech perception in infants. *Science*, *171*, 303–306.

Gleitman, L., & Wanner, E. (1982). Language acquisition: The state of the art. In E. Wanner & L. Gleitman (Eds.), *Language acquisition: The state of the art* (pp. 3–48). Cambridge, UK: Cambridge University Press.

Hazan, V., & Barrett, S. (2000). The development of phonemic categorization in children aged 6–12. *Journal of Phonetics, 28*, 377–396.

Jusczyk, P. W. (1995). Language acquisition: Speech sounds and the beginning of phonology. In J. L. Miller & P. D. Eimas (Eds.), *Speech, language, and communication* (pp. 263–301). San Diego, CA: Academic Press.

Jusczyk, P. W. (1997). *The discovery of spoken language*. Cambridge, MA: The MIT Press.

Kuhl, P. K. (1980). Perceptual constancy for speech sound categories in early infancy. In G. H. Yeni-Komshian, J. F. Kavanagh, & C. A. Ferguson (Eds.), *Child phonology* (vol. 2, pp. 199–261). New York: Academic Press.

Liberman, A. M., Cooper, F. S., Shankweiler, D. P., & Studdert-Kennedy, M. (1967). Perception of the speech code. *Psychological Review, 74*, 431–461.

Liberman, I. Y., Shankweiler, D., Fischer, F. W., & Carter, B. (1974). Explicit syllable and phoneme segmentation in the young child. *Journal of Experimental Child Psychology, 18*, 201–212.

Mann, V. A., & Liberman, A. M. (1983). Some differences between phonetic and auditory modes of perception. *Cognition, 14*, 211–235.

McGurk, H., & MacDonald, J. (1976). Hearing lips and seeing voices. *Nature, 264*, 746–748.

Mintz, T. H. (2003). Frequent frames as a cue for grammatical categories in child directed speech. *Cognition, 90*, 91–117.

Morgan, J. L., & Demuth, K. (1996). *Signal to syntax*. Mahwah, NJ: Erlbaum.

Nittrouer, S. (2001). Challenging the notion of innate phonetic boundaries. *Journal of the Acoustical Society of America, 110*, 1598–1605.

Nittrouer, S. (2006). Children hear the forest. *Journal of the Acoustical Society of America, 120*, 1799–1802.

Nittrouer, S., Lowenstein, J. H., & Packer, R. (2009). Children discover the spectral skeletons in their native language before the amplitude envelopes. *Journal of Experimental Psychology: Human Perception and Performance, 35*, in press (August).

Pennington, B. F., Van Orden, G. C., Smith, S. D., Green, P. A., & Haith, M. M. (1990). Phonological processing skills and deficits in adult dyslexics. *Child Development, 61*, 1753–1778.

Rauschecker, J. P. (1998). Cortical processing of complex sounds. *Current Opinion in Neurobiology, 8*, 516–521.

Rauschecker, J. P., Tian, B., & Hauser, M. (1995). Processing of complex sounds in the macaque nonprimary auditory cortex. *Science, 268*, 111–114.

Remez, R. E., Rubin, P. E., Berns, S. M., Pardo, J. S., & Lang, J. M. (1994). On the perceptual organization of speech. *Psychological Review, 101*, 129–156.

Remez, R. E., Rubin, P. E., Pisoni, D. B., & Carrell, T. D. (1981). Speech perception without traditional speech cues. *Science, 212*, 947–949.

Rizzolatti, G., & Craighero, L. (2004). The mirror-neuron system. *Annual Review of Neuroscience, 27*, 169–192.

Samuel, A. G. (1996). Does lexical information influence the perceptual restoration of phonemes? *Journal of Experimental Psychology: General, 125*, 28–51.

Scott, S. K., Blank, C. C., Rosen, S., & Wise, R. J. (2000). Identification of a pathway for intelligible speech in the left temporal lobe. *Brain, 123*, 2400–2406.

Shahin, A. J., Bishop, C. W., & Miller, L. M. (2009). Neural mechanisms for illusory filling-in of degraded speech. *NeuroImage, 44*, 1133–1143.

Shahin, A. J., & Miller, L. M. (2009). Multisensory integration enhances phonemic restoration. *Journal of the Acoustical Society of America, 125*, 1744–1750.

Shannon, R. V., Zeng, F. G., Kamath, V., Wygonski, J., & Ekelid, M. (1995). Speech recognition with primarily temporal cues. *Science, 270*, 303–304.

Soderstrom, M., Seidl, A., Kemler Nelson, D. G., & Jusczyk, P. W. (2003). The prosodic bootstrapping of phrases: Evidence from prelinguistic infants. *Journal of Memory and Language, 49,* 249–267.

Todd, N. D. M., Lee, C. S., & O'Boyle, D. J. (2006). A sensorimotor theory of speech perception: Implications for learning, organization, and recognition. In S. Greenberg & W. A. Ainsworth (Eds.), *Listening to speech: An auditory perspective* (pp. 351–373). Mahwah, NJ: Lawrence Erlbaum.

Wagner, R. K. (1986). Phonological processing abilities and reading: Implications for disabled readers. *Journal of Learning Disabilities, 19,* 623–630.

Wagner, R. K., & Torgesen, J. K. (1987). The nature of phonological processing and its causal role in the acquisition of reading skills. *Psychological Bulletin, 101,* 192–212.

Werker, J. F. (1991). The ontogeny of speech perception. In I. G. Mattingly & M. Studdert-Kennedy (Eds.), *Modularity and the motor theory of speech perception* (pp. 91–109). Hillsdale, NJ: Lawrence Erlbaum Associates.

Werker, J. F. (1994). Cross-language speech perception: Developmental change does not involve loss. In J. C. Goodman & H. C. Nusbaum (Eds.), *The development of speech perception* (pp. 93–120). Cambridge, MA: MIT.

Werker, J. F., & Yeung, H. H. (2005). Infant speech perception bootstraps word learning. *Trends in Neurosciences, 9,* 519–527.

Zeng, F. G. (2008). Combining hearing aids and cochlear implants to solve the cocktail party problem [Abstract]. *Journal of the Acoustical Society of America, 123,* 3167.

Appendix A

Educational and Occupational Indices for Socioeconomic Status

Occupational Index

1 = maid, parking lot attendant, cafeteria worker, welfare recipient

2 = fast food worker, meter reader, housekeeper, deliveryman, garbage man, packer, housewife, bill collector, telemarketer, waiter/waitress (e.g., bars), butler, factory worker, taxi driver, telephone operator, assembly line worker, data entry, nanny, bartender, painter (e.g., house), dishwasher

3 = daycare worker, construction worker, dispatcher, home appliance repairman, truck driver, bus driver, print room operator, gardener, machine operator, roofer, sales clerk, waiter/waitress (higher), brewer, camp counselor, dry cleaner, butcher, chef at a diner, exterminator, telephone company technician, mailman, car salesman, retail sales, military

enlisted, post office clerks, welder, auto body repairman, bank teller/clerk, engraver, mechanic, beautician, service technician, janitor, carpet installer, brick mason, security guard, maintenance worker

4 = barber, travel agent, proofreader, baker, plumber, insurance agent, farmer, florist, sales representative, court reporter, fast food manager, electrician, tailor, locksmith, jeweler, bookkeeper, undergraduate student, carpenter, corrections officer, piano teacher, loan officer, factory supervisor

5 = advertising agent, actor/actress, construction foreman, librarian, interior decorating, real estate broker, missionary, funeral director, artist, laboratory technician, chef at a good restaurant, insurance adjustor, manufacturer, oral hygienist, musician, tavern owner, electrical contractor, L.P.N., public

relations, social worker, executive assistant, office manager, radio/TV announcer, store manager (chain), executive secretary, personnel manager, accountant, contractor, graduate student, mortician, policeman, postmaster, fireman, medical technician, bank manager, firefighter

6 = computer programmer, restaurant owner, store or small business owner, elementary school teacher, research assistant, book or magazine editor, optician, real estate developer, stockbroker, high school teacher, military captain/lieutenant, chiropractor, registered nurse, military officer, lawyer, sheriff/police chief, clergyman, pharmacist, family therapist

7 = mayor, symphony conductor, engineer, large business owner, school principal, architect, judge, psychologist, veterinarian, company president, university professor, dentist

8 = university president, scientist, physician, surgeon

Educational Index

1.0 = Completed elementary school

2.0 = Completed junior high

2.5 = Received Graduate Education Equivalence

3.0 = Completed high school

3.5 = Completed 1 or more years of technical/vocational school

4.0 = Completed technical/vocational school

5.0 = Completed 1 or more years of university/college

6.0 = Bachelor's degree

6.5 = Completed 1 or more years of graduate school

7.0 = Master's degree

7.5 = Course work completed for PhD, but no dissertation; law degree without bar; medical degree without internship completed

8.0 = PhD; law degree with bar; medical degree with internship completed

Appendix B

Decision Tree for Scoring Children's Language Samples

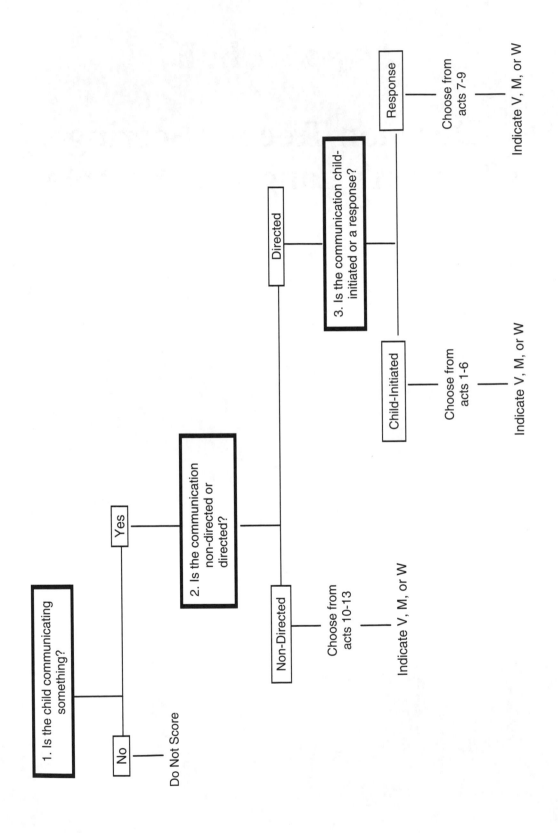

330

Appendix C

Communicative Acts Scored in Children's Language Samples

Each behavior is marked according to its number and then indicated as either *M* for manual only (including signs), *V* for vocalization, or *W* for word.

Child-Initiated (and Directed) Communications

To qualify as directed or addressed communication, a child's behavior must satisfy the following criteria: It must be directed to the adult. The child must look at, refer to, or address the adult directly in some way as part of the act. It must have the effect, or at least the obviously intended effect, of influencing the adult's behavior, focus of attention, or state of knowledge. The child must obviously be trying to get a message across to the adult. The child must be persistent in the attempt to convey a message if the adult fails to respond or responds in a way the child had not intended.

1. **Request for Objects:** Solicitation of an item, usually out of reach.

2. **Request for Action:** Solicitation to get an action done or to have the adult reinitiate an action that has stopped, including a persistent indication (an overt action or verbalization/word) for the adult to do something.

3. **Rejections or Protests:** Expression of disapproval of a speaker's utterance or action, of an item, or of something that is happening. Must be definite. May include fussing or crying.

4. **Directed Comment:** Attempt to get an adult to focus on an object or event by such acts as showing or pointing at objects or pictures, for the purposes of establishing social interaction, joint attention, or bringing some aspect of the object or event to the adult's attention. This category also includes smiling at the adult during interaction (should last at least 2 seconds), clearly indicating pleasure with an object or action.

5. **Inquiry:** Use of language to learn about the world. At the earliest stages, the requesting information

function can take the form of requests for the names of things. Later, it may include a wh- word, *can*, *how*, a rising intonation contour, or both a word and rising intonation. Includes questions from child to adult.

6. **Routines:** This category includes any universal routine, including nursery rhymes (e.g., "Mary Had a Little Lamb"), children's songs (e.g., "The Itsy Bitsy Spider"), and games (e.g., peek-a-boo). Initiating or joining in routines and rhymes started by the adult fits into this category. This category does not include book sharing, eating sounds, animal noises, *hi* and *bye-bye*, car noises, and so on.

Child Responses

To qualify as a response, the child's behavior must immediately follow (within 3 seconds) a statement or question posed by the adult. It must be made in such a way that there is a reasonable expectation that the adult will notice the child's response.

7. **Acknowledgment:** Response to a comment or request indicating the utterance was received and processed. In young children this is often accomplished verbally by mimicking the adult's intonation pattern. When the parent makes a *statement*, head nods from the child to the adult can also communicate this intention, as can performing the action indicated by the adult, but must immediately follow (within 3 seconds) the adult's

statement, request, or action. The difference between an *Acknowledgment* and an *Imitation* is that if the communication is within the realm of the child's understanding, it is an acknowledgment.

8. **Answer:** Response to a question using a semantically or pragmatically appropriate verbal remark. If the child answers incorrectly, but his/her response is semantically or pragmatically correct, then score it. "Yes" or "no" responses are scored as acknowledgments.

9. **Imitation:** A *verbal* imitation of the adult's speech with no apparent processing on the part of the child. Imitation of an action is not included in this category. Often this will follow a directive from the adult such as "Say _____."

Nondirected Communication

To qualify as nondirected or nonaddressed communication, the child's behavior should not be directed to the adult.

10. **Nondirected Comment:** A statement that is not directed to anyone in particular or that is directed to an object. Comment needs to be at least word length (single syllable) and moderate amplitude and have a resonating characteristic.

11. **Nondirected Request:** A nonaddressed or nondirected request, for example reaching for and focusing only on the object, not looking at the adult.

12. **Object Address:** Talking to or addressing an object, such as talking to a doll: "Do you want to go to sleep, baby?"

13. **Talk Through:** Uses an object as a conduit for speaking to another person, either real or imaginary. This can involve either speaking through a telephone, for example, or having one doll speak to another. Must be initiated by the child.

Appendix D

Communicative Acts Scored in Parental Language Samples

1. **Inquiry:** The parent asks the child a question that can reasonably require a verbal reply or a nonverbal action. This is a question initiated by the parent, not a response to a child's question or comment. Includes a comment paired with a question (i.e., elliptical sentences and also statements with a "huh?" at the end).

2. **Directive:** The parent verbally commands the child to pursue a given course of action. This category must include a command structure such as *say, look, find, put, watch, let's*. Also included are statements that indicate a child's action is incorrect, but not that the parent is displeased.

3. **Encourage/Approve:** The parent verbally indicates to the child to continue with the course of action, and/or expresses praise or approval aloud to the child.

4. **Visual Cue:** The parent attracts the child's attention to a given aspect of the task, without verbal utterance. This category includes pointing and physically manipu-

lating the object to draw attention to a part of it or physically helping the child do something. The Visual Cue should last at least 2 seconds. This category does not include the parent clapping his or her hands to get the child's attention. That is considered precommunicative and is not scored.

5. **Verbal Response:** The parent verbally responds to a *question, statement,* or *action* by the child clearly directed to the parent. This includes recasts and requests for clarification. The parent is providing information at the request or initiation of the child. Short utterances such as *OK* or *Uh-huh* are scored only if they are clearly responses to something the child has said to the parent. *Thank you* would be included in this category if the parent responds to something the child does.

6. **Nonverbal Response:** The parent nonverbally responds to a question, statement, or action by the child (e.g., the parent performs an

action the child requested or performs an action on an object following a statement by the child). Does not include moving the child.

7. **Nonverbal Approval:** The parent expresses favorable feelings by smiling or physically making contact with the child. Does not include moving the child.

8. **Verbal Disapproval:** The parent reprimands the child or verbally indicates displeasure with the child or the child's action. Unlike category 2, no instruction of appropriate action is provided. Displeasure is clearly indicated.

9. **Nonverbal Disapproval:** This category includes parental actions generally considered physical punishment, such as a slap to the hand.

10. **Nonverbal Manipulation/ Modeling:** The parent engages in an activity, with the child not engaged in the process. This does not include when the child and parent play parallel to each other, but does include modeling (child watching parent do something).

11. **Commentary:** The parent talks to herself, using language not intended for the child, with no expectation of a response from the child. This includes comments aloud to which the child could not respond. This category may include rhetorical questions, but not short phrases such as *OK, Oops,* or *Uh-huh.*

12. **Explanation/Description:** This category describes explanations above and beyond the immediate task or outside of the immediate context. It also includes the parent's acknowledgment of a statement or behavior of the child. The parent also describes something to the child, including speaking directly to the child with the purpose of clarifying or explaining something about the task at hand. Should be in child-directed tone and should be a statement the child is expected to understand. May involve a "constant state of description" by the parent to the child. May include animal sounds.

13. **Failure to Respond:** The child makes a clear and direct request to which the parent does not respond either verbally or with an action.

14. **Imitation:** The parent imitates the child's word or statement exactly as the child said it. This also includes imitation of babbling or animals sounds. It does not include imitation of sighs, grunts, or vegetative noises the child makes.

15. **Routine:** This category includes any universal routine, including nursery rhymes (e.g., "Mary Had a Little Lamb"), children's songs (e.g., "The Itsy Bitsy Spider"), and games (e.g., peek-a-boo). This category does not include book sharing, eating sounds, or *hi* and *bye.*

16. **Talk Through:** Uses an object as a conduit for speaking to another person, either real or imaginary. This can involve having one doll speak to another.

Appendix E

Modified Version of Figure 12–1

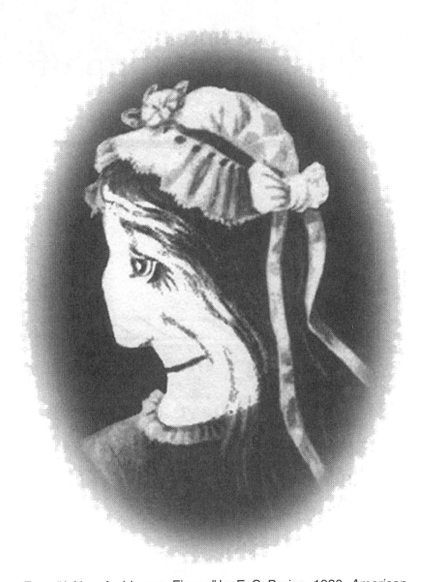

From "A New Ambiguous Figure," by E. G. Boring, 1930, *American Journal of Psychology*, *42*, pp. 444–445. Adapted by L. L. Lohr, 2003, *Creating Graphics for Learning and Performance: Lessons in Visual Literacy*. Upper Saddle River, NJ: Pearson. Copyright 1930, University of Illinois. Reproduced with permission.

Index